Rare Respiratory Diseases: A Personal and a Public Health Problem

Rare Respiratory Diseases: A Personal and a Public Health Problem

Editor

Francisco Dasí

MDPI • Basel • Beijing • Wuhan • Barcelona • Belgrade • Manchester • Tokyo • Cluj • Tianjin

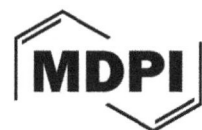

Editor
Francisco Dasí
University of Valencia
Spain

Editorial Office
MDPI
St. Alban-Anlage 66
4052 Basel, Switzerland

This is a reprint of articles from the Special Issue published online in the open access journal *Journal of Clinical Medicine* (ISSN 2077-0383) (available at: https://www.mdpi.com/journal/jcm/special_issues/Rare_Respiratory_Diseases).

For citation purposes, cite each article independently as indicated on the article page online and as indicated below:

LastName, A.A.; LastName, B.B.; LastName, C.C. Article Title. *Journal Name* **Year**, *Volume Number*, Page Range.

ISBN 978-3-0365-3669-9 (Hbk)
ISBN 978-3-0365-3670-5 (PDF)

© 2022 by the authors. Articles in this book are Open Access and distributed under the Creative Commons Attribution (CC BY) license, which allows users to download, copy and build upon published articles, as long as the author and publisher are properly credited, which ensures maximum dissemination and a wider impact of our publications.
The book as a whole is distributed by MDPI under the terms and conditions of the Creative Commons license CC BY-NC-ND.

Contents

About the Editor ix

María Magallón, Lucía Bañuls, Silvia Castillo, María Mercedes Navarro-García, Cruz González and Francisco Dasí
Special Issue: Rare Respiratory Diseases: A Personal and Public Health Issue
Reprinted from: *J. Clin. Med.* **2021**, *10*, 5906, doi:10.3390/jcm10245906 1

Miguel Armengot-Carceller, Ana Reula, Manuel Mata-Roig, Jordi Pérez-Panadés, Lara Milian-Medina and Carmen Carda-Batalla
Understanding Primary Ciliary Dyskinesia: Experience From a Mediterranean Diagnostic Reference Centre
Reprinted from: *J. Clin. Med.* **2020**, *9*, 810, doi:10.3390/jcm9030810 5

María Ángeles Requena-Fernández, Francisco Dasí, Silvia Castillo, Rafael Barajas-Cenobi, María Mercedes Navarro-García and Amparo Escribano
Knowledge of Rare Respiratory Diseases among Paediatricians and Medical School Students
Reprinted from: *J. Clin. Med.* **2020**, *9*, 869, doi:10.3390/jcm9030869 17

Kiyoharu Fukushima, Seigo Kitada, Yuko Abe, Yuji Yamamoto, Takanori Matsuki, Hiroyuki Kagawa, Yohei Oshitani, Kazuyuki Tsujino, Kenji Yoshimura, Mari Miki, Keisuke Miki and Hiroshi Kida
Long-Term Treatment Outcome of Progressive *Mycobacterium avium* Complex Pulmonary Disease
Reprinted from: *J. Clin. Med.* **2020**, *9*, 1315, doi:10.3390/jcm9051315 27

Zuzanna Stachowiak, Irena Wojsyk-Banaszak, Katarzyna Jończyk-Potoczna, Beata Narożna, Wojciech Langwiński, Zdzisława Kycler, Paulina Sobkowiak, Anna Bręborowicz and Aleksandra Szczepankiewicz
MiRNA Expression Profile in the Airways Is Altered during Pulmonary Exacerbation in Children with Cystic Fibrosis—A Preliminary Report
Reprinted from: *J. Clin. Med.* **2020**, *9*, 1887, doi:10.3390/jcm9061887 43

José Luis López-Campos, Laura Carrasco Hernandez and Candelaria Caballero Eraso
Implications of a Change of Paradigm in Alpha1 Antitrypsin Deficiency Augmentation Therapy: From Biochemical to Clinical Efficacy
Reprinted from: *J. Clin. Med.* **2020**, *9*, 2526, doi:10.3390/jcm9082526 55

Lucía Bañuls, Daniel Pellicer, Silvia Castillo, María Mercedes Navarro-García, María Magallón, Cruz González and Francisco Dasí
Gene Therapy in Rare Respiratory Diseases: What Have We Learned So Far?
Reprinted from: *J. Clin. Med.* **2020**, *9*, 2577, doi:10.3390/jcm9082577 75

Myrofora Goutaki, Florian S. Halbeisen, Angelo Barbato, Suzanne Crowley, Amanda Harris, Robert A. Hirst, Bülent Karadag, Vendula Martinu, Lucy Morgan, Christopher O'Callaghan, Ugur Ozçelik, Sergio Scigliano, Santiago Ucros, Panayiotis Yiallouros, Sven M. Schulzke and Claudia E. Kuehni
Late Diagnosis of Infants with PCD and Neonatal Respiratory Distress
Reprinted from: *J. Clin. Med.* **2020**, *9*, 2871, doi:10.3390/jcm9092871 105

Noelia Baz-Redón, Sandra Rovira-Amigo, Mónica Fernández-Cancio, Silvia Castillo-Corullón, Maria Cols, M. Araceli Caballero-Rabasco, Óscar Asensio, Carlos Martín de Vicente, Maria del Mar Martínez-Colls, Alba Torrent-Vernetta, Inés de Mir-Messa, Silvia Gartner, Ignacio Iglesias-Serrano, Ana Díez-Izquierdo, Eva Polverino, Esther Amengual-Pieras, Rosanel Amaro-Rodríguez, Montserrat Vendrell, Marta Mumany, María Teresa Pascual-Sánchez, Belén Pérez-Dueñas, Ana Reula, Amparo Escribano, Francisco Dasí, Miguel Armengot-Carceller, Marta Garrido-Pontnou, Núria Camats-Tarruella and Antonio Moreno-Galdó
Immunofluorescence Analysis as a Diagnostic Tool in a Spanish Cohort of Patients with Suspected Primary Ciliary Dyskinesia
Reprinted from: *J. Clin. Med.* **2020**, *9*, 3603, doi:10.3390/jcm9113603 . . . . **115**

Janice L. Coles, James Thompson, Katie L. Horton, Robert A. Hirst, Paul Griffin, Gwyneth M. Williams, Patricia Goggin, Regan Doherty, Peter M. Lackie, Amanda Harris, Woolf T. Walker, Christopher O'Callaghan, Claire Hogg, Jane S. Lucas, Cornelia Blume and Claire L. Jackson
A Revised Protocol for Culture of Airway Epithelial Cells as a Diagnostic Tool for Primary Ciliary Dyskinesia
Reprinted from: *J. Clin. Med.* **2020**, *9*, 3753, doi:10.3390/jcm9113753 . . . . **129**

José María Hernández Pérez, Ignacio Blanco, Agustín Jesús Sánchez Medina, Laura Díaz Hernández and José Antonio Pérez Pérez
Serum Levels of Glutamate-Pyruvate Transaminase, Glutamate-Oxaloacetate Transaminase and Gamma-Glutamyl Transferase in 1494 Patients with Various Genotypes for the Alpha-1 Antitrypsin Gene
Reprinted from: *J. Clin. Med.* **2020**, *9*, 3923, doi:10.3390/jcm9123923 . . . . **145**

Carolin Leoni Dobler, Britta Krüger, Jana Strahler, Christopher Weyh, Kristina Gebhardt, Khodr Tello, Hossein Ardeschir Ghofrani, Natascha Sommer, Henning Gall, Manuel Jonas Richter and Karsten Krüger
Physical Activity and Mental Health of Patients with Pulmonary Hypertension during the COVID-19 Pandemic
Reprinted from: *J. Clin. Med.* **2020**, , 4023, doi:10.3390/jcm9124023 . . . . **153**

Ana Reula, Daniel Pellicer, Silvia Castillo, María Magallón, Miguel Armengot, Guadalupe Herrera, José-Enrique O'Connor, Lucía Bañuls, María Mercedes Navarro-García, Amparo Escribano and Francisco Dasí
New Laboratory Protocol to Determine the Oxidative Stress Profile of Human Nasal Epithelial Cells Using Flow Cytometry
Reprinted from: *J. Clin. Med.* **2021**, *10*, 1172, doi:10.3390/jcm10061172 . . . . **167**

María Magallón, Ana Esther Carrión, Lucía Bañuls, Daniel Pellicer, Silvia Castillo, Sergio Bondía, María Mercedes Navarro-García, Cruz González and Francisco Dasí
Oxidative Stress and Endoplasmic Reticulum Stress in Rare Respiratory Diseases
Reprinted from: *J. Clin. Med.* **2021**, *10*, 1268, doi:10.3390/jcm10061268 . . . . **183**

Anna Annunziata, Ilaria Ferrarotti, Antonietta Coppola, Maurizia Lanza, Pasquale Imitazione, Sara Spinelli, Pierpaolo Di Micco and Giuseppe Fiorentino
Alpha-1 Antitrypsin Screening in a Selected Cohort of Patients Affected by Chronic Pulmonary Diseases in Naples, Italy
Reprinted from: *J. Clin. Med.* **2021**, *10*, 1546, doi:10.3390/jcm10081546 . . . . **209**

Mònica Pons, Alexa Núñez, Cristina Esquinas, María Torres-Durán, Juan Luis Rodríguez-Hermosa, Myriam Calle, Ramón Tubio-Pérez, Irene Belmonte, Francisco Rodríguez-Frías, Esther Rodríguez, Joan Genescà, Marc Miravitlles and Miriam Barrecheguren
Utility of Transient Elastography for the Screening of Liver Disease in Patients with Alpha1-Antitrypsin Deficiency
Reprinted from: *J. Clin. Med.* **2021**, *10*, 1724, doi:10.3390/jcm10081724 . . . . **217**

About the Editor

Francisco Dasí is Associate Professor of Human Physiology at the University of Valencia and leads the research group on Rare Respiratory Diseases (RRD) at the IIS INCLIVA (Valencia, Spain). He obtained his degree in Biology at the University of Valencia. Dr. Dasí received his Ph.D. degree in Pharmacology from the University of Valencia. He has been a research scholar at the Lineberger Cancer Center at the UNC-CH (USA) and the Karolinska Institutet (Sweden). Dr. Dasi's scientific interests are focused on: characterizing the molecular mechanisms (especially those aspects related to REDOX regulation) involved in the pathophysiology of alpha-1 antitrypsin deficiency; evaluating the diagnostic and prognostic value of circulating nucleic acids; developing new therapeutic strategies based on gene therapy; and generating social awareness of RRD, through the scientific dissemination of biomedical advances and social and health policies aimed at improving the quality of life of patients.

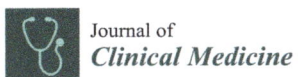

Editorial

Special Issue: Rare Respiratory Diseases: A Personal and Public Health Issue

María Magallón [1,2], Lucía Bañuls [1,2], Silvia Castillo [1,3], María Mercedes Navarro-García [1], Cruz González [1,4] and Francisco Dasí [1,2,*]

1. Research Group on Rare Respiratory Diseases (ERR), Instituto de Investigación Sanitaria INCLIVA, Fundación Investigación Hospital Clínico Valencia, Avda. Menéndez y Pelayo, 4, 46010 Valencia, Spain; mariamagallon94@gmail.com (M.M.); lucia.banyuls.soto@gmail.com (L.B.); sccorullon@gmail.com (S.C.); mer_navarro2002@yahoo.es (M.M.N.-G.); Cruz.Gonzalez@uv.es (C.G.)
2. Research Group on Rare Respiratory Diseases (ERR), Department of Physiology, School of Medicine, University of Valencia, Avda. Blasco Ibáñez, 15, 46010 Valencia, Spain
3. Paediatrics Unit, Hospital Clínico Universitario de Valencia, Avda. Blasco Ibáñez, 17, 46010 Valencia, Spain
4. Pneumology Unit, Hospital Clínico Universitario de Valencia, Avda. Blasco Ibáñez, 17, 46010 Valencia, Spain
* Correspondence: Francisco.Dasi@uv.es

Citation: Magallón, M.; Bañuls, L.; Castillo, S.; Navarro-García, M.M.; González, C.; Dasí, F. Special Issue: Rare Respiratory Diseases: A Personal and Public Health Issue. *J. Clin. Med.* **2021**, *10*, 5906. https://doi.org/10.3390/jcm10245906

Received: 13 December 2021
Accepted: 14 December 2021
Published: 16 December 2021

Publisher's Note: MDPI stays neutral with regard to jurisdictional claims in published maps and institutional affiliations.

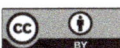

Copyright: © 2021 by the authors. Licensee MDPI, Basel, Switzerland. This article is an open access article distributed under the terms and conditions of the Creative Commons Attribution (CC BY) license (https://creativecommons.org/licenses/by/4.0/).

In the 1970s, the term "rare disease" was coined to describe a category of inherited metabolic diseases with low prevalence and a wide range of symptoms. The majority of rare diseases are life-threatening and have a considerable impact on a patient's quality of life. Many of them are fatal. Although rare diseases are uncommon, they affect millions of people worldwide, and the available information on them is often insufficient, consisting of a few isolated clinical cases. The term "low prevalence" is defined differently in different countries. A disease is considered rare in the European Union when the prevalence is fewer than 5 cases per 10,000 people. In the United States, the Orphan Drug Act defines a rare disease as one that affects fewer than 200,000 people. Other countries, such as Japan, prefer to employ a stricter threshold, such as fewer than 4 cases per 10,000 people. The number of rare diseases is estimated to be between 5000 and 8000, with the majority of them being genetic and having a hereditary component, while some occur due to exposure to infectious agents, toxins, or severe treatment side-effects. Between 3.5% and 5.9% of the world's population is affected by rare diseases, translating into 18–30 million in the European Union and 263–446 million worldwide. The figures for uncommon respiratory disorders are also significant. Even with a reasonable estimate of 5% of rare diseases with a respiratory component, 1–2 million Europeans are likely to be affected by a rare respiratory disease. As a result, rare (respiratory) disorders are a public health and social issue [1–3].

The pathophysiology of rare diseases is unclear due to a lack of research, making the creation of safe and efficient medications, biologics, and medical technologies to prevent, diagnose, treat, or cure these diseases extremely difficult. All of this translates into significant challenges in obtaining public or private funding for rare disease research and assembling a sufficient number of patients for ensuring conclusive results from which health authorities could authorize the use of safe and effective pharmaceutical products to treat rare diseases. Collaboration is always required to increase the understanding and development of innovative medicines for these uncommon diseases. In recent years, health authorities worldwide have collaborated closely to solve these issues with the help of pharmaceutical corporations, scientists, and healthcare professionals. As a result of this partnership, new methods for improving the diagnosis, prognosis, and treatment of uncommon diseases have been established [3]. Patient organizations play a significant role in this regard [4]. The physical, emotional, and financial impacts of rare diseases on affected people and their families explain why those affected join groups dedicated to supporting research into the origins or causes of their illness and the development of effective medicines. A growing number of patient organizations promote and fund research projects, learn about and follow up on their findings, and partner with government agencies, the pharmaceutical sector, and clinical and academic researchers. To name a few, the American Association of patients with alpha-1 antitrypsin deficiency (AATD) has been funding research on this disease for years [5]. The Alpha-1 Spanish Association has recently announced the first edition of the Amadeu Monteiro Fellowships to encourage younger researchers to initiate new research projects on AATD [6].

As is the case with most rare diseases, patients with rare respiratory diseases face several problems, including underdiagnosis and delayed diagnosis, which, in many cases, have a detrimental influence on the prognosis of patients. In addition, the lack of prognostic biomarkers and disease-specific treatments are also challenges. These problems have been addressed in this special issue on rare respiratory diseases that cover, among others, conditions such as AATD, primary ciliary dyskinesia (PCD), pulmonary hypertension, and cystic fibrosis (CF).

Alpha-1 antitrypsin deficiency (AATD) is a potentially deadly hereditary type of chronic obstructive pulmonary disease (COPD). Precise diagnostic criteria are lacking and might take years to arrive, and late diagnosis is an almost impossible challenge. Over 3 million individuals worldwide have deficient allele combinations leading to AATD, with over 120,000 Europeans expected to have severe forms of the disease. Because the symptoms and signs are similar, AATD is easily confused with smoking-induced COPD or asthma. The average time between the onset of pulmonary symptoms and diagnosis is 8.3 years, and patients visit an average of 2.7 doctors before receiving a definitive diagnosis, which translates into more than 90% of AATD patients being undiagnosed. These figures are unacceptable because there is a specific treatment for the disease. Augmentation therapy, the only approved therapy to treat the disease, slows down the progression of the pulmonary disease and improves survival rates significantly [7].

Lack of awareness is one reason that accounts for underdiagnosis and delayed diagnosis. In this special issue, several strategies are described that may help to improve AATD diagnosis. Requena et al. showed significant gaps in knowledge about AATD and PCD among medical students and paediatricians. The authors suggest that all physicians responsible for detecting and diagnosing rare respiratory diseases should get additional training—allowing for early diagnosis, the implementation of preventive measures, and appropriate treatment in the early stages [8].

Expert centres on rare respiratory diseases that focus on both the experience and the number of patients will lead to a more effective approach in managing these patients, as described in the article by Lopez-Campos et al [9].

Annunziatta et al. studied rare variants in the geographic area of Naples (Italy). The authors' findings may be useful for understanding the prevalence of AATD and its rare mutations, promoting early diagnosis and treatment for patients with chronic pulmonary disease and frequent exacerbations, and challenging the link between environmental causes of pulmonary damage, such as tobacco use [10].

Similar to AATD, the underdiagnosis of PCD is common. PCD symptoms are similar to those of other respiratory diseases [11]. To overcome these challenges, Armengot-Carceller et al. developed a diagnostic decision tree based on pansinusitis, situs inversus, periodicity, rhinorrhea, bronchiectasis, and chronic wet cough to classify new individuals. The authors concluded that the presence of all of these clinical symptoms in the same patient indicates a high risk of developing PCD [12]. However, validation of this diagnostic algorithm is still missing.

In addition, there is no gold standard for diagnosing PCD, and the currently available diagnostic methods are complex and not available in all hospital centres, leading to underdiagnosis in many cases. Several methods are currently being studied that will improve PCD diagnosis. Coles et al. have set up a new air–liquid culture procedure that produces high ciliation rates across three centers, minimizing patient recall for repeat brushing biopsies and improving diagnostic certainty. In addition, cryostorage of diagnostic samples was successful, facilitating PCD research [13]. Baz-Redon et al. demonstrated that an immunofluorescence-based method is a quick, low-cost, and reliable diagnostic test for PCD and is available in most hospitals. However, it cannot be used as an independent test [14].

Several authors have also studied the availability of prognostic biomarkers. Hernandez-Perez et al. demonstrated that the presence of a PI*Z allele seemed to be a risk factor for developing hepatic damage. Deficient AAT genotypes were linked to changes in liver enzymes, and low AAT levels were associated with high liver enzyme levels [15]. Pons et al. showed that abnormal liver enzymes are common in patients with AATD; however, most patients do not have significant liver fibrosis. The authors proposed using transient elastography to identify AATD patients with liver fibrosis, even if they have normal liver enzymes; this technique should be performed in all individuals with the Z allele to screen for liver disease [16].

In CF children, Stachowiak et al. discovered a profile of miRNAs, the expressions of which change during pulmonary exacerbations, and which are strongly linked to clinical outcomes [17].

The role of oxidative stress in the pathophysiology of rare respiratory diseases has also been discussed. In a review paper, Magallon et al. showed oxidative stress and increased biomarkers of oxidative damage in patients with AATD, idiopathic pulmonary fibrosis, and CF. As a result, targeting oxidative stress with antioxidant therapies is a rational approach to delaying disease progression and improving patient quality of life in all three conditions. In the case of PCD, the available data are limited, and further research is needed to determine the pathophysiological role of oxidative stress in the disease and, as a result, the possibility of administering antioxidant supplements [18]. A new method based on flow cytometry has been developed to investigate a comprehensive set of oxidative parameters in nasal epithelial cells, which might be useful in investigating respiratory diseases. This method has the benefit of using small samples and a non-invasive sampling technique [19].

Finally, the potential for new therapeutic strategies based on gene therapy has been explored, since no curative treatments are available for these diseases. As evidenced by the encouraging results in the preclinical and clinical phases, gene therapy is a promising alternative for the current therapies. However, further research is needed to ensure treatment safety and efficacy. In addition, new gene-editing tools used to correct mutations and enable cures for these diseases have been discussed [20].

In conclusion, this series of articles highlights some of the major problems that patients with rare diseases face and the need for further cooperative research between basic and clinical researchers to solve these problems.

Author Contributions: M.M., L.B., S.C., C.G., and F.D. wrote the manuscript. M.M.N.-G. edited and critically reviewed the manuscript. All authors have read and agreed to the published version of the manuscript.

Funding: This work was funded by the 2020 Sociedad Valenciana de Neumología, 2021 SEPAR and ISCIII #PI17/01250 grants and European Regional Development Funds (FEDER). M.M. is funded by 2021 Amadeu Monteiro grant. L.B. is supported by GVA grant number ACIF/2019/231.

Institutional Review Board Statement: Not applicable.

Informed Consent Statement: Not applicable.

Data Availability Statement: Not applicable.

Acknowledgments: We would like to thank the Spanish association of patients with alpha-1 antitrypsin deficiency for donations of research funds to our research group on rare respiratory diseases at IIS INCLIVA/UVEG.

Conflicts of Interest: The authors declare no conflict of interest.

References

1. Harari, S.; Lau, E.M.T.; Tamura, Y.; Cottin, V.; Simonneau, G.; Humbert, M. Rare (Pulmonary) Disease Day: "Feeding the Breath, Energy for Life!". *Eur. Respir. J.* **2015**, *45*, 297–300. [CrossRef] [PubMed]
2. Harari, S.; Humbert, M. Toward Better Management of Rare and Orphan Pulmonary Diseases. *Eur. Respir. J.* **2016**, *47*, 1334–1335. [CrossRef] [PubMed]
3. Humbert, M.; Wagner, T.O. Rare Respiratory Diseases Are Ready for Primetime: From Rare Disease Day to the European Reference Networks. *Eur. Respir. J.* **2017**, *49*, 1700085. [CrossRef] [PubMed]
4. Eurordis. Available online: https://www.eurordis.org (accessed on 9 December 2021).
5. Alpha-1 Web Page. Available online: https://www.alpha1.org/investigators/grants/grant-opportunities/ (accessed on 9 December 2021).
6. Alfa-1 España. Available online: https://alfa1.org.es/alfa-1-espana-concede-la-beca-amadeu-monteiro-a-dos-proyectos-que-investigan-esta-condicion-genetica-rara/ (accessed on 9 December 2021).
7. Torres-Duran, M.; Lopez-Campos, J.L.; Barrecheguren, M.; Miravitlles, M.; Martinez-Delgado, B.; Castillo, S.; Escribano, A.; Baloira, A.; Navarro-Garcia, M.M.; Pellicer, D.; et al. Alpha-1 Antitrypsin Deficiency: Outstanding Questions and Future Directions. *Orphanet J. Rare Dis.* **2018**, *13*, 114. [CrossRef] [PubMed]
8. Requena-Fernández, M.Á.; Dasí, F.; Castillo, S.; Barajas-Cenobi, R.; Navarro-García, M.M.; Escribano, A. Knowledge of Rare Respiratory Diseases among Paediatricians and Medical School Students. *J. Clin. Med.* **2020**, *9*, 869. [CrossRef] [PubMed]
9. López-Campos, J.L.; Carrasco Hernandez, L.; Caballero Eraso, C. Implications of a Change of Paradigm in Alpha1 Antitrypsin Deficiency Augmentation Therapy: From Biochemical to Clinical Efficacy. *J. Clin. Med.* **2020**, *9*, 2526. [CrossRef] [PubMed]
10. Annunziata, A.; Ferrarotti, I.; Coppola, A.; Lanza, M.; Imitazione, P.; Spinelli, S.; Micco, P.D.; Fiorentino, G. Alpha-1 Antitrypsin Screening in a Selected Cohort of Patients Affected by Chronic Pulmonary Diseases in Naples, Italy. *J. Clin. Med.* **2021**, *10*, 1546. [CrossRef] [PubMed]
11. Goutaki, M.; Halbeisen, F.S.; Barbato, A.; Crowley, S.; Harris, A.; Hirst, R.A.; Karadag, B.; Martinu, V.; Morgan, L.; O'Callaghan, C.; et al. Late Diagnosis of Infants with PCD and Neonatal Respiratory Distress. *J. Clin. Med.* **2020**, *9*, 2871. [CrossRef] [PubMed]
12. Armengot-Carceller, M.; Reula, A.; Mata-Roig, M.; Pérez-Panadés, J.; Milian-Medina, L.; Carda-Batalla, C. Understanding Primary Ciliary Dyskinesia: Experience From a Mediterranean Diagnostic Reference Centre. *J. Clin. Med.* **2020**, *9*, 810. [CrossRef] [PubMed]
13. Coles, J.L.; Thompson, J.; Horton, K.L.; Hirst, R.A.; Griffin, P.; Williams, G.M.; Goggin, P.; Doherty, R.; Lackie, P.M.; Harris, A.; et al. A Revised Protocol for Culture of Airway Epithelial Cells as a Diagnostic Tool for Primary Ciliary Dyskinesia. *J. Clin. Med.* **2020**, *9*, 3753. [CrossRef] [PubMed]
14. Baz-Redón, N.; Rovira-Amigo, S.; Fernández-Cancio, M.; Castillo-Corullón, S.; Cols, M.; Caballero-Rabasco, M.A.; Asensio, Ó.; Martín de Vicente, C.; Martínez-Colls, M.d.M.; Torrent-Vernetta, A.; et al. Immunofluorescence Analysis as a Diagnostic Tool in a Spanish Cohort of Patients with Suspected Primary Ciliary Dyskinesia. *J. Clin. Med.* **2020**, *9*, 3603. [CrossRef] [PubMed]
15. Hernández Pérez, J.M.; Blanco, I.; Jesús Sánchez Medina, A.; Díaz Hernández, L.; Antonio Pérez Pérez, J. Serum Levels of Glutamate-Pyruvate Transaminase, Glutamate-Oxaloacetate Transaminase and Gamma-Glutamyl Transferase in 1494 Patients with Various Genotypes for the Alpha-1 Antitrypsin Gene. *J. Clin. Med.* **2020**, *9*, 3923. [CrossRef] [PubMed]
16. Pons, M.; Núñez, A.; Esquinas, C.; Torres-Durán, M.; Rodríguez-Hermosa, J.L.; Calle, M.; Tubio-Pérez, R.; Belmonte, I.; Rodríguez-Frías, F.; Rodríguez, E.; et al. Utility of Transient Elastography for the Screening of Liver Disease in Patients with Alpha1-Antitrypsin Deficiency. *J. Clin. Med.* **2021**, *10*, 1724. [CrossRef] [PubMed]
17. Stachowiak, Z.; Wojsyk-Banaszak, I.; Jończyk-Potoczna, K.; Narożna, B.; Langwiński, W.; Kycler, Z.; Sobkowiak, P.; Bręborowicz, A.; Szczepankiewicz, A. MiRNA Expression Profile in the Airways Is Altered during Pulmonary Exacerbation in Children with Cystic Fibrosis—A Preliminary Report. *J. Clin. Med.* **2020**, *9*, 1887. [CrossRef] [PubMed]
18. Magallón, M.; Carrión, A.E.; Bañuls, L.; Pellicer, D.; Castillo, S.; Bondía, S.; Navarro-García, M.M.; González, C.; Dasí, F. Oxidative Stress and Endoplasmic Reticulum Stress in Rare Respiratory Diseases. *J. Clin. Med.* **2021**, *10*, 1268. [CrossRef] [PubMed]
19. Reula, A.; Pellicer, D.; Castillo, S.; Magallón, M.; Armengot, M.; Herrera, G.; O'Connor, J.-E.; Bañuls, L.; Navarro-García, M.M.; Escribano, A.; et al. New Laboratory Protocol to Determine the Oxidative Stress Profile of Human Nasal Epithelial Cells Using Flow Cytometry. *J. Clin. Med.* **2021**, *10*, 1172. [CrossRef] [PubMed]
20. Bañuls, L.; Pellicer, D.; Castillo, S.; Navarro-García, M.M.; Magallón, M.; González, C.; Dasí, F. Gene Therapy in Rare Respiratory Diseases: What Have We Learned So Far? *J. Clin. Med.* **2020**, *9*, 2577. [CrossRef] [PubMed]

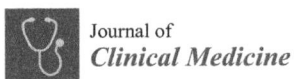

Article

Understanding Primary Ciliary Dyskinesia: Experience From a Mediterranean Diagnostic Reference Centre

Miguel Armengot-Carceller [1,2,3], Ana Reula [3,4,*], Manuel Mata-Roig [4], Jordi Pérez-Panadés [5], Lara Milian-Medina [4] and Carmen Carda-Batalla [4]

1. Surgery Department, Faculty of Medicine, University of Valencia, 46010 Valencia, Spain; miguel.armengot@uv.es
2. ENT Service, University and Polytechnic Hospital La Fe, 46026 Valencia, Spain
3. Grupo de Biomedicina Molecular, Celular y Genómica IIS La Fe, 46026 Valencia, Spain
4. Pathology Department, Faculty of Medicine, University of Valencia, 46010 Valencia, Spain; Manuel.Mata@uv.es (M.M.-R.); lara.milian@uv.es (L.M.-M.); carmen.carda@uv.es (C.C.-B.)
5. Subdirección General de Epidemiología, Vigilancia de la Salud y Sanidad Ambiental, Conselleria de Sanitat Universal i Salut Pública, Generalitat Valenciana, 46010 Valencia, Spain; perez_jorpan@gva.es
* Correspondence: Ana.Reula@uv.es

Received: 31 January 2020; Accepted: 10 March 2020; Published: 16 March 2020

Abstract: Background: Due to the lack of a gold standard diagnostic test, reference centres with experienced personnel and costly procedures are needed for primary ciliary dyskinesia (PCD) diagnostics. Diagnostic flowcharts always start with clinical symptoms. Therefore, the aim of this work is to define differential clinical criteria so that only patients clinically compatible with PCD are referred to reference centres. Materials and methods: 18 variables from 476 Mediterranean patients with clinically suspicious PCD were collected. After analysing cilia function and ultrastructure, 89 individuals were diagnosed with PCD and 387 had a negative diagnosis. Simple logistic regression analysis, considering PCD as a dependent variable and the others as independent variables, was done. In order to define the variables that best explain PCD, a step-wise logistic regression model was defined. Aiming to classify individuals as PCD or PCD-like patients, based on variables included in the study, a classification and regression tree (CART) was designed. Results and conclusions: Simple logistic regression analysis shows statistically significant association between age at the beginning of their symptomatology, periodicity, fertility, situs inversus, recurrent otitis, atelectasis, bronchiectasis, chronic productive cough, rhinorrea, rhinusinusitis and recurrent pneumonias, and PCD. The step-wise logistic regression model selected situs inversus, atelectasis, rhinorrea, chronic productive cough, bronchiectasis, recurrent pneumonias, and otitis as PCD predictive variables (82% sensitivity, 88% specificity, and 0.92 Area Under the Curve (AUC)). A decision tree was designed in order to classify new individuals based on pansinusitis, situs inversus, periodicity, rhinorrea, bronchiectasis, and chronic wet cough.

Keywords: standard diagnosis; reference centres; clinical presentation; cilia; primary ciliary dyskinesia

1. Introduction

Primary ciliary dyskinesia (PCD) is a rare disease with an estimated prevalence of 1/20,000–40,000 births (Code Orphanet: ORPHA244). It is a genetically determined condition, characterized by abnormal or absent mobility of motile cilia and flagella. Consequently, PCD patients present a deficient clearance of secretions and detritus from upper and lower airways. Thus, these patients have infections and chronic inflammation of airways, as well as reduced fertility and situs inversus in 40–50% of cases (Kartagener syndrome) [1]. As PCD presents clinical similarities with other chronic respiratory diseases, its diagnostic is often delayed and, consequently, its evolution and prognosis worsen. Symptoms often start from birth, and a daily wet cough, persistent rhinitis, and serous otitis are the most frequent manifestations in children [1].

At present, there is no "gold standard" diagnostic test. However, according to the European Respiratory Society Task Force guidelines [2], PCD patients are diagnosed based on their clinical manifestations, cilia motility pattern, and frequency, measured by high-speed video microscopy (HSVM) [3], cilia ultrastructure, analysed by transmission electron microscopy (TEM) [4], and genetic testing. Nasal nitric oxide (nNO) levels are used as a screening test [1,5], but other diseases, such as adenoid hypertrophy, could also cause low nNO levels in non-PCD patients [6]. Recently, immunofluorescence staining of specific ciliary structure proteins is becoming a potential test that needs to be validated [7,8], and poor sensitivity means that genotyping cannot be used in isolation [6].

PCD testing is expensive and time-consuming and requires an experienced team of clinicians and scientists. It is, therefore, necessary to define specific and differential clinical criteria regarding other causes of chronic respiratory disease, so that only patients clinically compatible with PCD are referred to diagnostic centres [1,2,9]. In this paper, we define a clinical PCD profile, based on the comparison between data from PCD-diagnosed patients and others clinically suspicious of PCD but with negative diagnostic tests ("PCD like"). With this work, we aim to help to identify patients that require PCD testing.

The definition of a specific clinical profile together with the decision tree based on clinical manifestations will help clinicians to know when do they have to refer a patient to a PCD diagnostic reference centre. Although there already exist other studies that aim to identify candidate patients for PCD diagnostic studies [10,11], our work complements studies by defining specific parameters that allow us to differentiate between a group of patients clinically similar to PCD from those who are PCD-confirmed by diagnostic tests.

2. Materials and Methods

Samples of nasal epithelial cells for diagnostics and clinical data from patients were collected for the study after informed consent. The study protocol complied with the ethical guidelines of the 1975 Declaration of Helsinki [12]. Before starting the PCD diagnostic pathway, cystic fibrosis and alpha-1-antitrypsin deficiency were discarded. Diagnostics were established with the study of ciliary motility using HSMV and ciliary structure by TEM, according to the criteria established by the European Respiratory Society guidelines[2]. PCD patients were considered positive when having abnormal ciliary motility by HSVM and presented a TEM defect. Additionally, patients without the obvious TEM defect, who presented abnormal ciliary motility in three different HSVM analyses (when patients were free of infection), with strong clinical history, and low nNO in (those who had the measure), were also considered in the PCD group. In contrast, patients with normal HSVM and TEM tests were considered in PCD-like group.

2.1. Study Population and Clinical Data

A total of 18 variables from 476 Mediterranean patients clinically suspicious of PCD were collected in the Valencian PCD Reference Centre from 2005 to 2018: gender, age at the beginning of their clinical symptomatology (younger or older than 2 years old), familiar history of respiratory diseases, periodicity, fertility problems, situs inversus, otitis, immunodeficiency, asthma, atelectasis, bronchiectasis, chronic productive cough, rhinorrhea, rhinosinusitis, pansinusitis, pneumonias, and nasal polyposis. Additionally, tobacco was included in the study as it is a standard variable included in the majority of respiratory disease studies. After studying ciliary motility frequencies and patterns and ciliary ultrastructure, 89 PCD cases were confirmed and 387 PCD-like cases were obtained.

Male infertility was determined, only in adults, by a spermiogram after obtaining patients' informed consent. By contrast, females were considered infertile after 3 years of failure in their attempts to become pregnant [3,13]. Immunodeficiency was considered by immunoglobulins, blood cell counting, and C3 and C4 complement determination. Functional tests, such as vaccine titers, were not considered for immunodeficiency diagnostics. Asthma was considered, according to GEMA 4.4 Guide (Spanish Guide for asthma management) [14]. Family history of respiratory diseases were considered when they presented chronic bronchopulmonary or rhinosinusal disease with unclear aetiology. Bronchiectasis and atelectasis were characterized according to Kennedy et al., 2007, [15] and rhinosinusitis, according to the European Position Paper on Rhinosinusitis and Nasal Polyps [16]. A partial or total occupation of all sinus, what is known as pansinusitis, was categorized according to the Beguinon et al., 2019, evaluation of PCD patients [17].

2.2. Data Analysis

Statistical analysis was carried out with R for windows software (R Foundation for Statistical Computing, Vienna, Austria) [18]. A 5% probability of rejecting a null hypothesis when it is true ($\alpha = 0.05$) was established in all tests. For all categorical variables, contingency tables were used, which reflected the number of data observed in each category and each group. Simple logistic regression (SLR) analysis, considering PCD as the dependent variable and the others as independent variables, was done with all variables. In some variables, there were missed values because particular clinical data from some patients are unknown. These missed values were not taken into account for statistical analysis.

2.3. Multivariate Logistic Regression Model

A multivariate logistic regression analysis was carried out. All variables were entered into the model individually, and a step-wise selection was made to identify and select the significant predictors of PCD. Moreover, the influence of each significant variable on PCD diagnosis was assessed. Finally, a receiver operating characteristic (ROC) curve showing sensitivity, specificity, and overall accuracy was used to interpret significant predictors [19]. Discrimination was considered moderate if Area Under the Curve (AUC) 0.6–0.8 and good if AUC > 0.8 [20]. The Hosmer–Lemeshow goodness-of-fit test was used to assess the calibration of the model, indicating a result of <0.05, which the predicted probabilities, and the current outcome agrees poorly [21].

2.4. Classification and Regression Tree (CART)

Aiming to classify individuals as PCD or PCD-like patients based on variables included in the study, a multivariate data analysis was carried out [22]. A classification and regression tree (CART) was designed, which is based on decision rules that appear in a binary tree manner [23,24]. The leaf nodes of the tree contain an output variable, which is used to make a decision. In order to search for the best algorithm, the program starts by growing an overly large tree using forward selection. At each step, it finds the best split and grows until reaching all terminal nodes. It then prunes the tree back, creating a nested sequence of trees, decreasing in complexity [25].

3. Results

3.1. Study Population

3.1.1. Demographic Characteristics

From the initial population of 476 PCD clinically suspicious cases, 89 individuals were diagnosed with PCD (19%) and 387 (81%) had a negative diagnosis (Table 1). The age range and the median value was 19 (0–76) for the PCD group and 13 (2–83) for the PCD-like group. Additionally, we had 116 adults in the PCD-like group and 45 adults in the PCD group.

Table 1. Demographical and clinical symptom characteristics of the study populations.

	Total	PCD	PCD-Like	Adjusted OR (95% CI)	p-Value
Subjects (n)	476 (1)	89 (0.19)	387 (0.81)	-	-
Gender					
Male	250 (0.53)	46 (0.52)	204 (0.53)	1.04 (0.66–1.65)	0.861
Female	226 (0.47)	43 (0,48)	183 (0,47)		
Tobacco					
Smoker	13 (0.03)	3 (0.03)	10 (0.03)	1.31 (0.35–4.87)	0.692
Non-smoker	462 (0.97)	86 (0.97)	376 (0.97)		
Age at the Beginning of Symptomatology					
Older than 2 years old	73 (0.16)	2 (0.02)	71 (0.19)	10.23 (2.46–42.54)	**<0.001**
Younger than 2 years old	389 (0.84)	87 (0.98)	302 (0.81)		
Family History of Respiratory Diseases					
Yes	185 (0.39)	42 (0.47)	143 (0.37)	1.52 (0.96–2.43)	0.076
No	291 (0.61)	47 (0.53)	244 (0.63)		
Periodicity					
Intermittent	186 (0.42)	7 (0.08)	179 (0.50)	11.65 (5.24–25.90)	**<0.001**
Perennial	262 (0.58)	82 (0.92)	180 (0.50)		
Fertility Problems					
Yes	61 (0.56)	19 (0.66)	42 (0.53)	1.67 (0.69–4.05)	0.029
No	47 (0.44)	10 (0.34)	37 (0.47)		
Situs Inversus					
Yes	40 (0.08)	26 (0.30)	14 (0.04)	11.17 (5.53–22.57)	**<0.001**
No	435 (0.92)	62 (0.70)	373 (0.96)		
Chronic Otitis Media					
Yes	185 (0.39)	58 (0.68)	127 (0.33)	4.38 (2.65–7.25)	**<0.001**
No	286 (0.61)	27 (0.32)	259 (0.67)		
Immunodeficiency					
Yes	12 (0.03)	0 (0)	12 (0.03)	-	-
No	464 (0.97)	89 (1)	375 (0.97)		
Asthma					
Yes	130 (0.28)	22 (0.27)	108 (0.28)	0.93 (0.54–1.59)	0.785
No	339 (0.72)	61 (0.73)	278 (0.72)		
Atelectasis					
Yes	47 (0.10)	21 (0.28)	26 (0.07)	5.27 (2.78–10.01)	**<0.001**
No	414 (0.90)	55 (0.72)	359 (0.93)		
Bronchiectasis					
Yes	165 (0.35)	54 (0.68)	111 (0.29)	5.37 (3.18–9.06)	**<0.001**
No	301 (0.65)	25 (0.32)	276 (0.71)		
Chronic Productive Cough					
Yes	342 (0.72)	86 (0.97)	256 (0.66)	14.56 (4.52–46.92)	**<0.001**
No	133 (0.28)	3 (0.03)	130 (0.34)		
Rhinorrhea					
Yes	255 (0.54)	83 (0.93)	172 (0.45)	17.21 (7.34–40.37)	**<0.001**
No	220 (0.46)	6 (0.07)	214 (0.55)		
Rhinosinusitis					
Yes	120 (0.25)	53 (0.62)	67 (0.17)	7.65 (4.60–12.71)	**<0.001**
No	352 (0.75)	33 (0.38)	319 (0.83)		
Pansinusitis					
Yes	20 (0.18)	20 (0.95)	0 (0)	-	-
No	90 (0.82)	1 (0.05)	89 (1)		
Pneumonias					
Yes	217 (0.46)	65 (0.73)	152 (0.39)	4.19 (2.51–6.98)	**<0.001**
No	259 (0.54)	24 (0.27)	235 (0.61)		
Nasal Polyposis					
Yes	16 (0.03)	2 (0.02)	14 (0.04)	0.61 (0.14–2.74)	0.497
No	460 (0.97)	87 (0.98)	373 (0.96)		

Primary Ciliary Dyskinesia (PCD), bold format means the statistically significant p-values.

In our PCD population, 18.6% had immotile cilia, 34.6% had stiff ciliary movement, and 46.8% had low frequency and uncoordinated movement when analysing using HSVM. Additionally, 20% of our PCD patients had normal ultrastructure, 14.1% undetermined defects (ciliary ultrastructure was unable to be determined because there were insufficient ciliary numbers, inadequate orientation, bad quality of the simple, etc. after sampling repetition), 18.6% combined Inner Dynein Arm (IDA) and Outer Dynein Arm (ODA) defects, 38.6% partial IDA, ODA, and short arms defects, and 9.2% presented other abnormalities (such as axoneme disorganization) when studying ciliary ultrastructure by TEM.

A total of 53% of PCD-like individuals were males, while 47% were females. A total of 52% of PCD patients were males, whereas 48% were females. SLR has a p-value of 0.861, indicating that gender is not significantly related to PCD.

3.1.2. Tobacco

A total of 97% PCD-like patients were non-smokers, having the same percentages as the PCD patients group. As expected, SLR had a p-value of 0.692, so was not significantly related to PCD.

3.1.3. Age at the Beginning of Symptomatology

Based on the age of the patients at the beginning of their clinical manifestations, two groups were made: younger than 2 years old and older than 2 years old. A tota, of 81% of PCD-like patients were under 2 years, whereas 19% were older than 2 years. A total of 98% of PCD patients were under 2 years and 2% of them were older than 2 years. A p-value of <0.001 in SLR shows that, in the great majority of PCD patients, symptoms started before they were 2 years old.

3.1.4. Family History of Respiratory Diseases

A total of 63% PCD-like individuals had no familiar history of respiratory diseases and 53% of PCD ones also had no familiar history of respiratory diseases. SLR had a p-value of 0.076, indicating that familiar history is not significantly related to PCD.

3.1.5. Periodicity

While 92% of PCD patients presented their clinical symptoms in a perennial manner, in PCD-like cases, 50% of them presented their symptoms perennially. A p-value of <0.001 indicates that the variable periodicity is significantly related with PCD; the risk of having perennial symptoms being 11 times higher in PCD patients than in PCD-like patients.

3.1.6. Fertility Problems

Out of 89 PCD patients, 60 did not proceed with any information about their fertility due to the fact that they were minors or they did not consent to spermiogram realization. Therefore, in our cohort, we had 66% with and 34% without fertility problems. On the other hand, 53% of PCD like-patients presented fertility problems and 47% of them had no problems related to fertility. A p-value of 0.029 indicated that fertility is significantly related with PCD, and the risk of having fertility problems in PCD patients was 67% higher than in PCD-like patiens.

3.1.7. Situs Inversus

While 30% of PCD patients presented situs inversus, only 4% of PCD-like patients presented this characteristic. SLR had a p-value of <0.001, indicating that the probability of having situs inversus is 11 times higher in PCD patients than in PCD-like patients.

3.1.8. Chronic Otitis Media

Results show that 33% of PCD-like patients suffered from chronic otits media during their life. In contrast, 68% of PCD patients presented chronic otitis media. SLR had a p-value of <0.001, indicating that variable otitis is significantly related to PCD and the probability of having otitis in PCD patients is 4.38 times higher than in PCD-like patients.

3.1.9. Immunodeficiency

A total of 3% of PCD-like patients had immunodeficiency. However, as none of the PCD patients presented immunodeficiency, SLR analysis did not make sense.

3.1.10. Asthma

A total of 28% of PCD-like patients had asthma. Similarly, 27% of PCD patients presented with asthma. SLR had a p-value of 0.785, indicating that asthma is not significantly related to PCD.

3.1.11. Atelectasis

Our results show that 7% of PCD-like patients presented atelectasis at any time. In contrast, 28% of PCD patients had atelectasis. SLR had a p-value of < 0.001, indicating that atelectasis is significantly related to PCD, and the risk of having atelectasis in PCD patients was 5.27 times higher than in PCD-like patients.

3.1.12. Bronchiectasis

A total of 29% of PCD-like patients presented bronchiectasis. In contrast, 68% of PCD patients had bronchiectasis. SLR analysis had a p-value of <0.001, indicating that the variable bronchiectasis is significantly related to PCD. The risk of suffering bronchiectasis is 5.37 times higher in PCD-diagnosed patients.

Bronchiectasis are clinical manifestations that are not present from birth and appear with age [1]. Our cohort of PCD-confirmed patients support this fact, as the mean age of PCD patients with bronchiectasis was 31.2, and for PCD patients without this clinical symptom, the mean age was 15.8. The p-value of the t-test was <0.001, indicating that the mean age of PCD-patients with bronchiectasis was significantly higher than PCD-patients without bronchiectasis.

3.1.13. Chronic Productive Cough

Results show that 66% of PCD-like patients suffered a chronic productive cough. In contrast, 97% of PCD patients presented a chronic productive cough. SLR with a p-value of <0.001 indicates that a chronic productive cough is significantly related to PCD. The risk of presenting a chronic productive cough was 14.56 times higher in PCD patients than in PCD-like patients.

3.1.14. Rhinorrhea

A total of 45% of PCD-like patients presented rhinorrhea. In contrast, 93% of PCD diagnosed patients presented this clinical manifestation. A p-value of <0.001 in the SLR indicates that rhinorrhea is significantly related to PCD and is 17 times higher in PCD diagnosed patients.

3.1.15. Rhinosinusitis

A total of 17% of PCD-like patients had chronic rhinosinusitis. On the other hand, 62% of PCD patients had chronic rhinosinusitis. SLR analysis had a p-value of <0.001, indicating that rhinosinusitis is significantly related with PCD, and the risk was 7.65 times higher in PCD patients than in PCD-like patients.

3.1.16. Pansinusitis

From 89 PCD patients, 68 patients had no information about pansinusitis (children under 14 do not have a complete sinus formation and, therefore, maxillofacial computed axial tomography does not proceed in these patients). Of 21 patients with pansinusitis information, our cohort had 95% of PCD patients with pansinusitis. In contrast, none of the 89 analyzed PCD-like patients presented pansinusitis. In this case, SLR does not make sense because of the disequilibrium and low number of PCD patients.

3.1.17. Pneumonias

Results show that 39% of PCD-like patients and 73% of PCD patients suffered recurrent pneumonias. SLR with a p-value of <0.001 indicates that recurrent pneumonias are significantly related to PCD. The risk of this clinical manifestation was 4.19 times higher in PCD patients than in PCD-like patients.

3.1.18. Nasal Polyposis

Results show that only 4% of PCD-like patients and 2% of PCD patients presented nasal polyposis. SLR had a p-value of 0.497, indicating that nasal polyposis is not significantly related to PCD.

3.2. Stepwise Logistic Regression Model

Only individuals that started their symptomatology from infancy were considered for the step-wise logistic regression model, as there were not enough individuals that started in adulthood. From the 18 variables included in the program, 7 were selected for the best logistic regression model (Table 2). These predictors were situs inversus, atelectasis, rhinorrhea, chronic productive cough, bronchiectasis, recurrent cases of pneumonia, and otitis (ordered by the odds ratio value); p-values indicate that all variables were statistically significant.

Table 2. Factors that best predict primary ciliary dyskinesia selected by step-wise logistic regression. Regression coefficient, adjusted odds ratio (by the others variables included), and test p-value are included.

	Regression Coefficient	Adjusted OR (95% CI)	p-Value
Situs Inversus	3.835	46.29 (12.51–171.33)	<0.001
Chronic Otitis Media	0.723	2.06 (1.02–4.15)	0.043
Atelectasis	2.380	10.81 (3.9–29.97)	<0.001
Bronchiectasis	1.394	4.03 (1.85–8.76)	<0.001
Chronic Productive Cough	1.419	4.13 (0.98–17.34)	0.032
Rhinorrhea	2.328	10.26 (3.63–29.03)	<0.001
Pneumonias	1.253	3.5 (1.66–7.38)	<0.001

The Hosmer–Lemeshow test showed a good agreement between the predicted probabilities and the actual outcome ($p = 0.1182$). The sensitivity (proportion of PCD patients correctly identified) and specificity (proportion of PCD-like patients correctly identified) of the model were 80% and 88%, respectively. The discriminant ability (AUC) of this model was 0.92, indicating a good discriminative capacity (Figure 1).

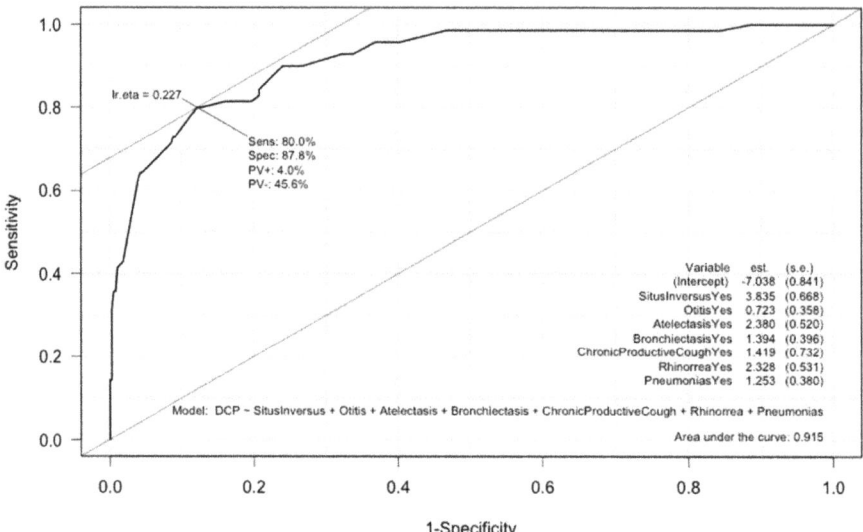

Figure 1. Receiver operating characteristic (ROC) curve for the best prediction model. Sensitivity 80%, specificity 88%, Area Under the Curve (AUC) 0.92.

3.3. Classification and Regression Tree Model

From all the variables included in the program, six were selected for the best decision tree (pansinusitis, situs inversus, periodicity, rhinorrhea, bronchiectasis, and chronic wet cough). Only individuals who started their symptomatology from infancy were considered for the CART design, as there were not enough individuals that started in adulthood. Based on these mentioned variables, an individual could be classified as a PCD patient or a PCD-like patient. As previously mentioned, pansinusitis only can be applied in patients older than 14 years old, as computed axial tomography findings could only be considered from this age. In each node (y = p1, p2), the probability of being PCD-like (p1) or PCD (p2) is specified (Figure 2). The number of patients belonging to each final group is also written.

- An individual with pansinusitis will be classified in group 13 ($n = 20$), with a 100% probability of being PCD and 0% probability of being PCD-like.
- An individual without pansinusitis that has situs inversus and intermittent periodicity will be classified in group 11 ($n = 7$) with a 100% probability of being PCD-like.
- An individual without pansinusitis that presents situs inversus and a perennial periodicity will be classified in group 12 ($n = 20$), with a 10% probability of being PCD-like and a 90% probability of being PCD.
- An individual without pansinusitis, situs inversus, and rhinorrhea will be classified in the fourth group ($n = 154$), with a 97.4% probability of being PCD-like and a 2.6% probability of being PCD.
- An individual without pansinusitis and situs inversus who presents rhinorrhea and bronchiectasis will be classified in the sixth group ($n = 62$), with a 59.7% probability of being PCD-like and a 40.3% probability of being PCD.
- An individual without pansinusitis, situs inversus, bronchiectasis, and chronic wet cough who presents rhinorrhea will be classified in group 8 ($n = 36$), with a 100% probability of being PCD-like.
- An individual without pansinusitis, situs inversus, and bronchiectasis who presents rhinorrhea and chronic wet cough will be classified in group 9 ($n = 90$), with a 77.8% probability of being PCD-like and a 22.2% probability of being PCD.

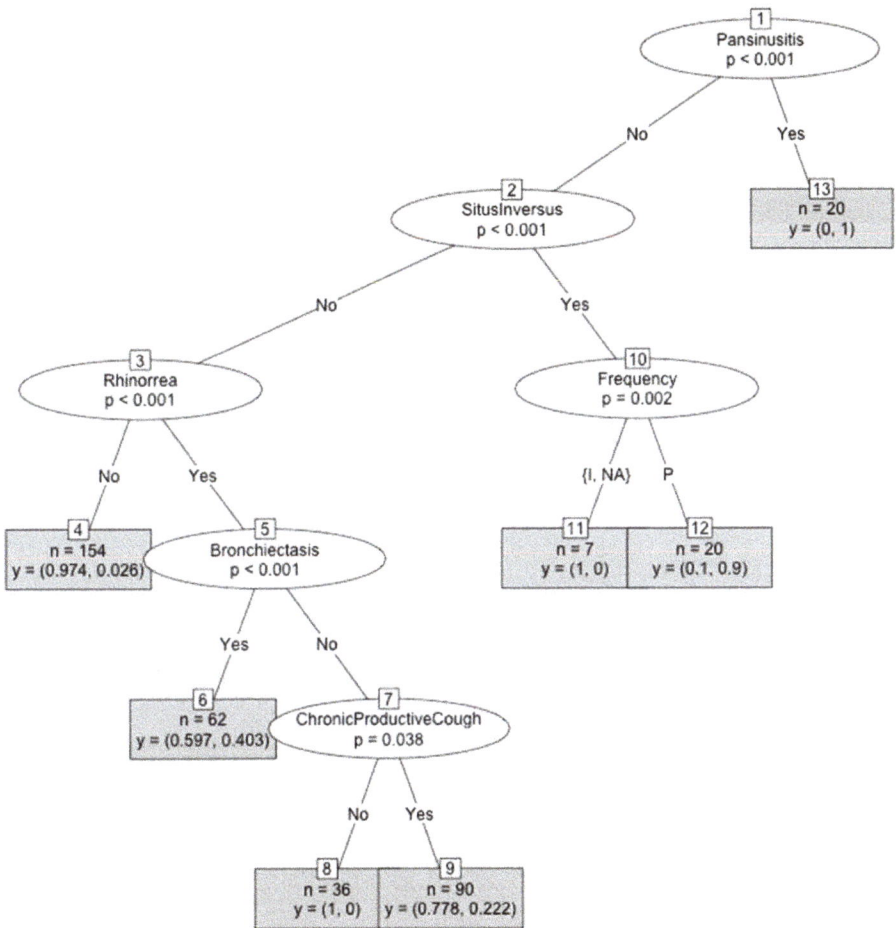

Figure 2. Classification and regression tree (CART) for the classification of individuals as PCD or PCD-like by using clinical variables as classificatory criteria. Intermittent (I), perennial (P), and not-applicable (NA).

4. Discussion

From our experience as a reference centre, we strongly believe that patient clinics are determinant for diagnostics. As mentioned before, expert personnel and expensive techniques are required, so only a compatible clinical history justifies the study [26]. Therefore, it is necessary that primary care clinicians, paediatricians, Ear, Nose and Throat clinicians (ENTs), and pulmonologists know PCD clinical compatible symptoms, in order to select which patients to refer to PCD centres. With this aim, we defined a clinical PCD profile, focused on symptoms that are significantly different in PCD-confirmed cases and PCD-like cases.

The main limitations of the study are that some data were missing for some variables, decreasing statistical test power. Due to the low number of individuals in some groups, we have no comparison between adults and patients groups to demonstrate if there were differences in the logistic regression model and the CART diagram between these age populations. Additionally, all data come from a Spanish reference centre, which can lead to bias.

We demonstrated that the great majority of PCD patients started their symptoms under 2 years old (2 years were selected as a cut-off point because patients had doubts about the neonatal clinic [22]) and they present edtheir symptomatology perennially (it did not differ between seasons). This fact is supported by Leigh et al. [10], who propose the early onset of symptoms and perennial periodicity as characteristics of PCD. Additionally, situs inversus, recurrent otitis, atelectasis, chronic productive cough, rhinorrhea, rhinosinusitis, and recurrent pneumonias are more frequent in PCD patients than in PCD-like patients, indicating that patients with these symptoms are highly suspicious of having PCD.

Immunodeficiency in some moments of its evolution could manifest with symptomatology similar to PCD, and thus we included it in our work to highlight it is an important criterion to discard before referring a patient to PCD diagnostics.

Fertility problems are significantly greater in PCD patients than in PCD-like patients. However, as our cohort was majorly composed of children, these problems were unknown in a great number of patients, which gives us inconclusive results when comparing differences between sexes. Additionally, fertility was the variable with more missing data because many patients did not consent to spermiogram realization for personal reasons. Thus, this variable was not included in the logistic regression model and the CART diagram as it was a variable that introduced bias in our data.

Bronchiectasis is also significantly more frequent in PCD patients than in PCD-like patients, being another PCD-clinical suggesting symptom. However, this clinical manifestation does not appear from birth, and our data demonstrated that this symptom became more frequent in adults than in children with PCD. Thus, bronchiectasis are helpful for PCD-suspicious adults, but it is a manifestation that is less informative in children.

One critical aspect before starting the diagnostic flowchart in a PCD reference centre is to define which are the key clinical manifestations [27,28]. With this aim, the step-wise logistic regression analysis of this work associates situs inversus, atelectasis, rhinorrhea, chronic productive cough, bronchiectasis, recurrent cases of pneumonia, and otitis as PCD predictive variables. These results agree with the four clinical features proposed by Leigh et al. [10] for PCD clinical characterisation, despite differing in the methodology used for diagnostics and statistical analysis.

Behan et al. in the PICADAR (PrImary CiliARy DyskinesiA Rule) study used a similar statistical approach to decide seven variables significantly associated with PCD. They found associations between PCD and situs inversus, neonatal chest symptoms, and hearing problems [11]. Our results are in the same line, but we considered symptoms presenting before 2 years old and chronic otitis media. However, we did not assess admission to the neonatal unit, rhinitis, gestational age, and congenital heart defects in our Mediterranian cohort.

Complementary to our work, Behan et al. [11] in PICADAR and Leigh et al. [10] defined clinical variables that help clinicians suspect PCD. On the one hand, Leigh et al. only included children and adolescents in their study. On the other hand, the PICADAR algorithm design is not sufficient for diagnosing PCD in adult patients as three of their considered items are related to neonates (scoring 6 points out of a maximum of 14). Our diagnostic diagrams arise not only in new-borns or paediatric patients, but also in adult clinics. This is a relevant point, as there are still many adults with PCD without a correct diagnostic and not all of them remember to register or have registered their manifestations when they born, so our method, which was also based in exploratory findings (such as rhinosinusal and pulmonary Computed Tomgraphy (CT)), is a valuable tool for adult patients. Additionally, in this work, we defined a classificatory tree that could help clinicians to know the probability of having a PCD patient, according to their clinical manifestations, based on our experience [23].

5. Conclusions

- SLR analysis shows a statistically significant association between some explicative variables and PCD: age at the beginning of their symptomatology, periodicity, fertility, situs inversus, recurrent otitis, atelectasis, bronchiectasis, chronic productive cough, rhinorrhea, rhinosinusitis, and recurrent pneumonias.

- Bronchiectasis is significantly more frequent in adults than in children with PCD.
- A step-wise logistic regression model selected situs inversus, atelectasis, rhinorrhea, chronic productive cough, bronchiectasis, recurrent pneumonias, and otitis as PCD predictive variables (from the most to the least important predicting factor), designing a model with 82% sensitivity, 88% specificity, and 0.92 AUC. Combination of all these clinical symptoms in the same patient determines a high probability of having PCD.
- A decision tree was designed in order to classify new individuals based on different clinical manifestations: pansinusitis, situs inversus, periodicity, rhinorrhea, bronchiectasis, and chronic wet cough.

Author Contributions: M.A.-C. recruited patients' clinical information and informed consents and contributed to diagnosis. A.R. contributed to high-speed video microscopy (HSVM) analysis and wrote the manuscript. M.M.-R., L.M.-M., and C.C.-B. contributed to transmission electron microscopy (TEM) analysis and database creation. J.P.-P. carried out the statistical analysis. All authors critically reviewed the manuscript. All authors have read and agreed to the published version of the manuscript.

Acknowledgments: Authors are grateful for the professional English language editing of Mr Arash Javadinejad, English Instructor and Publication Editor at the IIS La Fe, Valencia, Spain.

Conflicts of Interest: The authors declare no conflict of interest.

References

1. Reula, A.; Lucas, J.S.; Moreno-Galdó, A.; Romero, T.; Milara, X.; Carda, C.; Armengot-Carceller, M. New insights in primary ciliary dyskinesia. *Expert Opin. Orphan Drugs* **2017**, *5*, 537–548. [CrossRef]
2. Lucas, J.S.; Barbato, A.; Collins, S.A.; Goutaki, M.; Behan, L.; Caudri, D.; Hogg, C. European Respiratory Society guidelines for the diagnosis of primary ciliary dyskinesia. *Eur. Respir. J.* **2017**, *49*. [CrossRef] [PubMed]
3. Armengot, M.; Milara, J.; Mata, M.; Carda, C.; Cortijo, J. Cilia motility and structure in primary and secondary ciliary dyskinesia. *Am. J. Rhinol. Allergy* **2010**, *24*, 175–180. [CrossRef] [PubMed]
4. Carda, C.; Armengot, M.; Escribano, A.; Peydro, A. Ultrastructural patterns of primary ciliar dyskinesia syndrome. *Ultrastruct. Pathol.* **2005**, *29*, 3–8. [CrossRef] [PubMed]
5. Bush, A.; Chodhari, R.; Collins, N.; Copeland, F.; Hall, P.; Harcourt, J.; O'Callaghan, C. Primary ciliary dyskinesia: Current state of the art. *Arch. Dis. Child.* **2007**, *92*, 1136–1140. [CrossRef] [PubMed]
6. Rubbo, B.; Shoemark, A.; Jackson, C.L.; Hirst, R.; Thompson, J.; Hayes, J.; Reading, I. Accuracy of High-Speed Video Analysis to Diagnose Primary Ciliary Dyskinesia. *Chest* **2019**, *155*, 1008–1017. [CrossRef]
7. Baz-Redón, N.; Rovira-Amigo, S.; Camats-Tarruella, N.; Fernández-Cancio, M.; Garrido-Pontnou, M.; Antolín, M.; Moreno-Galdó, A. Role of Immunofluorescence and Molecular Diagnosis in the Characterization of Primary Ciliary Dyskinesia. *Arch. Bronconeumol.* **2019**, *55*, 439–441, in press. [CrossRef]
8. Shoemark, A.; Frost, E.; Dixon, M.; Ollosson, S.; Kilpin, K.; Patel, M.; Hogg, C. Accuracy of immunofluorescence in the diagnosis of primary ciliary dyskinesia. *Am. J. Respir. Crit. Care Med.* **2017**, *196*, 94–101. [CrossRef]
9. Knowles, M.R.; Daniels, L.A.; Davis, S.D.; Zariwala, M.A.; Leigh, M.W. Primary ciliary dyskinesia: Recent advances in diagnostics, genetics, and characterization of clinical disease. *Am. J. Respir. Crit. Care Med.* **2013**, *188*, 913–922. [CrossRef]
10. Leigh, M.W.; Ferkol, T.W.; Davis, S.D.; Lee, H.S.; Rosenfeld, M.; Dell, S.D.; Zariwala, M.A. Clinical Features and Associated Likelihood of Primary Ciliary Dyskinesia in Children and Adolescents. *Ann. Am. Thorac. Soc.* **2016**, *13*, 1305–1313. [CrossRef]
11. Behan, L.; Dimitrov, B.D.; Kuehni, C.E.; Hogg, C.; Carroll, M.; Evans, H.J.; Lucas, J.S. PICADAR: A diagnostic predictive tool for primary ciliary dyskinesia. *Eur. Respir. J.* **2016**, *47*, 1103–1112. [CrossRef] [PubMed]
12. World Medical Association. Declaration of Helsinki. *Br. Med. J.* **1996**, *313*, 1448–1449. [CrossRef]
13. Vanaken, G.J.; Bassinet, L.; Boon, M.; Mani, R.; Honore, I.; Papon, J.F.; Escudier, E. Infertility in an adult cohort with primary ciliary dyskinesia: Phenotype-gene association. *Eur. Respir. J.* **2017**, *50*, 1700314. [CrossRef] [PubMed]

14. Barranco Sanz, P.; Del Cuvillo, A.; Delgado-Romero, J.; Entrenas-Costa, L.M.; Ginel-Mendoza, L.; Giner-Donaire, J.; Korta-Murua, J.; Llauger-Rosselló, M.A.; Lobo-Álvarez, M.A.; Martín-Pérez, P.J.; et al. *4.4.Spanish Guide for Asthma Management*; Luzán5: Madrid, Spain, 2019.
15. Kennedy, M.P.; Noone, P.G.; Leigh, M.W.; Zariwala, M.A.; Minnix, S.L.; Knowles, M.R.; Molina, P.L. High-resolution CT of patients with primary ciliary dyskinesia. *Am. J. Roentgenol.* **2007**, *188*, 1232–1238. [CrossRef]
16. Fokkens, W.J.; Lund, V.J.; Mullol, J.; Bachert, C.; Alobid, I.; Baroody, F.; Georgalas, C. EPOS 2012: European position paper on rhinosinusitis and nasal polyps 2012. A summary for otorhinolaryngologists. *Rhinology* **2012**, *50*, 1–12. [CrossRef]
17. Bequignon, E.; Dupuy, L.; Zerah-Lancner, F.; Bassinet, L.; Honoré, I.; Legendre, M.; Escudier, E. Critical Evaluation of Sinonasal Disease in 64 Adults with Primary Ciliary Dyskinesia. *J. Clin. Med.* **2019**, *8*, 619. [CrossRef]
18. R Core Team. *R: A Language and Environment for Statistical Computing*; R Foundation for Statistical Computing: Vienna, Austria, 2018.
19. Carstensen, B.; Plummer, M.; Laara, E.; Hills, M. *Epi: A Package for Statistical Analysis in Epidemiology*, R package version 2.35; R Foundation for Statistical Computing: Vienna, Austria, 2019.
20. Kumar, A.; Indrayan, R. Receiver operating characteristic (ROC) curve for medical researchers. *Indian Pediatrics* **2011**, *48*, 277–287. [CrossRef]
21. Steyerberg, E. *Clinical Prediction Models: A Practical Approach to Development, Validation and Updating*; Springer: Berlin, Germany, 2009.
22. Peña, D. *Análisis de Datos Multivariantes*; McGraw-Hill: New York, NY, USA, 2013.
23. *Classification and Regression Trees*; Routledge: Abingdon, UK, 2017.
24. Kamiński, P.; Jakubczyk, B.; Szufel, M. A framework for sensitivity analysis of decision trees. *Cent. Eur. J. Oper. Res.* **2018**, *26*, 135–159. [CrossRef]
25. Horthorn, T.; Hornik, K. Unbiased Recursive Partitioning: A Conditional Inference Framework. *J. Comput. Graph. Stat.* **2006**, *15*, 651–674. [CrossRef]
26. Halbeisen, F.S.; Shoemark, A.; Barbato, A.; Boon, M.; Carr, S.; Crowley, S.; Lucas, J.S. Time trends in diagnostic testing for PCD in Europe. *Eur. Respir. J.* **2019**, *54*, 1900528. [CrossRef]
27. Contarini, M.; Shoemark, A.; Rademacher, J.; Finch, S.; Gramegna, A.; Gaffuri, M.; Blasi, F. Why, when and how to investigate primary ciliary dyskinesia in adult patients with bronchiectasis. *Multidiscip. Respir. Med.* **2018**, *13*, 26. [CrossRef] [PubMed]
28. Dalrymple, R.A.; Kenia, P. European Respiratory Society guidelines for the diagnosis of primary ciliary dyskinesia: A guideline review. *Arch. Dis. Child. Educ. Pract. Ed.* **2018**, 1–5. [CrossRef] [PubMed]

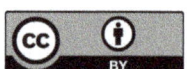

© 2020 by the authors. Licensee MDPI, Basel, Switzerland. This article is an open access article distributed under the terms and conditions of the Creative Commons Attribution (CC BY) license (http://creativecommons.org/licenses/by/4.0/).

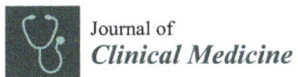

Article

Knowledge of Rare Respiratory Diseases among Paediatricians and Medical School Students

María Ángeles Requena-Fernández [1], Francisco Dasí [2,3,*], Silvia Castillo [2,4], Rafael Barajas-Cenobi [2], María Mercedes Navarro-García [2] and Amparo Escribano [2,4,5]

1. Paediatrics Unit, Hellín Hospital, 02400 Albacete, Spain; ma.reke@hotmail.com
2. Fundación Investigación Hospital Clínico Universitario de Valencia/Instituto de Investigación Sanitaria INCLIVA, 46010 Valencia, Spain; castillo_sil@gva.es (S.C.); rbarajas@incliva.es (R.B.-C.); mer_navarro2002@yahoo.es (M.M.N.-G.); aescribano@separ.es (A.E.)
3. Department of Physiology, School of Medicine, University of Valencia, 46010 Valencia, Spain
4. Paediatrics Pulmonology Unit, Hospital Clínico Universitario Valencia, 46010 Valencia, Spain
5. Department of Paediatrics, Obstetrics and Gynaecology, School of Medicine, University of Valencia, 46010 Valencia, Spain
* Correspondence: Francisco.Dasi@uv.es

Received: 10 March 2020; Accepted: 18 March 2020; Published: 22 March 2020

Abstract: Alpha-1-antitrypsin deficiency (AATD) and primary ciliary dyskinesia (PCD) are underdiagnosed rare diseases showing a median diagnostic delay of five to ten years, which has negative effects on patient prognosis. Lack of awareness and education among healthcare professionals involved in the management of these patients have been suggested as possible causes. Our aim was to assess knowledge of these diseases among paediatricians and medical school students to determine which knowledge areas are most deficient. A survey was designed with questions testing fundamental aspects of the diagnosis and treatment of AATD and PCD. A score equal to or greater than 50% of the maximum score was set as the level necessary to ensure a good knowledge of both diseases. Our results indicate a profound lack of knowledge of rare respiratory diseases among paediatric professionals and medical students, suggesting that it is necessary to increase rare respiratory diseases training among all physicians responsible for suspecting and diagnosing them; this will allow early diagnosis and the setup of preventive measures and appropriate early-stage treatment. The first step in closing this knowledge gap could be to include relevant material in the medical syllabus.

Keywords: alpha-1 antitrypsin deficiency; primary ciliary dyskinesia; rare respiratory diseases

1. Introduction

Alpha1-antitrypsin deficiency (AATD) is a rare hereditary condition characterised by low plasma levels of alpha1-antitrypsin (AAT), a serine protease inhibitor synthesised and secreted mainly by hepatocytes, of which the primary role is to protect the lung parenchyma from proteolytic enzymes such as neutrophil elastase (NE) and proteinase 3. The disease is caused by mutations in the *SERPINA1* gene. Clinical manifestations include pulmonary emphysema; liver cirrhosis; and, in rare cases, necrotising panniculitis and antineutrophil cytoplasmic antibody (C-ANCA)-positive vasculitis [1]. Current American Thoracic Society (ATS) and European Respiratory Society (ERS) guidelines recommend testing plasma AAT levels in individuals with Chronic Obstructive Pulmonary Disease (COPD), unexplained chronic liver disease, bronchiectasis, panniculitis, or granulomatosis with polyangiitis, along with the parents, siblings, and children of individuals with a mutated AAT allele. Despite these recommendations, AATD is highly underdiagnosed [2]. AATD is one of the most common inherited disorders [3], with a prevalence of 1–5/10,000. It is estimated that about 3.4 million individuals worldwide have deficient allele genotypes that lead to AAT deficiency [4]; nevertheless, more than 90% of affected subjects remain underdiagnosed [3,5]. A diagnostic delay is observed with an average interval of 8.3 years between onset of pulmonary symptoms and diagnosis and consultations with several clinicians before diagnosis [5] (an average of 2.7 physicians), leading to irreversible lung function impairment, which could be delayed by establishing clinical controls and healthy lifestyle habits in childhood or early stages of the disease.

Primary ciliary dyskinesia (PCD) is a rare hereditary disorder with autosomal recessive inheritance, characterised by altered or absent ciliary movement, which generates mucociliary clearance deficit [6]. Prevalence is estimated at around 1/10,000 live births [7]. Clinical manifestations include neonatal respiratory distress of unknown cause; presence of *situs inversus*, ventriculomegaly, constant rhinorrhoea, chronic productive cough, or bronchiectasis of unknown cause; immobile sperm in adult males; and recurrent ectopic pregnancies in women [8,9]. Symptoms are early and recurrent from the first years of life, but as they are linked to respiratory infections, frequent in childhood, it is easy to underestimate the existence of this disease. In addition, diagnostic tests involve complex studies of ciliary motility, electron microscopy, and genetic tests, which are inaccessible in many centres and yield difficult-to-interpret results.

Prompt diagnosis is important in both diseases because early treatment helps slow progression. Therefore, the aim of the present work was to evaluate whether the under- and delayed diagnosis observed was due to a lack of knowledge of these diseases by medical doctors who manage these patients at the paediatric age (primary care paediatricians and paediatric specialists in pulmonology and gastroenterology). To this end, a series of surveys assessing physicians' knowledge of these rare diseases were prepared. Medical students were also included in the survey to ascertain whether the problem is due to insufficient medical school training (since education in medical schools is generalist and based primarily on knowledge of highly prevalent diseases) or to the impossibility of gaining experience in clinical practice because of the rarity of these pathologies together with limited training recycling in this area.

2. Materials and Methods

2.1. Study Design, Setting, and Participants

An analytical, observational, and cross-sectional study was carried out using anonymous surveys at the Paediatric Pulmonology Unit of the Hospital Clínico Universitario Valencia (HCUV) from January 2015 to January 2017.

All members of the Valencian Society of Paediatrics (SVP) (1241 members); Spanish Society of Paediatric Pulmonology (SENP) (275); and Spanish Paediatric Gastroenterology, Hepathology and Nutrition Society (SEGHNP) (400) were invited to participate in the study, as were all students enrolled in the final year of the Faculty of Medicine of the University of Valencia (271 students). The Supplementary file shows the specific questionnaires developed for AATD and for PCD, respectively. Both questionnaires were validated by four experts in both pathologies (see Supplementary file for further explanations on validation). After project approval from the Boards of Directors of the Scientific Societies involved and by the Dean of Valencia School of Medicine, a letter of invitation was sent by e-mail to all members of the institutions and to final-year medical school students requesting their participation.

A separate online data-collection questionnaire was used for each of the two diseases studied, using a web platform called *Typeform*, which permits centralised data collection. Members of the SEGHNP answered a 12-question AATD survey (Supplementary file), while members of the SVP and SENP and medical students completed a test on both diseases, which consisted of 21 questions (Supplementary file). The surveys included four questions on professional profile (years of clinical experience, type and location of work centre, and paediatric medical speciality) and on the number of children diagnosed. Questions on self-assessment and a test of diagnostic and therapeutic competence in both diseases were also included. Overall, maximum scores were set at 7 points for the AATD and at 17 for the PCD tests. Both surveys took place in parallel. Correct answers are shown in Supplementary file.

Data were collected on an individual basis. Confidentiality was maintained in all surveys in accordance with Spanish personal data protection laws. After requesting approval from the societies' boards of directors and the Dean of the University of Valencia medical school, an invitation letter was sent by e-mail (through the medical societies and the medical school, which have legitimate access to such mailings) to the members of the aforementioned societies and to the students, requesting their participation in the study. No personal data were collected in the questionnaires. Answers collected from the online form were automatically stored in a database and then converted to a numerical scale for processing.

2.2. Statistical Analysis

Data recorded on the *Typeform* web platform were exported to the statistical software "IBM SPSS Statistics for Windows, Version 20.0" (IBM Corp, Armonk, NY, USA) for further analysis. A descriptive study of the sample was conducted, separating the results for the two diseases. Qualitative variables are shown as frequency and percentages, while for quantitative variables, data are shown as mean and standard deviation (SD). Assessment of normality was performed using the D'Agostino–Pearson normality test. Comparison between clinical specialities was performed using chi-square or Fisher test for qualitative variables and by ANOVA or by Student's t-test (normal distribution) or Mann–Whitney U test (non-normal distribution) for quantitative variables. Differences were considered statistically significant when p was <0.05.

3. Results

3.1. AATD Knowledge

The demographic characteristics and professional experience of the individuals participating in the AATD/PCD knowledge survey are shown in Table 1; 618 surveys were completed on AATD with the following distribution by groups: (i) 193 General Paediatricians (GP); (ii) 123 Paediatric Pneumologists (PP); (iii) 166 Paediatric Gastroenterologists (PG); and iv) 136 Medical School students (MS).

Regarding years of clinical practice, about one-quarter of GP (25.3%) and PG (28.3) and 7.3% of PP had less than five years' clinical experience. Characteristics of respondents with 5–15 years of clinical practice were more homogeneous between groups, showing similar percentages in GP (35.2%) and PG (32.0%) with a higher percentage of PP (43.1%). Similar results were observed in the group with more than 15 years of clinical practice, in which GP (39.3%) and PG (39.7%) showed similar percentages, with a higher percentage of PP (49.6%).

Regarding the type of healthcare practice, 57.5% of the GPs who completed the survey worked in primary care, while around 64.2% of the PPs and 63.2% of PGs worked in public tertiary hospitals. Paediatric pneumologists were considered the paediatric specialists best prepared to diagnose AATD by all the groups that participated in the survey (selected by 59% of paediatricians, 86.1% of gastroenterologists, 93.5% of pneumologists, and 35.2% of medical students). Medical doctors were notably unaware of the existence both of reference units for AATD (unknown to 70% of PPs and 77.1% of PGs) and of the Spanish Register of AATD (REDAAT) (unknown to 67.8% of those surveyed).

In the self-evaluation section, 61.7% of MSs and 45.6% of GPs admitted to having a very basic knowledge of the disease, while the majority of paediatric specialists (78.8% of pulmonologists and 62% of gastroenterologists) positively self-evaluated on diagnostic procedures. The professionals surveyed reported screening serum levels of AAT in children with hepatopathy or transaminase elevation (40.9%), repeat pneumonias (39.9%), or bronchiectasis (34.1%).

Regarding level of expertise on clinical manifestations of the disease [1] (Table 2), 39.8% of PPs and 31.9% of PGs got two or three answers correct, compared to 16% of GPs and 2.1% of

MSs. Responses regarding the most severe AATD phenotype [1] were quite satisfactory: 93.5% of PPs, 86.1% of PGs, and 59.1% of GPs answered correctly, whereas 35.3% of MSs got it right. The results are definitively unbalanced in the third question about treatment/management of AATD in children [1,10–15]. Only 25.9% of GPs, 25.2% of PPs, and 21.7% of PGs choose the three correct options. This percentage was reduced to 14.7% in MSs (Table 2).

When analysing the average score of the four groups surveyed, the highest score corresponds to the group PP (3.12 points) which, nonetheless, failed to reach the theoretical 50% set as the minimum level to "pass", a fact that reveals the respondents' low AATD knowledge level (Figure 1A).

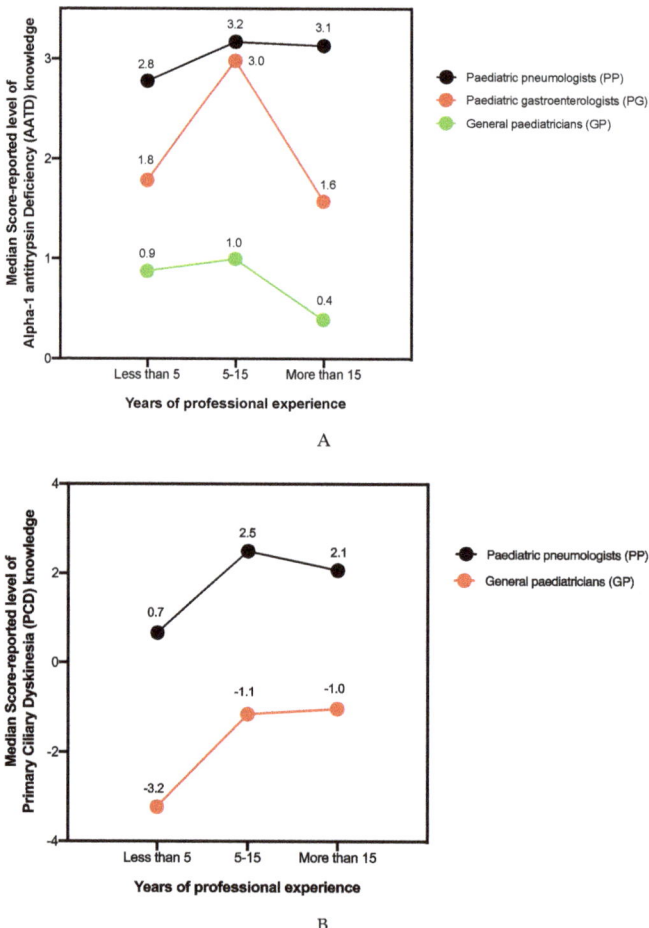

Figure 1. Alpha-1 Antitrypsin Deficiency (AATD) and Primary Ciliary Dyskinesia (PCD) knowledge in paediatric specialists in relation to years of professional experience: No group reached the minimum score required to make an early diagnosis and to adopt the appropriate measurements for correct management of patients with AATD (**A**) or PCD (**B**) regardless of years of professional experience. Maximum scores were 7 points for the AATD and 17 for the PCD tests.

A statistically significant relationship between professional profile and AATD test score ($p < 0.001$) was observed, with PPs achieving a significantly higher average than the rest. Also significant is the relationship between years of experience and score achieved ($p = 0.045$), with the particularity that the group of professionals with intermediate experience (between 5 and 15 years) were shown to be the most up-to-date on AATD, with higher average scores than those with greater or lesser experience. No significant relationship was found between subjective perception of competence by the different groups analysed (self-evaluation) and results obtained in the test ($p = 0.139$) or between degree of awareness the disease and type of healthcare practice, with the exception of the PP group ($p = 0.008$).

Finally, experience of treating patients with AATD correlated significantly with the average score obtained in the test on this pathology in PPs and PGs ($p = 0.029$ and $p < 0.001$, respectively), in contrast with the GP group ($p = 0.329$).

3.2. PCD Knowledge

Of the 457 respondents to the PCD survey, 190 were GPs, 123 were PPs, and 135 were MSs (Table 1). Professional experience was also very disparate, being more homogeneous among GPs (<5 years of experience: 25.78%; 5–15 years: 35.78%; and >15 years: 38.42%) and longer among PPs (43% 5 to 15 years and 49.6% over 15 years). As for the type of healthcare practice, 57.3% of GPs worked in health centres and 64.2% of PPs worked in tertiary public hospitals.

The professionals considered most suitable for diagnosing PCD were also paediatric specialists; specifically, the paediatric pulmonologist was chosen by 243 of those surveyed.

In the study, 66.6% of PPs stated that they knew where to refer this type of patient for more specialised diagnosis and/or follow-up. However, 78.9% of GPs and 91.1% of MSs were unaware of the existence of referral units for this disease. These data are inconsistent with their own self-evaluation, since around 50% of the three populations analysed (49.5% of GPs, 58.5% of PPs, and 54.4% of MSs) claimed to know PCD.

Based on a total score of 0–7, more than one-half of the GPs (52.6%) and MSs (77.7%) obtained a score of less than 50% (Table 3), nowhere near the results of PPs (49.59% correctly identified all early symptoms). However, this apparently excellent result is overshadowed by a not inconsiderable percentage (38.2%) that considered some late clinical manifestations such as bronchiectasis to be early ones or that incorrectly identified others as characteristic symptoms of PCD (e.g., recurrent bronchial obstructive crisis).

In the section on diagnostic options (Table 3), with a maximum score of 10 points, 27.36% and 26% of GPs and MSs, respectively, obtained more than 50% of correct options, whereas 43.9% of PPs obtained five or more correct answers [16–22].

After penalising respondents for incorrectly selected options, the average scores obtained by GPs, PPs, and MSs were −1.64, 2.15, and −2.47 points, respectively, out of a total 17 possible points, denoting very low overall PCD knowledge (Figure 1B).

Not unexpectedly, the results are closely related to the respondent's professional profile ($p < 0.001$), with PPs showing the greatest knowledge of the disease, despite not reaching the minimum 8.5 points (50% of the maximum score) required to pass. The overall test score does not correlate with years of professional experience ($p = 0.778$), self-assessment ($p = 0.687$), or work centre ($p = 0.132$). Only the GP group showed a significant correlation with having diagnosed patients with PCD ($p = 0.023$), absent in PPs ($p = 0.163$).

Table 1. Demographic characteristics and professional experience of the individuals participating in the alpha-1 antitrypsin deficiency/primary ciliary dyskinesia (AATD/PCD) knowledge study.

Groups	Number of Surveys Completed	Years of Clinical Practice			Healthcare Practice Type						AATD/PCD Patient Management		Awareness of Reference Units	
		<5	5-15	>15	Primary Care (Clinic)	Private Hospital	Public Tertiary Hospital	District Hospital	Private Practice	Public Secondary Hospital	Yes	No	Yes	No
General paediatricians (GP)	A: 193	25.3%	35.2%	39.3%	57.5%	2.6%	19.7%	17.1%	2.1%	1.0%	48.7%	51.3%	14.5%	85.5%
	B: 190	25.7%	35.7%	38.4%	57.3%	2.6%	19.4%	17.3%	2.1%	1.3%	46.8%	52.1%	19.7%	80.3%
Paediatric pneumologists (PP)	A: 123	7.3%	43.1%	49.6%	-	3.2%	64.2%	24.4%	2.4%	5.7%	52.0%	48.0%	30.0%	70.0%
	B: 123	7.4%	43.0%	49.6%	-	3.2%	64.2%	24.3%	2.4%	5.7%	47.1%	52.9%	66.6%	33.3%
Paediatric gastroenterologists (PG)	A: 166	28.3%	32.0%	39.7%	-	8.4%	63.2%	26.5%	1.2%	0.6%	66.9%	33.1%	22.9%	77.1%
Medical students (MS)	A: 136	-	-	-	-	-	-	-	-	-	32.3%	67.7%	9.5%	90.4%
	B: 135	-	-	-	-	-	-	-	-	-			8.9%	91.1%

A: AATD knowledge survey. B: PCD knowledge survey.

Table 2. Correct answers to the alpha-1 antitrypsin deficiency (AATD) knowledge questionnaire.

Groups	Number of Correct Answers on the Clinical Manifestations of the Disease				Correct Answers about the Phenotype of the Disease	Number of Correct Answers about the Treatment of the Disease			
	0	1	2	3		0	1	2	3
General paediatricians (GP)	44.5%	38.5%	15.5%	1.50%	59.1%	16.1%	24.9%	33.2%	25.8%
Paediatric pneumologists (PP)	12.2%	47.9%	37.4%	2.4%	93.5%	9.8%	26.8%	38.2%	25.2%
Paediatric gastroenterologists (PG)	18.6%	49.4%	30.1%	1.8%	86.1%	21.7%	25.3%	31.3%	21.7%
Medical students (MS)	77.9%	19.8%	1.4%	0.7%	35.3%	32.4%	23.5%	29.4%	14.7%

Correct symptoms [1]: neonatal jaundice; transaminases elevation; no expression. Correct phenotype [1]: most severe phenotype = ZZ. Correct treatment [1,10–15]: balanced diet rich in antioxidants; early prevention/control of respiratory infections and bronchial inflammation; avoiding active/passive smoking and environmental pollution.

Table 3. Correct answers to primary ciliary dyskinesia (PCD) knowledge questionnaire.

Groups	Correct clinical Manifestations									Correct Diagnostic Options										
	0	1	2	3	4	5	6	7		0	1	2	3	4	5	6	7	8	9	10
General paediatricians (GP)	2.6%	13.1%	21.0%	15.7%	14.2%	13.6%	11.5%	7.8%		0.5%	4.7%	20.0%	28.4%	18.9%	15.7%	10.0%	1.05%	-	0.5%	-
Paediatric pneumologists (PP)	-	1.6%	6.5%	8.1%	4.8%	13.0%	16.2%	49.5%		-	1.6%	8.1%	21.9%	24.3%	25.5%	8.9%	8.1%	3.5%	-	-
Medical students (MS)	17.0%	22.9%	25.1%	12.5%	8.8%	9.6%	1.4%	2.2%		4.4%	8.1%	18.5%	19.2%	23.7%	18.5%	5.1%	1.4%	0.7%	-	-

Correct clinical manifestations: onset of symptoms in neonatal period, *situs inversus*; neonatal respiratory distress with no apparent cause; constant/persistent rhinorrhoea; recurrent or chronic moist cough; recurrent otitis; repeat pneumonia.

Correct diagnostic options in childhood:

- Not definitive for PCD diagnosis: audiometry [17], sperm motility [18], saccharin test [17].
- Partially diagnostic: chest and/or sinus x-ray [16,19], pulmonary CT, spirometry and/or plethysmography and/or diffusion test [20].

Diagnostic screening tests: nasal nitric oxide [16], mucociliary clearance test with radioisotopes [21]. Determining diagnostic tests: ciliary motility (pattern and speed) and ciliary ultrastructure [16,21,23].

4. Discussion

In rare diseases, early diagnosis is key and represents one of the main problems faced by patients and their families. Underdiagnosis and delayed diagnosis are relatively constant, probably due to the insufficient academic training on this subject in medical schools, where teaching focuses mainly on the most prevalent pathologies.

Identifying the cause of a problem is the first step towards a possible solution. Various studies have shown that lack of knowledge of rare diseases by medical doctors is a cause of under- and delayed diagnosis [5,23,24]. However, despite the fact that, in a high percentage of cases, paediatricians are at the front line in attending this type of patient/pathology, no study so far has evaluated their knowledge level in these areas, hence our proposition focusing on two of the most prevalent rare respiratory diseases, AATD and PCD, and also including students in their final year at the School of Medicine of the University of Valencia (Spain) in order to assess the level of academic training received.

We collected a total of 1081 surveys, 624 on AATD and 457 on PCD, widely surpassing the number of participants in other previous studies and focusing on previously unstudied populations: paediatricians, paediatric specialists, and final-year degree students.

The results of the two surveys showed that both MSs and GPs are unfamiliar with most of the signs or symptoms on which diagnostic suspicion of both diseases is based and are also unaware of the steps to be taken to arrive at a definitive diagnosis or to enter the relevant healthcare circuit.

As expected, familiarity with these processes is higher among PP who also have greater work experience (49.6% practicing for more than 15 years); however, the difference cannot be explained by this circumstance alone, since the number of cases diagnosed or treated by each professional is very low, regardless of their years of professional service.

No group reached the minimum score required to be able to make an early diagnosis and to adopt the appropriate measures for correct management of patients with AATD or PCD. This low formation contradicts the self-evaluations of respondents who overestimated their knowledge of both diseases; this further aggravates the problem because unawareness of shortcomings precludes learning. In the case of AATD, 45.6% of GPs and 61.7% of MS claimed to know the disease, while 78.8% of PPs and 62% of PGs believed they knew the diagnostic procedure. In PCD, half of those surveyed (49.5% of GPs, 54.4% of MSs, and 58.5%, of PPs) considered themselves competent in the disease.

In light of the above, it is particularly striking that half of the GP surveyed claimed to have attended patients with AATD (50.6%) and/or PCD (41.6%) when the low prevalence of these rare diseases limits this possibility. In the case of PCD, GP would not be the ones to diagnose these patients due to the specialised and complex techniques required for diagnosis only available at two centres in Spain (Valencia and Barcelona). This also raises doubt as to whether many PCD cases are correctly classified by GPs. This is not an issue among PPs because their specialty requires a greater degree of information/training on PCD and they do not rely exclusively on having diagnosed patients.

Analysing the responses to questions 9 and 16, PPs are the physicians considered most suitable for diagnosing both clinical entities, which is fully in line with ATS/ERS recommendations on AATD [2,25] and PCD [17], which advocate arriving at an early diagnosis during childhood.

Paediatricians' lack of awareness about reference units for either disease is also noteworthy. This could be due in the case of AATD to the scarce/null expression of the disease during paediatric age but not in PCD, since one of the two Spanish referral units is in Valencia, where this study was carried out.

It is even more surprising considering that 425 of the 457 surveyed viewed PCD as a complex disease requiring diagnostic confirmation and management in specialised centres.

Turning to screening, since the initial AATD diagnosis is performed by measuring AAT plasma levels, it was interesting to know in which cases the participating paediatricians requested this test, a question previously posed only to doctors attending adult populations [5,23,24]. It is accepted that AATD should always be ruled out in the blood relatives of patients with this diagnosis even if they are asymptomatic and in cases of neonatal jaundice or hypertransaminasemia, regardless of age, especially if there is a previous history of jaundice or liver disease. The association between AATD and asthma is controversial, with contradictory publications regarding the presence of Z alleles in asthma patients. The ATS–ERS-published consensus [2,25] recommends testing in adults with nonatopic asthma and in individuals with unexplained liver disease, including neonates and children. In our study, more than 50% of the physicians surveyed claim to request AAT levels in the clinical circumstances mentioned (Table 3) and almost 25% of PPs routinely include it when requesting any other blood test from their patients. If so, one would expect that early diagnosis of this disease would be less uncommon than it has been to date.

Contrary to expectations, working in tertiary hospitals does not seem to improve awareness of AATD and PCD. As far as the latter is concerned, the fact that most Spanish hospitals are not equipped to carry out the complete diagnosis probably explains why professionals are not familiar with the disease.

Finally, medical students were the worst performers in all questions raised about both diseases. This highlights the limited information received on rare diseases during their university studies and the need to rectify this situation. On this note, it is worth mentioning that the first course on rare diseases in Spain has been included in the Valencia School of Medicine syllabus [26]. The main objective of this course is not that students know ALL rare diseases, which would not be realistic (since there are between 6000 and 8000 rare diseases), but to generate an academic and formative space which provides tools for students and future health professionals to cope with an orphan disease. More specifically, the aim is to familiarise the student with aspects such as what a rare disease is, how and when to suspect that a patient suffers from a rare disease, the main problems faced by rare disease patients, the problems of underdiagnosis and delayed diagnosis, where to find information once the patient has been diagnosed, the lack of specific treatments, the need to boost research on rare diseases, the importance of patient associations, etc. In other words, it is intended to fill the gap in specific training in this field by developing general competencies in the field of rare diseases without focusing on individual rare diseases. Importantly, rare diseases are an opportunity, as they serve as models for diseases of high prevalence. There are numerous examples. In particular, research on familial hypercholesterolemia has contributed to the development of statins, drugs used daily by millions of people worldwide to lower high cholesterol levels and to prevent the development of cardiovascular diseases. In our view, this undoubtedly commendable initiative should be adopted in other universities worldwide.

5. Conclusions

There are significant knowledge gaps regarding AATD and PCD among medical students and paediatricians—the physicians responsible for diagnosing these diseases early—and this shortcoming is not even recognised by the majority. Our results indicate that it is necessary to increase rare respiratory diseases training among all physicians responsible for suspecting and diagnosing them, which will allow early diagnosis and the setup of preventive measures and appropriate early-stage treatment.

Supplementary Materials: The following are available online at http://www.mdpi.com/2077-0383/9/3/869/s1, Supplementary file: AATD Survey with Answers and PCD Survey with Answers and Validation Procedures.

Author Contributions: Requena had full access to all of the data in the study and takes responsibility for the integrity of the data and the accuracy of the data analysis. Conceptualization, F.D. and A.E.; Methodology, F.D. and A.E. and R.B.-C.; Software, R.B.-C.; Validation, M.Á.R.-F. and F.D. and S.C. and A.E.; Formal analysis, M.Á.R.-F.;

Investigation, M.Á.R.-F.; Resources, F.D. and A.E.; Data curation, M.Á.R.-F.; Writing, F.D.; Writing-review-editing, M.Á.R.-F. and F.D. and S.C. and R.B.-C. and M.M.N.-G. and A.E.; Visualization, M.M.N.-G.; Supervision, F.D. and A.E.; Project administration, M.M.N.-G.; Funding acquisition, F.D. and A.E. All authors have read and agreed to the published version of the manuscript.

Funding: This research received no external funding.

Conflicts of Interest: The authors declare no conflict of interest.

References

1. Torres-Durán, M.; Lopez-Campos, J.L.; Barrecheguren, M.; Miravitlles, M.; Martinez-Delgado, B.; Castillo, S.; Escribano, A.; Baloira, A.; Navarro-Garcia, M.M.; Pellicer, D.; et al. Alpha-1 antitrypsin deficiency: Outstanding questions and future directions. *Orphanet J. Rare Dis.* **2018**, *13*, 114. [CrossRef]
2. Miravitlles, M.; Dirksen, A.; Ferrarotti, I.; Koblizek, V.; Lange, P.; Mahadeva, R.; McElvaney, N.G.; Parr, D.; Piitulainen, E.; Roche, N.; et al. European Respiratory Society statement: Diagnosis and treatment of pulmonary disease in alpha1-antitrypsin deficiency. *Eur. Respir. J.* **2017**, *30*, 50. [CrossRef]
3. Greulich, T.; Vogelmeier, C.F. Alpha-1-antitrypsin deficiency: Increasing awareness and improving diagnosis. *Ther. Adv. Respir. Dis.* **2016**, *10*, 72–84. [CrossRef]
4. Stoller, J.K.; Aboussouan, L.S. A Review of 1-Antitrypsin Deficiency. *Am. J. Respir. Crit. Care Med.* **2012**, *185*, 246–259. [CrossRef] [PubMed]
5. Greulich, T.; Ottaviani, S.; Bals, R.; Lepper, P.M.; Vogelmeier, C.; Luisetti, M.; Ferrarotti, I. Alpha1-antitrypsin deficiency—Diagnostic testing and disease awareness in Germany and Italy. *Respir. Med.* **2013**, *107*, 1400–1408. [CrossRef] [PubMed]
6. Reula, A.; Lucas, J.S.; Moreno-Galdó, A.; Romero, T.; Milara, X.; Carda, C.; Mata-Roig, M.; Escribano, A.; Dasi, F.; Armengot-Carceller, M. New insights in primary ciliary dyskinesia. *Expert Opin. Orphan Drugs* **2017**, *5*, 537–548. [CrossRef]
7. Lobo, J.; Zariwala, M.A.; Noone, P.G. Primary ciliary dyskinesia. *Semin. Respir. Crit. Care Med.* **2015**, *36*, 169–179. [CrossRef]
8. Knowles, M.R.; Daniels, L.A.; Davis, S.D.; Zariwala, M.A.; Leigh, M.W. Primary ciliary dyskinesia: Recent advances in diagnostics, genetics, and characterization of clinical disease. *Am. J. Respir. Crit. Care Med.* **2013**, *188*, 913–922. [CrossRef]
9. Kuehni, C.E.; Frischer, T.; Strippoli, M.P.F.; Maurer, E.; Bush, A.; Nielsen, K.G.; Escribano, A.; Lucase, J.S.A.; Yiallouros, P.; Omran, H.; et al. Factors influencing age at diagnosis of primary ciliary dyskinesia in European children. *Eur. Respir. J.* **2010**, *36*, 1248–1258. [CrossRef]
10. Casas, F.; Blanco, I.; Martínez, M.T.; Bustamante, A.; Miravitlles, M.; Cadenas, S.; Hernández, J.M.; Lázaro, L.; Rodríguez, E.; Rodríguez-Frías, F.; et al. Actualización sobre indicaciones de búsqueda activa de casos y tratamiento con alfa-1 antitripsina por vía intravenosa en pacientes con enfermedad pulmonar obstructiva crónica asociada a déficit de alfa-1 antitripsina. *Arch. Bronconeumol.* **2015**, *51*, 185–192. [CrossRef]
11. Siri, D.; Farah, H.; Hogarth, D.K. Distinguishing alpha1-antitrypsin deficiency from asthma. *Ann. Allergy Asthma Immunol.* **2013**, *111*, 458–464. [CrossRef] [PubMed]
12. Stolk, J.; Seersholm, N.; Kalsheker, N. Alpha1-antitrypsin deficiency: Current perspective on research, diagnosis, and management. *Int. J. Chron. Obstruct. Pulmon. Dis.* **2006**, *1*, 151–160. [CrossRef] [PubMed]
13. Stolk, J. Case detection of α1-antitrypsin deficiency: Does it help the patient or the doctor? *Eur. Respir. J.* **2005**, *26*, 561–562. [CrossRef] [PubMed]
14. Tanash, H.A.; Nilsson, P.M.; Nilsson, J.Å.; Piitulainen, E. Clinical course and prognosis of never-smokers with severe alpha-1-antitrypsin deficiency (PiZZ). *Thorax* **2008**, *63*, 1091–1095. [CrossRef]
15. Teckman, J.H. Liver disease in alpha-1 antitrypsin deficiency: Current understanding and future therapy. *COPD J. Chronic Obstr. Pulm. Dis.* **2013**, *10*, 35–43. [CrossRef]
16. Bush, A.; Chodhari, R.; Collins, N.; Copeland, F.; Hall, P.; Harcourt, J.; Hariri, M.; Hogg, C.; Lucas, J.; Mitchison, H.M.; et al. Primary ciliary dyskinesia: Current state of the art. *Arch. Dis. Child.* **2007**, *92*, 1136–1140. [CrossRef]
17. Barbato, A.; Frischer, T.; Kuehni, C.E.; Snijders, D.; Azevedo, I.; Baktai, G.; Bartoloni, L.; Eber, E.; Escribano, A.; Haarman, E.; et al. Primary ciliary dyskinesia: A consensus statement on diagnostic and treatment approaches in children. *Eur. Respir. J.* **2009**, *34*, 1264–1276. [CrossRef]

18. Mittal, V.; Shah, A. Situs Inversus Totalis: The Association of Kartagener's Syndrome with Diffuse Bronchiolitis and Azoospermia. *Arch. Bronconeumol.* **2012**, *48*, 179–182. [CrossRef]
19. Magnin, M.L.; Cros, P.; Beydon, N.; Mahloul, M.; Tamalet, A.; Escudier, E.; Clément, A.; le Pointe, H.D.; Blanchon, S. Longitudinal lung function and structural changes in children with primary ciliary dyskinesia. *Pediatr. Pulmonol.* **2012**, *47*, 816–825.
20. Armengot, M.; Bonet, M.; Carda, C.; Gómez, M.J.; Milara, J.; Mata, M.; Cortijo, J. Development and Validation of a Method of Cilia Motility Analysis for the Early Diagnosis of Primary Ciliary Dyskinesia. *Acta Otorrinolaringol.* **2012**, *63*, 1–8. [CrossRef]
21. Carlén, B.; Stenram, U. Primary ciliary dyskinesia: A review. *Ultrastruct. Pathol.* **2005**, *29*, 217–220. [CrossRef] [PubMed]
22. Armengot, M.; Milara, J.; Mata, M.; Carda, C.; Cortijo, J. Cilia motility and structure in primary and secondary ciliary dyskinesia. *Am. J. Rhinol. Allergy* **2010**, *24*, 175–180. [CrossRef] [PubMed]
23. Taliercio, R.M.; Chatburn, R.L.; Stoller, J.K. Knowledge of alpha-1 antitrypsin deficiency among internal medicine house officers and respiratory therapists: Results of a survey. *Respir. Care* **2010**, *55*, 322–327. [PubMed]
24. Esquinas, C.; Barrecheguren, M.; Sucena, M.; Rodriguez, E.; Fernandez, S.; Miravitlles, M. Practice and knowledge about diagnosis and treatment of alpha-1 antitrypsin deficiency in Spain and Portugal. *BMC Pulm. Med.* **2016**. [CrossRef]
25. European, Respiratory Society, and American Thoracic Society. American Thoracic Society/European Respiratory Society statement: Standards for the diagnosis and management of individuals with alpha-1 antitrypsin deficiency. *Am. J. Respir. Crit. Care Med.* **2003**, *168*, 818–900. [CrossRef]
26. University of Valencia. School of Medicine Degree Programme. Available online: https://www.uv.es/uvweb/undergraduate-degree-medicine/en/what-can-study-/degree-programme/degree-programme/degree-medicine-1285938467926/Titulacio.html?id=1285847387054&p2=2 (accessed on 19 March 2020).

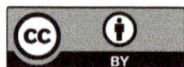

© 2020 by the authors. Licensee MDPI, Basel, Switzerland. This article is an open access article distributed under the terms and conditions of the Creative Commons Attribution (CC BY) license (http://creativecommons.org/licenses/by/4.0/).

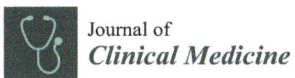
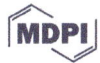

Article

Long-Term Treatment Outcome of Progressive *Mycobacterium avium* Complex Pulmonary Disease

Kiyoharu Fukushima [1,2], Seigo Kitada [3], Yuko Abe [2], Yuji Yamamoto [1], Takanori Matsuki [1], Hiroyuki Kagawa [1], Yohei Oshitani [1], Kazuyuki Tsujino [1], Kenji Yoshimura [1], Mari Miki [1], Keisuke Miki [1] and Hiroshi Kida [1,2,*]

1. Department of Respiratory Medicine, National Hospital Organization Osaka Toneyama Medical Centre, 5-1-1 Toneyama, Toyonaka, Osaka 560-8552, Japan; fukushima@imed3.med.osaka-u.ac.jp (K.F.); yamamoto.yuji.yf@mail.hosp.go.jp (Y.Y.); matsuki.takanori.qn@mail.hosp.go.jp (T.M.); kagawa.hiroyuki.kx@mail.hosp.go.jp (H.K.); oshitani.yohei.fp@mail.hosp.go.jp (Y.O.); tsujino.kazuyuki.bh@mail.hosp.go.jp (K.T.); yoshimura.kenji.ka@mail.hosp.go.jp (K.Y.); miki.mari.bk@mail.hosp.go.jp (M.M.); miki.keisuke.pu@mail.hosp.go.jp (K.M.)
2. Department of Respiratory Medicine and Clinical Immunology, Osaka University Graduate School of Medicine, 2-2 Yamadaoka, Suita, Osaka 565-0871, Japan; y.abe@imed3.med.osaka-u.ac.jp
3. Department of Respiratory Medicine, Yao Tokusyuukai General Hospital, 1-17 Wakakusa-cho, Yao, Osaka 581-0011, Japan; kitadas1@mac.com
* Correspondence: hiroshi.kida@icloud.com; Tel.: +81-6-6853-2001; Fax: +81-6-6853-3127

Received: 2 March 2020; Accepted: 29 April 2020; Published: 2 May 2020

Abstract: Background: Multidrug therapy is essential for preventing respiratory failure in patients with highly progressive *Mycobacterium avium* complex pulmonary disease (MAC-PD). However, the prognosis and long-term outcome following combination therapy is poorly understood. Methods: We retrospectively evaluated the clinical characteristics and long-term outcomes in patients with chemo-naïve progressive MAC-PD, hospitalized for first-line multidrug therapy. Results: Among 125 patients, 86 (68.8%) received standardized treatment (rifampicin, ethambutol, clarithromycin), 25 (20.0%) received a fluoroquinolone (FQ)-containing regimen, and 53 (42.4%) received aminoglycoside injection. The sputum conversion rate was 80.0%, and was independently associated with standardized treatment. The incidence of refractory disease (45.6%) was independently and negatively associated with standardized regimen and aminoglycoside use. Choice of an FQ-containing regimen was not associated with positive outcome. Clarithromycin resistance occurred in 16.8% and was independently associated with refractory disease. MAC-PD-associated death occurred in 3.3% of patients with non-cavitary nodular bronchiectasis (NB) and 21.3% with cavitary MAC-PD over a median follow-up period of 56.4 months. The rates of MAC-PD-associated death were comparable between cavitary-NB and fibrocavitary disease. Concurrent chronic pulmonary aspergillosis (CPA) occurred in 13 (17.3%) patients with cavitary MAC-PD, and age, diabetes mellitus, and CPA were independent risk factors for mortality. Conclusions: Standardized intensive multidrug treatment reduces disease progression and persistence in progressive MAC-PD. Cavitary NB may differ from, rather than being just an advanced stage of, non-cavitary NB. The high incidence and significant mortality of CPA in cavitary MAC-PD highlight the need for early diagnosis and treatment.

Keywords: *Mycobacterium avium*; *Mycobacterium intracellulare*; nodular bronchiectasis; non-tuberculous mycobacteria; pulmonary aspergillosis; rare pulmonary disease

1. Introduction

Non-tuberculous mycobacterial pulmonary disease (NTM-PD) has been increasingly implicated in a broad range of infectious diseases both in Japan and worldwide [1,2]. *Mycobacterium avium* complex (MAC), predominantly comprising *M. avium* and *M. intracellulare*, is the most common etiology of NTM lung disease [3]. The correct diagnosis and management of this disease are extremely important. Although, multidrug combination therapy is considered essential for preventing respiratory failure in highly progressive MAC-PD, and rifampicin (RFP) + ethambutol (EB) + macrolides are considered to be the standardized regimen, no large studies have validated the appropriateness of current treatment guidelines for MAC-PD [4–6]. Fluoroquinolones (FQ) have also reportedly been effective and represent a promising alternative for MAC infection [7,8]; however, data regarding combination therapy including FQ are lacking. Furthermore, the addition of an aminoglycoside may also be recommended in patients with severe and advanced disease, but their long term benefits also remain unproven [9]. There is thus a need to determine the efficacy and long-term outcome of combination therapy in patients with progressive MAC-PD. In this study, we aimed to evaluate the clinical outcomes of patients treated with combined antimicrobial drugs for progressive MAC-PD, and examine the factors associated with refractory disease and mortality.

2. Material and Methods

2.1. Study Design and Patients

This retrospective study was performed in accordance with the Declaration of Helsinki and was approved by the institutional research ethics board of the National Hospital Organization Osaka Toneyama Medical Centre (TNH-2019033), which waived the requirement for informed consent due to the retrospective nature of the analysis. The medical records of patients with non-tuberculous mycobacterial pulmonary disease (NTM-PD) hospitalized at the National Hospital Organization Osaka Toneyama Medical Centre between January 2012 and April 2018 were retrospectively reviewed. None of the patients tested positive for human immunodeficiency virus (HIV). None of the patients received clarithromycin (CAM) monotherapy before hospitalization. All patients were followed until their last visit, death, or the end of study period (31 October 2019).

2.2. Data Collection

Clinical data were collected from medical records. Baseline clinical parameters were obtained within 1 month of the initial diagnosis. Patient data included age, sex, body mass index (BMI), smoking status, underlying diseases, acquired comorbidities, treatment durations, antimicrobial treatment for MAC-PD, results of bacterial culture, and chest computed tomography (CT) findings. The diagnosis of chronic pulmonary aspergillosis (CPA) was based on the European Respiratory Society (ERS) and European Society of Clinical Microbiology and Infectious Diseases (ESCMID) guidelines for the management of CPA combined with clinical symptoms, radiological findings, positive *Aspergillus* serology, or isolation of *Aspergillus* species from respiratory samples [10].

2.3. Radiological Evaluation

Radiographic abnormalities were classified according to distinct disease patterns on chest CT. Patients with fibrocavitary lesions and pleural thickening mainly in the upper lobes on CT were diagnosed with fibrocavitary (FC) disease, and patients with multiple nodules on CT and bronchiectasis were diagnosed with nodular bronchiectatic (NB) disease. Patients with no specific pattern on CT, such as solitary pulmonary nodules, were diagnosed with unclassifiable disease.

2.4. Antibiotic Therapy and Treatment Outcomes

All patients who began daily antibiotic therapy received standardized (rifampicin (RFP) + ethambutol (EB) + CAM) or modified combination antibiotic therapy with CAM, RFP, EB, and fluoroquinolones (gatifloxacin, sitafloxacin, moxifloxacin, garenoxacin, or levofloxacin) [6]. Aminoglycoside antibiotics were administered intramuscularly (kanamycin and streptomycin) or intravenously (amikacin). Streptomycin and kanamycin were administered intramuscularly three times a week for the first several months, at the discretion of the attending physician. Amikacin was administered daily for 28 days, followed by kanamycin or streptomycin for the first several months. The main treatment regimen was evaluated for 3 months after treatment initiation.

2.5. Sputum Examination

Sputum cultures were examined for acid-fast bacilli using 2% Ogawa egg medium (Japan BCG, Tokyo, Japan) or a mycobacteria growth indicator tube (Japan Becton, Dickinson and Company, Tokyo Japan). Nontuberculous mycobacterial species were identified using the AccuProbe (Gen-Probe Inc., San Diego, CA, USA) or COBAS AMPLICOR (Roche Diagnostic, Tokyo, Japan) systems or by DNA–DNA hybridization assay (Kyokuto Pharmaceutical Industrial, Tokyo, Japan) CAM susceptibility was determined by broth microdilution (BrothMIC NTM; Kyokuto Pharmaceutical Industrial, Tokyo, Japan), and CAM resistance was defined as a minimum inhibitory concentration ≥32 µg/mL [11].

2.6. Definition of Sputum Conversion, Recurrence, and Refractory Case

Patient status at the end of follow-up was recorded in terms of deceased or alive, microbiologic or radiologic recurrence, and cause of death, if applicable. Sputum conversion was defined as more than three consecutive negative sputum cultures over a period of 3 months. In patients who achieved sputum conversion, clinical recurrence was defined by at least two positive sputum cultures. Refractory cases were those with no negative sputum conversion, or recurrent cases as sustained positive sputum culture until the end of follow-up.

2.7. Statistical Analysis

All statistical analyses were performed using GraphPad Prism version 7 (GraphPad Software, San Diego, CA, USA) and JMP Pro 13 (SAS Institute Inc., Cary, NC, USA). Continuous variables were reported as mean and standard deviation, or median and interquartile range. Patient groups were compared using the Mann–Whitney U test for continuous variables, and χ^2 or Fisher's exact test for categorical variables. Potential independent factors identified as significant by univariate analysis were evaluated by multivariate logistic regression analysis, in addition to age, sex, BMI, and cavity. Cumulative rates of MAC-PD-associated death were estimated using the Kaplan–Meier method and compared using log-rank tests. A two-sided $p < 0.05$ was considered significant.

3. Results

3.1. Patient Selection and Treatment Modalities

A total of 331 patients with a main diagnosis of NTM-PD (international classification of disease (ICD)-10 code) were hospitalized during the study period. Among 331 patients, 313 met the American Thoracic Society/Infectious Diseases Society of America criteria for non-tuberculous mycobacterial pulmonary disease [6], and 252 met the diagnostic criteria for MAC-PD. Among these, 125 chemo-naïve patients were hospitalized for the induction of first-line combination antibiotic therapy in our hospital (Figure S1). The treatments regimens are shown in Table 1. Of the 125 patients, 86 (68.8%) were treated with an RFP + EB + CAM-based regimen, 21 (16.8 %) were treated with EB + CAM with or without FQ, 18 (14.4 %) were treated with another treatment regimen (CAM + RFP, $n = 4$; CAM + RFP + FQ, $n = 7$; EB + RFP, $n = 2$; CAM + FQ, $n = 4$; EB + FQ, $n = 1$), and 25 (20.0%) were treated with an FQ-containing regimen (RFP + EB + CAM + FQ, $n = 4$; EB + CAM + FQ, $n = 9$; CAM + RFP + FQ, $n = 7$; CAM + FQ, $n = 4$; EB + FQ, $n = 1$). Aminoglycoside injection was used in 53 (42.4%). All 125 patients were tested for drug susceptibility before treatment. Susceptibility to CAM was as follows: sensitive (minimum inhibitory concentration (MIC) ≤ 2, $n = 124$), resistant (MIC > 32, $n = 1$). Susceptibility to levofloxacin was as follows: sensitive (MIC < 2, $n = 84$), intermediate (MIC ≥ 2 to < 8, $n = 30$), resistant (MIC ≥ 8, $n = 11$). Susceptibility to moxifloxacin (MFLX) was tested in five levofloxacin-resistant patients and all five strains were resistant to MFLX (MIC 4, $n = 3$; MIC > 8, $n = 2$). Susceptibility to aminoglycosides was as follows: amikacin: sensitive (MIC < 4, n = 17), intermediate (MIC ≥ 4 to <16, n = 82), resistant (MIC ≥ 16, n = 26); kanamycin: sensitive (MIC < 4, n = 15), intermediate (MIC ≥ 4 to <16, n = 83), resistant (MIC ≥ 16, n = 26); streptomycin: sensitive (MIC < 4, n = 56), intermediate (MIC ≥ 4 to <8, n = 36), resistant (MIC ≥ 8, n = 32).

Table 1. Treatment regimen.

Treatment Regimen (n = 125)	No. (%)
RFP + EB + CAM	82 (65.6)
RFP + EB + CAM + FQ	4 (3.2)
EB + CAM + FQ	10 (8.0)
RFP + CAM + FQ	7 (5.6)
CAM + FQ	4 (3.2)
EB + FQ	1 (0.8)
EB + CAM	11 (8.8)
RFP + CAM	4 (3.2)
RFP + EB	2 (1.6)

RFP, rifampicin; EB, ethambutol; CAM, clarithromycin; FQ, fluoroquinolones.

3.2. Baseline Characteristics

The median age and BMI of the patients were comparable to previous reports [12]. The main underlying diseases were previous pulmonary tuberculosis (8.8%), chronic obstructive pulmonary disease (4.0%), and diabetes mellitus (6.4%). Of the bacterial species identified, *M. avium* was the most frequent, followed by *M. intracellulare* and both (Table 2).

3.3. Predictive Factors for Sputum Conversion

Of the 125 patients, 100 (80.0%) patients achieved sputum conversion. Univariate analysis identified diabetes mellitus as a risk factor for failure of sputum conversion, while a standardized (RFP + EB + CAM-based) regimen and aminoglycoside use were significantly associated with positive outcome. Multiple logistic regression analysis revealed that a standardized regimen (p = 0.0238) was significantly and independently associated with outcome (Table 2).

3.4. Risk Factors for Refractory Disease

Univariate analysis identified BMI, concurrent CPA, and acquired CAM resistance as risk factors for refractory disease, and standardized (RFP + EB + CAM-based) regimen and aminoglycoside use as significantly associated with positive outcome. Multiple logistic regression analysis revealed that BMI (p = 0.0162), standardized regimen (p = 0.0023), aminoglycoside use (p = 0.0056), and acquired CAM resistance (p = 0.0002) were independently associated with outcome (Table 3).

Table 2. Baseline characteristics and analysis of sputum conversion in patients with *Mycobacterium avium* complex pulmonary disease, no. (%) or median (IQR).

Characteristic	Total (n = 125)	Conversion (n = 100)	Non-Conversion (n = 25)	Univariate Analysis p-Value	OR (95%CI)	Multivariate Analysis p-Value	Adjusted OR (95%CI)
Sex, female	85 (68.0)	73 (73.0)	12 (48.0)	0.0292	0.34 (0.14–0.80)	0.0756	
Age, years	68 (60–73.5)	68 (60–73)	69 (63.5–75)	0.278		0.4364	
BMI	17.46 (16.16–19.77)	17.56 (16.32–20.3)	17.1 (15.9–19)	0.219		0.4012	
Underlying disease							
COPD	5 (4.0)	3 (3.0)	2 (8.0)	0.261			
Old Tb	11 (8.8)	7 (7.0)	4 (16.0)	0.228			
DM	8 (6.4)	2 (2.0)	6 (24.0)	0.0008		0.0586	
CRP	0.38 (0.1–2.26)	0.225 (0.1–1.05)	2.13 (0.81–4.88)	<0.0001		0.1424	
NB form	89 (71.2)	70 (70.0)	19 (76.0)	0.629			
Cavitation	80 (64.0)	63 (63.0)	17 (68.0)	0.816			
M. avium	71 (56.8)	57 (57.0)	14 (56.0)	>0.999			
Treatment duration, days	450 (294.5–825.5)	447.5 (345–756.3)	547 (167.5–1266)	0.8697		0.7808	
RFP + EB + CAM-containing regimen	86 (68.8)	75 (75.0)	11 (44.0)	0.0068	0.26 (0.10–0.63)	0.0238	0.298 (0.11–0.85)
FQ-containing regimen	25 (20.0)	19 (19.0)	6 (24.0)	0.5878	15.47 (3.40–77.25)		
Aminoglycoside use	53 (42.4)	47 (47.0)	6 (24.0)	0.0434	0.35 (0.13–0.98)	0.2158	

IQR, interquartile range; OR, odds ratio; CI, confidence interval; BMI, body mass index; COPD, chronic obstructive pulmonary disease; Tb, tuberculosis; DM, diabetes mellitus; CRP, C-reactive protein; NB, nodular bronchiectasis; RFP + EB + CAM, rifampicin + ethambutol + clarithromycin; FQ, fluoroquinolones.

Table 3. Treatment selection modified disease progression and persistence in patients with *Mycobacterium avium* complex pulmonary disease.

Characteristic	Treatment Success (n = 68)	Refractory Disease [a] (n = 57)	Univariate Analysis		Multivariate Analysis	
			p-Value	OR (95%CI)	p-Value	Adjusted OR (95%CI)
Sex, female	50 (73.5)	35 (61.4)	0.1792		0.0599	
Age, years	67 (60.5–72)	69 (60–74.5)	0.3995		0.3091	
BMI	18.25 (16.46–21.03)	17.05 (16.07–18.77)	0.0198		0.0162	
DM	5 (7.4)	7 (12.3)	0.3783			
CRP	0.27 (0.1–1)	0.64 (0.1–2.873)	0.1147			
NB form	46 (67.6)	43 (75.4)	0.4283			
Cavitation	42 (61.8)	38 (66.7)	0.5813		0.8641	
M. avium	36 (52.9)	35 (61.4)	0.7112			
Treatment duration, days	441 (351.3–694.5)	459 (220.5–1184)	0.5182			
RFP + EB + CAM-containing regimen	57 (83.8)	29 (50.9)	<0.0001	0.199 (0.091–0.457)	0.0023	0.244 (0.098–0.605)
FQ-containing regimen	12 (17.6)	13 (22.8)	0.8252			
Aminoglycoside use	39 (57.4)	14 (24.6)	0.0003	0.242 (0.114–0.537)	0.0056	0.304 (0.131–0.705)
Acquired condition						
CAM resistance	2 (2.9)	19 (33.3)	<0.0001	16.5 (4.23–73.37)	0.0002	20.12 (4.13–97.94)
Concurrent CPA	6 (8.8)	11 (19.3)	0.1171			

Values given as no. (%) or median (IQR). [a] Refractory case: no sputum conversion, or recurrence and persistent positive sputum status until the end of follow-up. OR, odds ratio; CI, confidence interval; IQR, interquartile range; BMI, body mass index; CPA, chronic pulmonary aspergillosis.

3.5. Analysis of FQ-Containing Regimens

FQ-containing regimens showed no additional benefit in terms of sputum conversion and preventing refractory disease (Tables 2 and 3). We further evaluated FQs as potential candidates of multidrug regimens by comparing RFP + EB + CAM and RFP/EB + CAM + FQ regimens (Table 4). The baseline characteristics and initial sputum conversion rates of the two regimens were comparable. However, the number of refractory cases and acquired CAM resistance were significantly higher in patients using the RFP/EB + CAM + FQ regimen.

Table 4. Comparison of RFP + EB + CAM and RFP/EB + CAM + FQ regimens.

	RFP + EB + CAM (n = 82)	RFP/EB + CAM + FQ (n = 17)	Univariate Analysis	
			p-Value	OR (95%CI)
Characteristic				
Sex, female	54 (64.9)	12 (70.6)	0.7845	
Age, years	69 (60–73)	70 (64.5–75.5)	0.3794	
BMI	17.56(16.61–20.11)	17.46 (16.1–19.93)	0.8433	
DM	8 (9.8)	1 (5.9)	>0.9999	
CRP	0.32 (0.1–1.93)	0.18 (0.1–3.505)	0.9702	
NB form	59 (72.0)	15 (88.2)	0.2248	
Cavitation	50 (61.0)	11 (64.7)	>0.9999	
M. avium	43 (52.4)	12 (70.6)	0.1921	
Treatment duration, days	441 (351.3–694.5)	459 (220.5–1184)	0.5182	
Aminoglycoside use	42 (51.2)	5 (29.4)	0.1171	
Sputum conversion	71 (86.6)	13 (76.5)	0.2831	
Refractory case	26 (31.7)	11 (64.7)	0.0141	3.95 (1.40–12.2)
Acquired condition				
CAM resistance	7 (8.5)	7 (41.2)	0.0022	7.5 (2.16–26.9)
Concurrent CPA	9 (11.0)	3 (17.6)	0.1171	0.4277

Values given as no. (%) or median (IQR). OR, odds ratio; CI, confidence interval; BMI, body mass index; DM, diabetes mellitus; CRP, C-reactive protein; NB, nodular bronchiectasis; IQR, interquartile range; RFP + EB + CAM, rifampicin + ethambutol + clarithromycin; FQ, fluoroquinolone; CAM, clarithromycin; CPA, chronic pulmonary aspergillosis.

3.6. Mortality

Death from any cause occurred in 27 (21.6%) patients over a median follow-up period of 56.4 months (38.1–82.9) (Figure S2). Among these, 18 patients died from MAC-PD-associated causes (progression of MAC-PD, $n = 14$; respiratory failure due to MAC-PD, $n = 2$; concomitant bacterial or fungal infection, $n = 2$) and nine patients died from other causes (interstitial pneumonia, $n = 2$; lung cancer, $n = 2$; chronic obstructive pulmonary disease, $n = 1$; heart failure $n = 1$; tuberculosis, $n = 1$; unknown, $n = 2$).

3.7. MAC-PD-Associated Death

The occurrence rate of MAC-PD-associated death according to radiographic features was estimated (Figure 1). MAC-PD-associated death occurred mainly in patients with cavitary disease (88.9%). There was a significant difference in survival curves between patients with non-cavitary and cavitary NB ($p = 0.0241$). However, the survival curves for cavitary NB and FC disease were comparable ($p = 0.7830$). The 5-year occurrence rates of MAC-associated death for patients with cavitary NB disease and FC disease were 16.6% and 16.7%, respectively. We also analysed the prognostic factors in patients with cavitary disease (Table 5). Among the 75 patients with cavitary MAC-PD, univariate analysis identified age, low BMI, high C-reactive protein, diabetes mellitus, concurrent CPA, and acquired CAM resistance as risk factors for death. In contrast, standardized RFP + EB + CAM-based regimen and aminoglycoside use were significantly associated with positive outcome. Multiple logistic regression analysis revealed that age ($p = 0.0136$), diabetes mellitus ($p = 0.041$), and concurrent CPA ($p = 0.0243$) were independently associated with outcomes.

Table 5. Risk factor analysis in patients with cavitary *Mycobacterium avium* complex pulmonary disease.

Characteristic	Censored (n = 59)	MAC-PD-Associated Death (n = 16)	Univariate Analysis p-Value	Univariate Analysis OR (95%CI)	Multivariate Analysis p-Value	Multivariate Analysis Adjusted OR (95%CI)
Sex, female	41 (69.5)	7 (43.8)	0.079		0.23	
Age, years	67 (58–71)	75 (69.5–77)	0.0002		0.033	
BMI	17.56 (16.77–20)	16.24 (14.9–18.83)	0.0150		0.084	
DM	2 (3.4)	4 (25.0)	0.0168	9.5 (1.94–52.01)	0.041	9.96 (1.10–90.09)
CRP	0.38 (0.1–1.463)	2.73 (1.09–5.46)	0.0021		0.82	
NB form	34 (57.6)	9 (56.3)	>0.9999			
M. avium	31 (52.5)	8 (50.0)	>0.9999			
Treatment duration, days	589 (387–1325)	476 (143.5–745.5)	0.1257			
RFP + EB + CAM-containing regimen	44 (74.6)	6 (37.5)	0.0079	0.2045 (0.062–0.67)	0.66	
FQ-containing regimen	12 (20.3)	5 (31.3)	0.501			
Aminoglycoside use	28 (47.5)	3 (18.8)	0.0478	0.2555 (0.072–0.96)	0.82	
Acquired condition						
CAM resistance	9 (15.3)	7 (43.8)	0.0335	4.321 (1.28–14.11)	0.115	
Concurrent CPA	5 (8.5)	8 (50.0)	0.0006	10.8 (2.84–40.94)	0.0235	8.552 (1.335–54.77)

MAC-PD, *Mycobacterium avium* complex pulmonary disease; OR, odds ratio; CI, confidence interval; BMI, body mass index; DM, diabetes mellitus; CRP, C-reactive protein; NB, nodular bronchiectasis; RFP + EB + CAM, rifampicin + ethambutol + clarithromycin; FQ, fluoroquinolone; CAM, clarithromycin; CPA, chronic pulmonary aspergillosis.

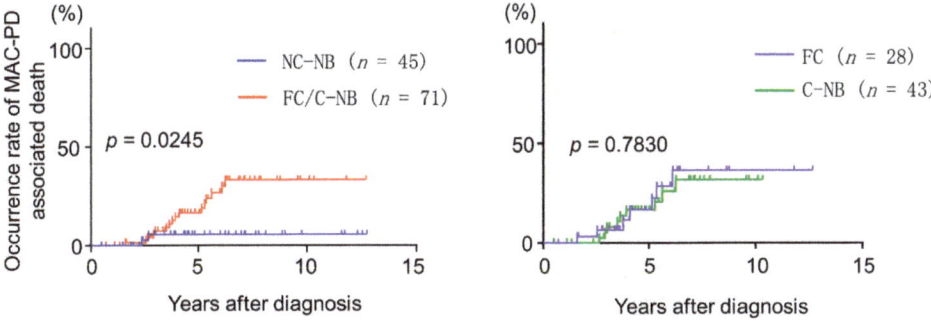

Figure 1. Occurrence rates of *Mycobacterium avium* complex pulmonary disease-associated death in patients with different forms of disease. The mortality rate of cavitary disease was high and different from that of non-cavitary disease. MAC-PD, *Mycobacterium avium* complex pulmonary disease; NC-NB, non-cavitary nodular bronchiectasis; FC, fibrocavitary form; C-NB, cavitary nodular bronchiectasis.

3.8. Occurrence Rate of CPA Diagnosis

CPA was diagnosed in 17 (13.6%) patients over a median follow-up period of 56.4 months (38.1–82.9) and the occurrence rate of CPA was estimated (Figure 2). There was a significant difference in CPA between patients with non-cavitary NB and cavitary NB/FC disease ($p = 0.0388$). The 5-year occurrence rates of CPA in patients with non-cavitary NB and cavitary NB/FC were 3.3 and 16.5%, respectively. Serial CT scans showed thickening of the cavitary wall with paracavity or extensive fibrosis (Figure 3).

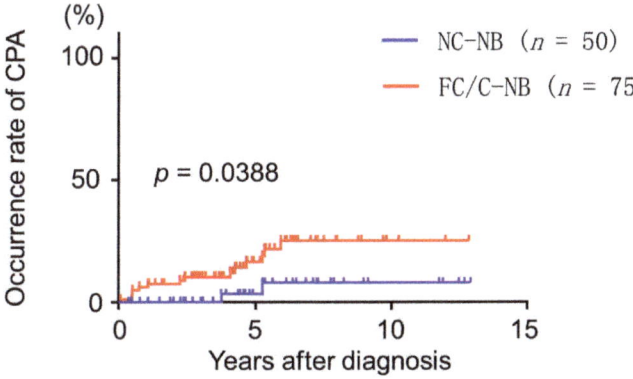

Figure 2. Occurrence rate of chronic pulmonary aspergillosis after diagnosis of *Mycobacterium avium* complex pulmonary disease. CPA, chronic pulmonary aspergillosis, NC-NB, non-cavitary nodular bronchiectasis; FC, fibrocavitary form; C-NB, cavitary nodular bronchiectasis.

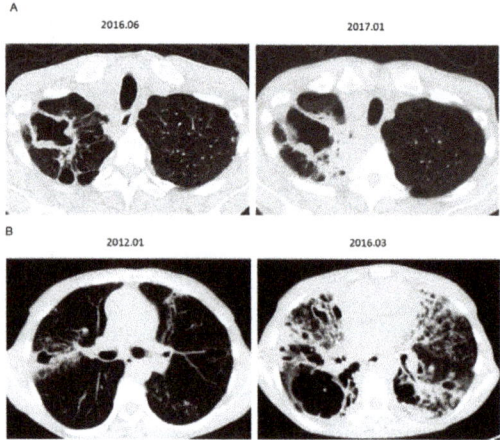

Figure 3. Serial computed tomography scans of patients with cavitary *Mycobacterium avium* complex pulmonary disease (MAC-PD) before and after diagnosis of chronic pulmonary aspergillosis (CPA). (**A**) Left: at the time of MAC-PD diagnosis (fibrocavitary form). *Aspergillus* galactomannan antigen 0.3, β-D glucan 8.8. Right: at the time of CPA diagnosis. *Aspergillus* galactomannan antigen 0.4, *Aspergillus* precipitating antibody-positive, β-D glucan 18.8 pg/mL, and isolation of *A. fumigatus* from sputum culture. (**B**) Left: at the time of MAC-PD diagnosis (cavitary nodular bronchiectasis). *Aspergillus* galactomannan antigen 0.2, β-D glucan 7.5. Right: at the time of CPA diagnosis. *Aspergillus* galactomannan antigen 5.0, *Aspergillus* precipitating antibody-positive, β-D glucan 300.0 pg/mL, and isolation of *A. fumigatus* from sputum culture.

4. Discussion

This study evaluated the prognosis and long-term outcome in 125 patients with chemo-naïve progressive MAC-PD hospitalized for the induction of multidrug combination therapy. In this study, the standardized RFP + EB + CAM-based regimen was shown to be an independent factor associated with negative-sputum conversion and a reduced rate of refractory disease, while aminoglycoside use was independently associated with a reduced rate of refractory disease.

Multidrug combination therapy is currently considered essential for preventing respiratory failure in patients with progressive MAC-PD, and RFP, EB, and macrolides are considered to be the standard multidrug regimen [6,13]. However, although macrolides are generally accepted as key drugs and a cornerstone of MAC treatment [14–16], no large studies have validated the appropriateness of current treatment guidelines for MAC-PD. Furthermore, even after successful treatment with antibiotic therapy, microbiological recurrence is relatively common [17,18]. However, most previous studies of combination therapy focused primarily on negative culture conversion with short-term observation periods [19–21], and the prognosis and long-term outcomes following combination therapy are thus poorly understood. In addition, FQs have been reported to be effective against MAC infection in vitro and in vivo and are widely and safely used, thus providing a promising alternative. However, data on the use of combination therapy including FQ are totally insufficient [22]. There is thus an urgent need to examine the efficacy and long-term outcomes of current standard regimens and other alternatives. The results of the current study are therefore important. In this study of 125 chemo-naïve patients with progressive MAC-PD, we showed that standardized regimens (RFP + EB + CAM containing at least three drugs), but not FQ-containing regimens, inhibited long-term disease progression, while the addition of an aminoglycoside inhibited refractory disease. In addition, although an FQ-containing three-drug regimen showed a comparable sputum-conversion rate to the RFP + EB + CAM regimen, the long-term disease-control rate was lower and CAM-resistant MAC strains were more frequent. This result coincides with a previous report that suggested the benefit of three-drug macrolide regimens including EB and RFP for protecting against macrolide resistance [23]. In contrast, a recent study showed that an EB + CAM-containing two-drug regimen was comparable to the standardized regimen (RFP + EB + CAM) in terms of the negative sputum-conversion rate [20]. However, the current results suggests that two-drug regimens should be selected cautiously in relation to long-term disease progression and persistence.

Numerous retrospective studies have reported on the prognostic factors of MAC-PD, and male sex, age, cavity, comorbidity, non-NB form, low BMI, and higher ESR have been associated with mortality [12,24,25]. *Aspergillus* coinfection was also reported in a small study involving patients with NTM-PD [26]. Furthermore, several issues remain to be clarified regarding MAC-PD disease type. The prognosis of cavitary NB has been suggested to differ from that of non-cavitary NB disease, rather than just being an advanced stage of the same disease [3]. However, many published studies failed to differentiate between these [20,27,28], and clarification of the prognostic difference between these two NB diseases is urgently needed to ensure the appropriate management of MAC-PD. This study, involving chemo-naïve 125 patients with progressive MAC-PD, showed that the risk of MAC-PD-associated death was higher in patients with cavitary disease, and age, diabetes mellitus, and CPA were independently associated with mortality among patients with cavitary MAC-PD. We also showed that mortality was significantly lower in patients with non-cavitary NB disease compared with patients with cavitary NB and FC disease. No patients changed from non-cavitary to cavitary NB in this study. These results suggested that cavitary disease, including cavitary NB, may be completely different from non-cavitary NB, rather than just an advanced stage. Indeed, fewer than 5% of patients with non-cavitary disease experienced MAC-PD-associated death, compared with about 25% of patients with cavitary MAC-PD, despite intensive antimicrobial therapy. However, we cannot exclude the possibility that the apparent lack of progression to cavitary disease may be ascribed to the effects of combination antimicrobial treatment. Future studies of the natural history of NB disease are necessary to confirm if cavitary NB disease is totally different from non-cavitary NB disease.

The incidence of refractory cases increased during the observation period, despite the use of multidrug combination therapy, finally accounting for almost half of all patients (45.6% in this study). The treatment of refractory MAC-PD presents a major clinical problem, requiring a thorough analysis of the factors associated with this condition. The current study revealed that BMI and acquired CAM resistance were independent risk factors for refractory disease. Notably, 21 (16.8%) patients acquired CAM resistance during the observation period, which led to poor treatment outcomes [23]. We also showed that use of a standardized RFP + EB + CAM-based regimen and the addition of an aminoglycoside inhibited future disease persistence. In contrast, FQ-containing regimens induced a significantly higher rate of acquired CAM resistance.

Risk factor analysis for mortality identified age, BMI, chronic systemic inflammation, and diabetes mellitus, which lead to reduced immune regulation, and cavitary form of the disease, which is a reflection of pulmonary parenchymal damage caused by MAC, as factors significantly associated with death. These factors predispose MAC-PD patients to the development of chronic Aspergillus infection, which is a severely debilitating disease often resulting in a shortened lifespan [29]. As a consequence, CPA was also an independent risk factor for death, especially in patients with cavitary MAC-PD. Overall, 17.3% of patients with cavitary MAC-PD were diagnosed with CPA, mainly 2–5 years after a MAC diagnosis, and 61.5% died during the observation period. The high incidence and significant mortality of CPA in patients with cavitary MAC-PD suggests the need for prophylactic measures in future practice.

Azoles such as voriconazole and itraconazole are important for the treatment of CPA, but the interactions of these drugs with RFP are well known. Interactions between such antifungal agents and RFP makes it difficult to select suitable therapeutic drugs, which, together with diagnostic difficulties, may contribute to the poor prognosis of MAC-PD patients complicated with CPA. Among 17 CPA patients, RFP was prescribed to eight patients at the diagnosis of CPA. Among these eight patients, two patients stopped RFP because of concerns regarding drug interactions, micafungin (MCFG) was used in five patients, and itraconazole (ITZ) and voriconazole (VRCZ) were used in one patient each. Among the other nine patients, caspofungin (CPFG) was used in three patients, MCFG in five, ITZ in two, VRCZ in one, and liposomal amphotericin B (L-AMB) in one patient. We did not check drug levels of antifungal agents. Interruption of RFP may result in inadequate MAC treatment, and continuation of RFP with avoidance of ITZ and VRCZ in light of drug interactions may result in inadequate CPA treatment, both of which could lead to a poor prognostic outcome. Difficulties in assessing the disease activity and severity of CPA in MAC-PD patients meant that intermittent administration of candins, such as CPFG and MCFG, was the main therapy in this study, and long-term oral anti-fungal agents were administered in less than a third of CPA patients (29.4%). Thus, considering the high frequency and mortality of this complication, treatment strategies for CPA and MAC co-infection need to be examined and determined.

Furthermore, MAC-PD and fungal PD in adult bronchiectasis patients are associated with airway clearance defects [30]. All patients with MAC-PD would therefore benefit from airway-clearance therapies, in addition to optimal combinations of antibiotics. Considering the high rate of refractory disease despite the use of multidrug combination therapy, airway-clearance therapy would improve the conversion rate to sputum negativity, reduce the relapse frequency, and reduce disease persistence and progression.

The current study had some limitations. First, it was a retrospective study and we therefore could not exclude potential confounding factors, such as microbiologic and other laboratory data. Second, this study included a heterogeneous population of progressive MAC-PD patients hospitalized for initial combination antimicrobial drug therapy. Given that patients who are hospitalized in a referral centre for first-line combination treatment tend to have advanced disease, this might have affected the clinical outcome following treatment, and these results therefore cannot be generally applied to all MAC-PD patients undergoing combination therapy. Prospective large-scale studies are therefore needed to evaluate the outcomes of first-line combination therapies, involving strict statistics and unbiased methods. Third, patients were only selected from one referral centre with experience in the management of MAC-PD, which might have led to selection bias. Finally, we did not evaluate the factors affecting decision-making by pulmonary physicians with regard to the timing and selection of antimicrobial therapy. Indeed, of 39 patients treated with a modified regimen, 12 were initially treated with a standardized regimen, which was modified soon after the start of treatment because of side effects (RFP: exanthema, $n = 3$, fever, $n = 3$, hepatotoxicity, $n = 2$; EB: visual impairment, $n = 2$; CAM: exanthema, $n = 1$, nausea + abdominal pain, $n = 1$). On the other hand, one patient treated with a standardized regimen developed exanthema and fever caused by RFP and underwent successful drug desensitization therapy, one patient stopped EB because of visual impairment more than 1 year after initiation of standard treatment, and one patient continued standardized treatment despite CAM-induced exanthema. Finally, no patients in this study were diagnosed with cystic fibrosis, although examinations to definitely exclude this disease, such as *CFTR* polymorphisms, deltaF508 heterozygosity, and sweat chloride tests, were not performed. However, a previous study reported that the incidence of cystic fibrosis in the Japanese population was much lower than other countries, and all the patients in the current study were Japanese, with an average age of 68 years at diagnosis (60–73.5 years) [31]. We therefore considered it unlikely that the lack of definite exclusion of cystic fibrosis would have affected the results of this study. However, a previous study in the United States involving adult patients with bronchiectasis, including MAC-PD, showed a significantly elevated prevalence of *CFTR* mutations when they were screened for an expanded range of polymorphisms. Further research applying clinical and genomic criteria based on our current knowledge of cystic fibrosis is therefore necessary to clarify the incidence of cystic fibrosis in Japan [32].

5. Conclusions

In conclusion, the present study clarified that the choice of first-line treatment was independently associated with sputum conversion and the development of refractory disease in patients with progressive MAC-PD. The use of an RFP + EB + CAM-based regimen was significantly and independently associated with negative sputum conversion and reduced disease progression, although the side effects were not acceptable in some patients. Aminoglycoside addition reduced the risk of refractory disease. Regarding the prognosis, cavitary NB was associated with a higher mortality than non-cavitary disease, and seems to be a totally different disease, rather than just an advanced form of non-cavitary NB. CPA was prevalent among patients with cavitary MAC-PD and was independently associated with increased mortality. Host factors affecting systemic immune regulation, and cavitary lesions reflecting pulmonary parenchymal damage, predispose MAC-PD patients to the development of chronic devastating Aspergillus infection. Intensive multidrug combination therapy including aminoglycosides should be administered to patients with progressive MAC-PD to inhibit disease progression and persistence. However, these results were based on patients with progressive MAC-PD hospitalized for the induction of first-line combination therapy, and further prospective, large-scale studies are therefore needed to validate these promising results.

Supplementary Materials: The following are available online at http://www.mdpi.com/2077-0383/9/5/1315/s1, Figure S1: Study design, Figure S2: Analysis of MAC-PD associated death.

Author Contributions: K.F. and S.K. designed the project. K.F. conducted clinical data extraction and analysis. Y.Y., T.M. and H.K. (Hiroyuki Kagawa) assisted with data extraction. Y.O., K.Y., M.M., K.M., Y.A. and K.T. assisted with data analysis. K.F. and S.K. wrote the manuscript. H.K. (Hiroshi Kida) supervised the project. All authors have read and agreed to the published version of the manuscript.

Funding: This work was supported by the "Establishment of epidemiological investigation, diagnostic tools, and therapeutics of non-tuberculous mycobacteria" from the Japan Agency for Medical Research and Development.

Acknowledgments: We thank E. Akiba for assistance with data collection and helpful discussions. We thank Susan Furness from Edanz Group (https://en-author-services.edanzgroup.com/) for editing a draft of this manuscript.

Conflicts of Interest: The authors declare competing financial interests. Details are available in the online version of the paper. The funders had no role in the design of the study; in the collection, analyses, or interpretation of data; in the writing of the manuscript, or in the decision to publish the results.

Abbreviations

BMI	body mass index
CAM	clarithromycin
CPA	chronic pulmonary aspergillosis
CT	computed tomography
EB	ethambutol
FC	fibrocavitary
FQ	fluoroquinolones
HIV	human immunodeficiency virus
MAC	*Mycobacterium avium* complex
MAC-PD	*Mycobacterium avium* complex pulmonary disease
NB	nodular bronchiectasis
NTM-PD	non-tuberculous mycobacterial pulmonary disease
RFP	rifampicin

References

1. Namkoong, H.; Kurashima, A.; Morimoto, K.; Hoshino, Y.; Hasegawa, N.; Ato, M.; Mitarai, S. Epidemiology of Pulmonary Nontuberculous Mycobacterial Disease, Japan. *Emerg. Infect. Dis.* **2016**, *22*, 1116–1117. [CrossRef] [PubMed]
2. Choi, Y.; Jhun, B.W.; Kim, J.; Huh, H.J.; Lee, N.Y. Clinical Characteristics and Outcomes of Surgically Resected Solitary Pulmonary Nodules Due to Nontuberculous Mycobacterial Infections. *J. Clin. Med.* **2019**, *8*, 1898. [CrossRef] [PubMed]
3. Koh, W.J.; Moon, S.M.; Kim, S.Y.; Woo, M.A.; Kim, S.; Jhun, B.W.; Park, H.Y.; Jeon, K.; Huh, H.J.; Ki, C.S.; et al. Outcomes of *Mycobacterium avium* complex lung disease based on clinical phenotype. *Eur. Respir. J.* **2017**, *50*, 1602503. [CrossRef] [PubMed]

4. Shafran, S.D.; Singer, J.; Zarowny, D.P.; Phillips, P.; Salit, I.; Walmsley, S.L.; Fong, I.W.; Gill, M.J.; Rachlis, A.R.; Lalonde, R.G. A comparison of two regimens for the treatment of *Mycobacterium avium* complex bacteremia in AIDS: Rifabutin, ethambutol, and clarithromycin versus rifampin, ethambutol, clofazimine, and ciprofloxacin. Canadian HIV Trials Network Protocol 010 Study Group. *New Engl. J. Med.* **1996**, *335*, 377–383. [CrossRef]
5. Dube, M.P.; Sattler, F.R.; Torriani, F.J.; See, D.; Havlir, D.V.; Kemper, C.A.; Dezfuli, M.G.; Bozzette, S.A.; Bartok, A.E.; Leedom, J.M.; et al. A randomized evaluation of ethambutol for prevention of relapse and drug resistance during treatment of *Mycobacterium avium* complex bacteremia with clarithromycin-based combination therapy. California Collaborative Treatment Group. *J. Infect. Dis.* **1997**, *176*, 1225–1232. [CrossRef]
6. Griffith, D.E.; Aksamit, T.; Brown-Elliott, B.A.; Catanzaro, A.; Daley, C.; Gordin, F.; Holland, S.M.; Horsburgh, R.; Huitt, G.; Iademarco, M.F.; et al. An official ATS/IDSA statement: Diagnosis, treatment, and prevention of nontuberculous mycobacterial diseases. *Am. J. Respir. Crit. Care Med.* **2007**, *175*, 367–416. [CrossRef]
7. Koh, W.J.; Hong, G.; Kim, S.Y.; Jeong, B.H.; Park, H.Y.; Jeon, K.; Kwon, O.J.; Lee, S.H.; Kim, C.K.; Shin, S.J. Treatment of refractory *Mycobacterium avium* complex lung disease with a moxifloxacin-containing regimen. *Antimicrob Agents Chemother.* **2013**, *57*, 2281–2285. [CrossRef]
8. Sano, C.; Tatano, Y.; Shimizu, T.; Yamabe, S.; Sato, K.; Tomioka, H. Comparative in vitro and in vivo antimicrobial activities of sitafloxacin, gatifloxacin and moxifloxacin against *Mycobacterium avium*. *Int. J. Antimicrob. Agents* **2011**, *37*, 296–301. [CrossRef]
9. Kobashi, Y.; Matsushima, T.; Oka, M. A double-blind randomized study of aminoglycoside infusion with combined therapy for pulmonary *Mycobacterium avium* complex disease. *Respir. Med.* **2007**, *101*, 130–138. [CrossRef]
10. Denning, D.W.; Cadranel, J.; Beigelman-Aubry, C.; Ader, F.; Chakrabarti, A.; Blot, S.; Ullmann, A.J.; Dimopoulos, G.; Lange, C. Chronic pulmonary aspergillosis: Rationale and clinical guidelines for diagnosis and management. *Eur. Respir. J.* **2016**, *47*, 45–68. [CrossRef]
11. Morimoto, K.; Namkoong, H.; Hasegawa, N.; Nakagawa, T.; Morino, E.; Shiraishi, Y.; Ogawa, K.; Izumi, K.; Takasaki, J.; Yoshiyama, T.; et al. Macrolide-Resistant *Mycobacterium avium* Complex Lung Disease: Analysis of 102 Consecutive Cases. *Ann. Am. Thorac. Soc.* **2016**, *13*, 1904–1911. [CrossRef] [PubMed]
12. Hayashi, M.; Takayanagi, N.; Kanauchi, T.; Miyahara, Y.; Yanagisawa, T.; Sugita, Y. Prognostic factors of 634 HIV-negative patients with *Mycobacterium avium* complex lung disease. *Am. J. Respir. Crit. Care Med.* **2012**, *185*, 575–583. [CrossRef] [PubMed]
13. Haworth, C.S.; Banks, J.; Capstick, T.; Fisher, A.J.; Gorsuch, T.; Laurenson, I.F.; Leitch, A.; Loebinger, M.R.; Milburn, H.J.; Nightingale, M.; et al. British Thoracic Society guidelines for the management of non-tuberculous mycobacterial pulmonary disease (NTM-PD). *Thorax* **2017**, *72*, 1–64. [CrossRef] [PubMed]
14. Dautzenberg, B.; Piperno, D.; Diot, P.; Truffot-Pernot, C.; Chauvin, J.P. Clarithromycin in the treatment of *Mycobacterium avium* lung infections in patients without AIDS. Clarithromycin Study Group of France. *Chest* **1995**, *107*, 1035–1040. [CrossRef]
15. Wallace, R.J., Jr.; Brown, B.A.; Griffith, D.E.; Girard, W.M.; Murphy, D.T.; Onyi, G.O.; Steingrube, V.A.; Mazurek, G.H. Initial clarithromycin monotherapy for *Mycobacterium avium-intracellulare* complex lung disease. *Am. J. Respir. Crit. Care Med.* **1994**, *149*, 1335–1341. [CrossRef]
16. Tanaka, E.; Kimoto, T.; Tsuyuguchi, K.; Watanabe, I.; Matsumoto, H.; Niimi, A.; Suzuki, K.; Murayama, T.; Amitani, R.; Kuze, F. Effect of clarithromycin regimen for *Mycobacterium avium* complex pulmonary disease. *Am. J. Respir. Crit. Care Med.* **1999**, *160*, 866–872. [CrossRef]
17. Lee, B.Y.; Kim, S.; Hong, Y.; Lee, S.D.; Kim, W.S.; Kim, D.S.; Shim, T.S.; Jo, K.W. Risk factors for recurrence after successful treatment of *Mycobacterium avium* complex lung disease. *Antimicrob. Agents Chemother.* **2015**, *59*, 2972–2977. [CrossRef]
18. Min, J.; Park, J.; Lee, Y.J.; Kim, S.J.; Park, J.S.; Cho, Y.J.; Yoon, H.I.; Lee, C.T.; Lee, J.H. Determinants of recurrence after successful treatment of *Mycobacterium avium* complex lung disease. *Int. J. Tuberc. Lung Dis.* **2015**, *19*, 1239–1245.
19. Kobashi, Y.; Matsushima, T. The effect of combined therapy according to the guidelines for the treatment of *Mycobacterium avium* complex pulmonary disease. *Intern. Med.* **2003**, *42*, 670–675. [CrossRef]

20. Miwa, S.; Shirai, M.; Toyoshima, M.; Shirai, T.; Yasuda, K.; Yokomura, K.; Yamada, T.; Masuda, M.; Inui, N.; Chida, K.; et al. Efficacy of clarithromycin and ethambutol for *Mycobacterium avium* complex pulmonary disease. A preliminary study. *Ann. Am. Thorac. Soc.* **2014**, *11*, 23–29. [CrossRef]
21. Kobashi, Y.; Matsushima, T. The microbiological and clinical effects of combined therapy according to guidelines on the treatment of pulmonary *Mycobacterium avium* complex disease in Japan—Including a follow-up study. *Respir. Int. Rev. Thorac. Dis.* **2007**, *74*, 394–400. [CrossRef] [PubMed]
22. Jacobson, M.A.; Yajko, D.; Northfelt, D.; Charlebois, E.; Gary, D.; Brosgart, C.; Sanders, C.A.; Hadley, W.K. Randomized, placebo-controlled trial of rifampin, ethambutol, and ciprofloxacin for AIDS patients with disseminated *Mycobacterium avium* complex infection. *J. Infect. Dis.* **1993**, *168*, 112–119. [CrossRef] [PubMed]
23. Griffith, D.E.; Brown-Elliott, B.A.; Langsjoen, B.; Zhang, Y.; Pan, X.; Girard, W.; Nelson, K.; Caccitolo, J.; Alvarez, J.; Shepherd, S.; et al. Clinical and molecular analysis of macrolide resistance in *Mycobacterium avium* complex lung disease. *Am. J. Respir. Crit. Care Med.* **2006**, *174*, 928–934. [CrossRef] [PubMed]
24. Kitada, S.; Uenami, T.; Yoshimura, K.; Tateishi, Y.; Miki, K.; Miki, M.; Hashimoto, H.; Fujikawa, T.; Mori, M.; Matsuura, K.; et al. Long-term radiographic outcome of nodular bronchiectatic *Mycobacterium avium* complex pulmonary disease. *Int. J. Tuberc. Lung Dis.* **2012**, *16*, 660–664. [CrossRef]
25. Gochi, M.; Takayanagi, N.; Kanauchi, T.; Ishiguro, T.; Yanagisawa, T.; Sugita, Y. Retrospective study of the predictors of mortality and radiographic deterioration in 782 patients with nodular/bronchiectatic *Mycobacterium avium* complex lung disease. *BMJ Open* **2015**, *5*, e008058. [CrossRef]
26. Zoumot, Z.; Boutou, A.K.; Gill, S.S.; van Zeller, M.; Hansell, D.M.; Wells, A.U.; Wilson, R.; Loebinger, M.R. *Mycobacterium avium* complex infection in non-cystic fibrosis bronchiectasis. *Respirology* **2014**, *19*, 714–722. [CrossRef]
27. Lam, P.K.; Griffith, D.E.; Aksamit, T.R.; Ruoss, S.J.; Garay, S.M.; Daley, C.L.; Catanzaro, A. Factors related to response to intermittent treatment of *Mycobacterium avium* complex lung disease. *Am. J. Respir. Crit. Care Med.* **2006**, *173*, 1283–1289. [CrossRef]
28. Jarand, J.; Davis, J.P.; Cowie, R.L.; Field, S.K.; Fisher, D.A. Long-term Follow-up of *Mycobacterium avium* Complex Lung Disease in Patients Treated With Regimens Including Clofazimine and/or Rifampin. *Chest* **2016**, *149*, 1285–1293. [CrossRef]
29. Takeda, K.; Imamura, Y.; Takazono, T.; Yoshida, M.; Ide, S.; Hirano, K.; Tashiro, M.; Saijo, T.; Kosai, K.; Morinaga, Y.; et al. The risk factors for developing of chronic pulmonary aspergillosis in nontuberculous mycobacteria patients and clinical characteristics and outcomes in chronic pulmonary aspergillosis patients coinfected with nontuberculous mycobacteria. *Med. Mycol.* **2016**, *54*, 120–127. [CrossRef]
30. Delliere, S.; Angebault, C.; Fihman, V.; Foulet, F.; Lepeule, R.; Maitre, B.; Schlemmer, F.; Botterel, F. Concomitant Presence of Aspergillus Species and Mycobacterium Species in the Respiratory Tract of Patients: Underestimated Co-occurrence? *Front. Microbiol.* **2019**, *10*, 2980. [CrossRef]
31. Yamashiro, Y.; Shimizu, T.; Oguchi, S.; Shioya, T.; Nagata, S.; Ohtsuka, Y. The estimated incidence of cystic fibrosis in Japan. *J. Pediatr. Gastroenterol. Nutr.* **1997**, *24*, 544–547. [CrossRef] [PubMed]
32. Ziedalski, T.M.; Kao, P.N.; Henig, N.R.; Jacobs, S.S.; Ruoss, S.J. Prospective analysis of cystic fibrosis transmembrane regulator mutations in adults with bronchiectasis or pulmonary nontuberculous mycobacterial infection. *Chest* **2006**, *130*, 995–1002. [CrossRef] [PubMed]

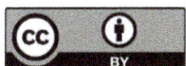

© 2020 by the authors. Licensee MDPI, Basel, Switzerland. This article is an open access article distributed under the terms and conditions of the Creative Commons Attribution (CC BY) license (http://creativecommons.org/licenses/by/4.0/).

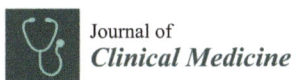
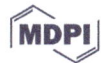

Article

MiRNA Expression Profile in the Airways Is Altered during Pulmonary Exacerbation in Children with Cystic Fibrosis—A Preliminary Report

Zuzanna Stachowiak [1], Irena Wojsyk-Banaszak [2], Katarzyna Jończyk-Potoczna [3], Beata Narożna [1], Wojciech Langwiński [1], Zdzisława Kycler [2], Paulina Sobkowiak [2], Anna Bręborowicz [2] and Aleksandra Szczepankiewicz [1],*

1. Molecular and Cell Biology Unit, Department of Paediatric Pulmonology, Allergy and Clinical Immunology, Poznan University of Medical Sciences, 60-572 Poznań, Poland; zuzastachowiak9@gmail.com (Z.S.); b.narozna@gmail.com (B.N.); wlangwinski654@gmail.com (W.L.)
2. Department of Paediatric Pulmonology, Allergy and Clinical Immunology, Poznan University of Medical Sciences, 60-572 Poznań, Poland; iwojsyk@ump.edu.pl (I.W.-B.); kyclerzdzislawa@interia.pl (Z.K.); paulina-25@tlen.pl (P.S.); abreborowicz@wp.pl (A.B.)
3. Department of Paediatric Radiology, Poznan University of Medical Sciences, 60-572 Poznań, Poland; potocznak@op.pl
* Correspondence: alszczep@gmail.com; Tel.: +48-618-547-643

Received: 26 May 2020; Accepted: 15 June 2020; Published: 16 June 2020

Abstract: MicroRNAs are small non-coding RNAs that regulate immune response and inflammation. We assumed that miRNAs may be involved in the immune response during cystic fibrosis pulmonary exacerbations (CFPE) and that altered expression profile in the airways and blood may underlie clinical outcomes in CF pediatric patients. Methods: We included 30 pediatric patients diagnosed with cystic fibrosis. The biologic material (blood, sputum, exhaled breath condensate) was collected during pulmonary exacerbation and in stable condition. The miRNA expression profile from blood and sputum ($n = 6$) was done using the next-generation sequencing. For validation, selected four miRNAs were analyzed by qPCR in exosomes from sputum supernatant and exhaled breath condensate ($n = 24$). NGS analysis was done in Base Space, correlations of gene expression with clinical data were done in Statistica. Results: The miRNA profiling showed that four miRNAs (miR-223, miR-451a, miR-27b-3p, miR-486-5p) were significantly altered during pulmonary exacerbation in CF patients in sputum but did not differ significantly in blood. MiRNA differently expressed in exhaled breath condensate (EBC) and sputum showed correlation with clinical parameters in CFPE. Conclusion: MiRNA expression profile changes in the airways during pulmonary exacerbation in CF pediatric patients. We suggest that miRNA alterations during CFPE are restricted to the airways and strongly correlate with clinical outcome.

Keywords: miRNA expression; exhaled breath condensate; sputum; severity; pulmonary exacerbation

1. Introduction

Cystic fibrosis (CF) is a common autosomal recessive disorder caused by mutations in the cystic fibrosis transmembrane conductance regulator (CFTR) gene. It is a multiorgan disease that affects the pancreas, gastrointestinal and reproductive tracts and lungs [1]. Common pulmonary symptoms include deposition of thick mucus that leads to severe airflow obstruction, chronic inflammation and chronic airway infection [2]. Lung disease is characterized by intermittent episodes of acute worsening of respiratory symptoms, pulmonary exacerbations (CFPE) [3] that cause lung function decline and contribute to disease progression, poor quality of life and shortened life expectancy in CF patients.

Retention of thick mucus in the airways facilitates frequent pulmonary infections (caused by such pathogens as *P. aeruginosa, S. aureus, H. influenzae*) [4]. However, pulmonary exacerbations do not usually result from increased bacterial density within the airways [5,6], and more severe symptoms are caused by chronic enhanced airway inflammation that may even precede infection. Chronic inflammation in the airways leads to airway epithelium damage and activates repair processes contributing to remodeling and subepithelial fibrosis that further impair lung function. Current CFPEs are the leading cause of morbidity and mortality [7,8], indicating the need for biomarker discovery.

Published data looking for CFPE biomarkers either in blood or the airways suggest many immunologically active molecules, such as TNFα, IL-8, myeloperoxidase (MPO), calprotectin, C reactive protein (CRP), correlated with clinical deterioration [9,10]. However, none of them were specific for CF pulmonary exacerbation. Moreover, peripheral biomarkers may not truly reflect the local inflammatory response in the lungs [11]. Available data suggest that sputum is a reliable source of inflammatory biomarkers, including circulating miRNA [12,13]. Less is known about the markers in exhaled breath condensate (EBC) [14].

MicroRNA are small (21–23 bp), non-coding RNAs that modulate the expression of various proteins via post-transcriptional inhibition of gene expression. They are well-known regulators of immune responses and chronic inflammation in respiratory diseases, including asthma, COPD or idiopathic pulmonary fibrosis (as reviewed by [15,16]). Moreover, they are expressed not only inside the cells but are also stably present in extracellular space i.e., body fluids such as plasma, sputum, bronchoalveolar lavage fluid (BALF) and EBC. Previous studies of miRNA in the course of CF reported a few miRNAs associated with CFTR activity (either decreased expression e.g., miR-509-3p, miR-145, miR-223 or increased expression, e.g., miR-138) [17] as well as a pulmonary exacerbation. Krause et al. studied the latter and found that the expression of the Mirc1/Mir17–92 cluster correlated with pulmonary exacerbation, but only in sputum samples and not in plasma [18]. Altered miRNA expression also affects innate immune responses in the CF lung. Previous reports showed that mir-126 was significantly downregulated in CF bronchial brushings and thus influenced the expression of Target of Myb1 (TOM1) membrane trafficking protein [19,20]. However, previous studies on the role of miRNA in the pediatric CF population are limited. The recent analysis focused on the miRNA expression profile and gender differences in CF children [21], but the studies investigating miRNA expression profile in CF pulmonary exacerbation are lacking.

Taking into account that miRNAs are regulators of immune inflammatory responses and that enhanced chronic inflammation plays a significant role in pulmonary exacerbations in cystic fibrosis, we aimed to investigate if miRNA expression differs between exacerbation and stable period of disease and if altered expression profile in the airways may underlie clinical outcome in CF pediatric patients.

2. Materials and Methods

2.1. Study Design

The prospective cohort of 30 pediatric patients, girls and boys aged 6–18 years diagnosed with cystic fibrosis and admitted to the Department of Pulmonology, Pediatric Allergy and Immunology, was enrolled in the project. Patients were either experiencing a pulmonary exacerbation or in a stable stage of disease (control visit). The Bioethics Committee approved the study (no. 386/17). All pediatric participants and their parents gave written consent.

2.2. Clinical Analysis

CF was diagnosed based on typical clinical presentation, two positive sweat chloride tests and the presence of two pathogenic mutations of CFTR. Pulmonary exacerbation was defined according to the EuroCareCF working group [22,23]. In all patients, we assessed: blood morphology, inflammatory proteins (CRP), microbiologic sputum culture, chest imaging (Brasfield score), spirometry and disease severity (with Shwachman–Kulczycki score). The data were collected, as described previously [24].

Sputum samples were collected during spontaneous expectoration. Samples were prepared by the addition of Sputolysin (Merck, Kenilworth, NJ, USA) and centrifuged to separate the cell pellet from the supernatant. For further analysis, sputum supernatant was used. We used the Turbo DECCS device (Medivac) to collect EBC according to ERS recommendation [25]. From all patients, the same amount (3 mL) of EBC was collected. Whole blood samples were drawn to tubes with EDTA anticoagulant, and after the immediate addition of Lysis Buffer (Macherey–Nagel, Düren, Germany), samples were frozen at −80 °C for further analysis.

2.3. Molecular Analysis

MiRNA samples from blood and sputum were extracted using NucleoSpin RNA blood kit (Macherey–Nagel). Exosomes from sputum supernatant and exhaled breath samples were precipitated using a miRCURY exosome cell/urine/CSF Isolation Kit (Qiagen, Hilden, Germany). MicroRNA was extracted using RNeasy mini kit (Qiagen) and RNeasy MinElute spin columns according to protocol to obtain miRNA fraction. The quantity of miRNA in the samples was measured using microRNA assay kit (Thermo Fisher Scientific, Waltham, MA, USA). The miRNA expression profile from the whole blood and sputum samples of 6 CF patients during exacerbation and stable period was performed using next-generation sequencing. Libraries were generated from 50 ng of miRNA sample using TruSeq small RNA library preparation kit (Illumina, San Diego, CA, USA) following the manufacturer's instructions. Libraries were validated and quantified using high sensitivity DNA screen tape (Agilent, Santa Clara, CA, USA) on Tape Station 2200 (Agilent) and run on MiniSeq sequencer (Illumina) with 50-nt single-end reads. Differential miRNA expression analysis was done in Base Space software. The miRNA genes that showed the most significant differences between CF exacerbation and stable period in miRNA expression profiling from sputum were analyzed using qPCR in the validation CF cohort (n = 24 samples) in sputum supernatants and exhaled breath condensate. For reverse transcription, we used MystiCq microRNA cDNA Synthesis Mix (Sigma-Aldrich, St. Louis, MO, USA). Quantitative PCR was done using MystiCq microRNA SYBR Green qPCR ReadyMix (Sigma Aldrich) and microRNA assays for miR-486-5p, miR-223, miR-451a, miR-27b. Expression analysis was conducted on the 7900HT fast-real time PCR system (Applied Biosystems, Foster City, CA, USA). Differential expression results from qPCR were compared using Data Assist software (Thermo Fisher Scientific) with a relative quantification method based on the global normalization algorithm.

2.4. Statistical Analysis

The data distribution was analyzed using the Shapiro–Wilk test. Normally distributed data were analyzed using parametric tests and data that deviated from normal distribution were analyzed using nonparametric tests. The correlation of miRNA expression and interval variables (lung function parameters, Shwachman–Kulczycki score, Brasfield score, neutrophil counts, CRP level) compared between exacerbation and stable period was done using the Spearman correlation test. The comparison of miRNA expression and nominal variables (presence of bacterial or fungal infection, presence of exacerbation) was performed using analysis of variance (one-way or two-way ANOVA) in Statistica v.12 (Statsoft, Cracow, Poland).

3. Results

3.1. A Clinical Description of the Analyzed Group

Clinical characteristics of the patients based on biologic material (exhaled breath condensate, sputum supernatant) are given in Tables 1 and 2. The exacerbation group was similar in age and gender to the patients during a stable period. Chronic *Pseudomonas aeruginosa* colonization was rarely observed in our population (≤25%) and not significantly different between exacerbation vs. stable groups. The lung function between groups was not significantly different, but the groups differed in clinical outcomes such as disease severity (SK score, Brasfield score). The treatment was uniform for the CF patients, depending on clinical symptoms. Patients chronically infected with *Pseudomonas aeruginosa* were treated with inhaled antibiotics, mostly colistimethate sodium, and two patients received inhaled tobramycin. All the patients received dornase alfa, all patients with pancreatic insufficiency received pancreatic enzymes and none were treated with CFTR modulators.

Table 1. Characteristics of the Cystic fibrosis (CF) patients (exhaled breath condensate (EBC) samples).

Variable	Mean (±SD) or Number (%)		
	Stable	Exacerbation	*p* Value
Number of subjects	12	12	-
Female	6 (50%)	7 (58%)	1.000
Age (years)	12.4 (±3.5)	13.0 (±3.4)	0.706
F508 del homozygous	4 (33%)	6 (50%)	0.680
F508del heterozygous	5 (42%)	2 (17%)	0.371
BMI (kg/m^2)	17.8 (±2.0)	17.1 (±2.3)	0.421
Diabetes (including under observation)	3 (25%)	5 (42%)	0.667
Pancreatic insufficiency	10 (83%)	11 (92%)	1.000
P. aergionsa colonization	2 (17%)	4 (33%)	0.365
P. aeruginosa current infection	0 (0%)	3 (25%)	0.217
S. aureus colonization	9 (75%)	11 (92%)	0.590
FEV$_1$% pred.	98.3 (±19.8)	82.8 (±14.9)	0.041
		84.8 (±12.5) *	0.058
FVC% pred.	96.6 (±14.5)	82.9 (±16.4)	0.041
		83.2 (±13.3) *	0.027
Shwachman–Kulczycki score (median)	90.0 (65.0–95.0)	65.0 (40.0–85.0)	0.001
Brasfield score (median)	23.0 (11.0–25.0)	13.0 (5.0–22.0)	0.009

* spirometry baseline result. BMI–body mass index; FEV1–forced expiratory volume in the first second, FVC–forced vital capacity.

Table 2. Characteristics of the CF patients (sputum samples).

Variable	Mean (±SD) or Number (%)		
	Stable	Exacerbation	*p* Value
Number of subjects	11	13	-
Female	5 (45%)	6 (43%)	1.000
Age (years)	11.8 (±3.1)	13.7 (±3.8)	0.200
F508 del homozygous	5 (45%)	10 (71%)	0.241
F508del heterozygous	3 (27%)	3 (21%)	1.000
BMI (kg/m^2)	18.5 (±3.1)	18.7 (±2.4)	0.885
Diabetes (including under observation)	4 (36%)	7 (50%)	0.689
Pancreatic insufficiency	9 (81%)	12 (92%)	0.615
P. aeruginosa colonization	2 (18%)	0 (0%)	0.113
P. aeruginosa current infection	2 (18%)	6 (43%)	0.234
S. aureus colonization	8 (73%)	13 (93%)	0.288
FEV$_1$% pred.	96.0 (±20.7)	79.6 (±24.6)	0.095
		84.2 (±22.2) *	0.194
FVC% pred.	94.8 (±15.1)	83.2 (±19.4)	0.121
		86.9 (±18.1) *	0.263
Shwachman–Kulczycki score (median)	90.0 (60.0–95.0)	70.0 (40.0–85.0)	0.009
Brasfield score	20.2 (±3.3)	15.4 (±3.9)	0.006

* spirometry baseline result. BMI–body mass index; FEV1–forced expiratory volume in the first second, FVC–forced vital capacity.

3.2. Comparison of miRNA Expression Profile between Exacerbation and Stable Period

Next-generation sequencing of the whole blood miRNA profile showed that out of 186 miRNAs expressed in blood, CF patients did not differ significantly between exacerbation and the stable period in (Figure 1a). Comparative analysis of the miRNA expression profile in sputum showed significant differences in the expression of 9 miRNAs (including mature miRNAs: miR-223-3p, miR-451a, miR-27b-3p and miR-486–5p and their isomiRs: 2 isomiRs of miR-486–5p, one of miR-451a and one of miR-223-3p.) between exacerbation and stable period out of 158 expressed in sputum (Figure 1b). Three of them, miR-27b, miR-223 and miR-19b, showed a decrease, whereas the other two (miR-486-5p, miR-451a) showed increased expression during exacerbation.

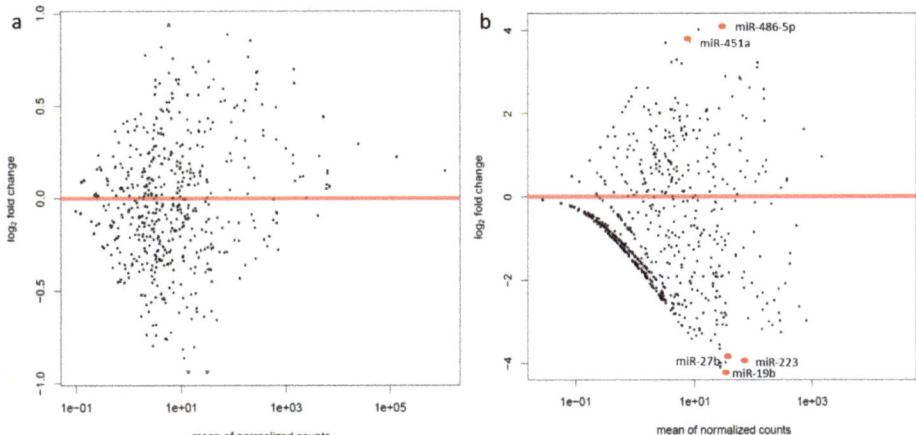

Figure 1. MA-plot between exacerbation and stable period of the gene expression counts (**a**) for the whole blood and (**b**) for sputum. Significantly altered miRNAs are marked as red dots (DeSeq).

Four mature miRNAs differentially expressed in sputum (miR-223-3p, miR-451a, miR-27b-3p and miR-486–5p) were selected for qPCR analysis in the sputum supernatant from 24 patients and exhaled breath condensate samples from 24 patients. One miRNA, miR-19b, showed very low expression in the sequencing experiment, so we excluded it from qPCR validation. During exacerbation, we observed the highest increase in expression for miR-486–5p in both EBC and sputum supernatant samples, but the difference compared to a stable period was not significant. For miR-223-3p, we found that decreased expression during exacerbation in the sequencing experiment was not confirmed in the validation cohort.

Expression of exosomal miR-223-3p was higher in CF patients during exacerbation in EBC and sputum samples, but the difference was not significant ($p > 0.05$). In EBC during exacerbation miR-451a was more abundant than in stable period, but the difference was not statistically significant ($p = 0.41$). In sputum supernatant, miR-451a was decreased during exacerbation than stable period, yet the difference did not reach significance. The only miRNA that showed decreased expression in both EBC and sputum samples during exacerbation was miR-27b, but this decrease was not significant. The results are shown in Table 3.

Table 3. MicroRNA (MiRNA) levels in patients during pulmonary exacerbation in reference to stable period.

miRNA	Expression (EBC)	p Value	Expression (Sputum)	p Value
miR-223-3p	↑	0.177	↑	0.411
miR-451a	↑	0.342	↓	0.406
miR-27b-3p	↓	0.160	↓	0.312
miR-486-5p	↑	0.656	↑	0.341

3.3. Correlation of miRNA Expression with Clinical Parameters

3.3.1. MiR-223-3p

The higher expression of this miRNA in EBC correlated with *Aspergillus* infection in the airways during pulmonary exacerbation in CF patients ($p = 0.02$). Similar to EBC, we observed higher levels of this miRNA in sputum supernatants in children infected with *Aspergillus* ($p = 0.08$) (Figure 2), but not with symptoms severity (Shwachman–Kulczycki score, Brasfield score) or lung function.

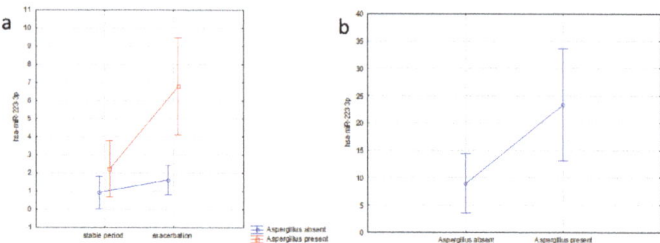

Figure 2. The association of miR-223-3p expression and clinical parameters in CF patients (**a**) in EBC in relation to *Aspergillus* infection and exacerbation (F = 5.953, $p = 0.024$, 2-way analysis of variance); (**b**) in sputum supernatant in relation to *Aspergillus* infection (F = 6.714, $p = 0.017$, one-way analysis of variance).

3.3.2. MiR-451a

We observed that CF patients infected with *H. influenzae* had significantly higher miR-451a EBC expression during exacerbation ($p = 0.02$). In contrast, the level of expression in uninfected CF patients was similar and independent of exacerbation. We also observed a significant inverse correlation between miR-451a EBC expression and the Brasfield score ($r^2 = -0.53$, $p = 0.01$) (Figure 3), but the other clinical parameters did not correlate with the expression of this miRNA. We found no significant differences in miR-451a expression with clinical parameters in sputum.

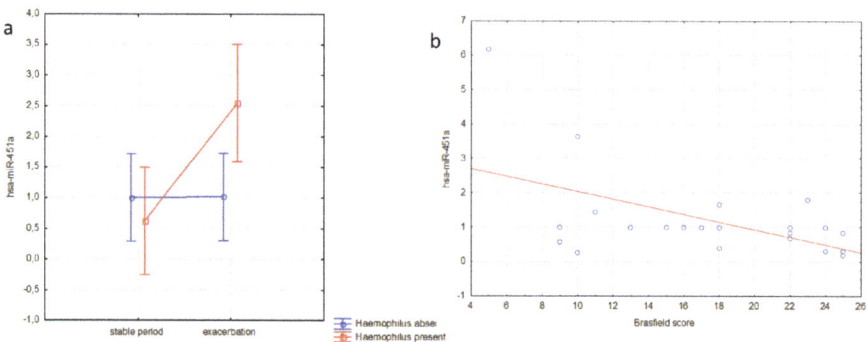

Figure 3. Association of miR-451a expression in EBC and clinical parameters in CF patients, (**a**) in relation to *Hemophilus* infection and exacerbation (F = 5.760; $p = 0.024$, 2-way analysis of variance); (**b**) correlation with the Brasfield score (r = −0.526; $p = 0.001$, Spearman correlation).

3.3.3. MiR-27b-3p

The expression of miR-27b in EBC positively correlated with lung function parameters: FEV1 ($r^2 = 0.669$, $p = 0.077$) and FVC ($r^2 = 0.637$, $p = 0.006$) during pulmonary exacerbation.

Current infection with *Pseudomonas aeruginosa* was associated with decreased expression of miR-27b-3p in sputum supernatant during exacerbation than the patients in a stable period ($p < 0.0001$). It remained unaltered in patients without *Pseudomonas* infection (Figure 4).

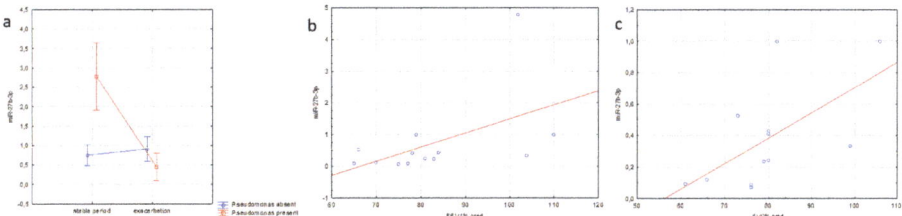

Figure 4. Association of miR-27b expression and clinical parameters in CF patients, (**a**) in sputum correlation with *Pseudomonas* infection during exacerbation ($F = 25.267$, $p < 0.001$, 2-way analysis of variance); (**b**) in EBC correlation with FEV1 ($r = 0.510$; $p = 0.077$) and (**c**) FVC ($r = 0611$; $p = 0.034$) during exacerbation (Spearman correlation).

3.3.4. MiR-486-5p

The expression of this miRNA in EBC did not correlate significantly with analyzed clinical parameters in CF patients. In sputum, miR-486-5p expression was higher in CF patients colonized with *Pseudomonas aeruginosa* ($p = 0.044$). Further analysis showed an inverse correlation between this miRNA and Shwachman–Kulczycki score ($r^2 = -0.419$, $p = 0.047$) as well as the Brasfield score ($r^2 = -0.459$, $p = 0.031$) and lung function (FVC) ($r^2 = -0.421$, $p = 0.046$). On the other hand, results for two parameters of peripheral inflammation, CRP and neutrophilia, positively correlated with miR-486-5p expression in CF patients during PE for CRP ($r^2 = 0.592$, $p = 0.027$) and neutrophilia ($r^2 = 0.772$, $p = 0.001$) (Figure 5).

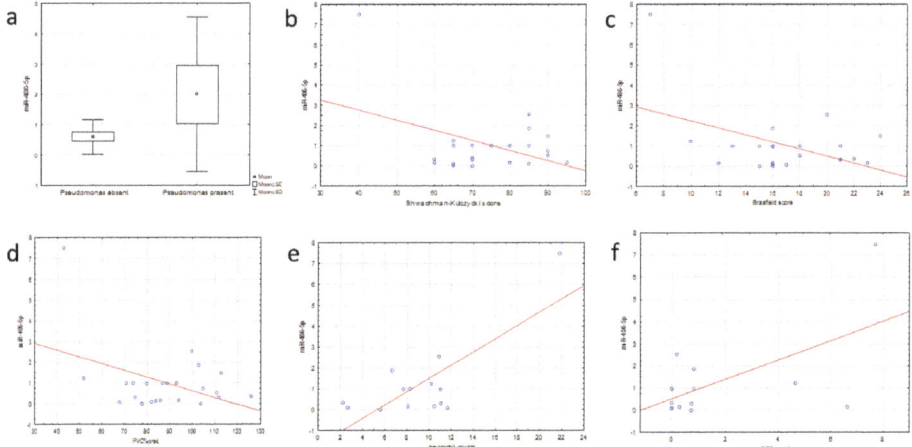

Figure 5. Association of miR-486-5p expression in sputum and clinical parameters in CF patients (**a**) in relation to *Pseudomonas* infection ($p = 0.044$, 1-way analysis of variance); (**b**) correlation with Shwachman–Kulczycki score ($r = -0.42$, $p = 0.048$), (**c**) correlation with Brasfield score ($r = -0.45$, $p = 0.031$); (**d**) Spearman correlation with FVC ($r = -0.451$, $p = 0.045$); correlation with peripheral markers of inflammation: (**e**) neutrophil counts ($r = 0.772$; $p = 0.001$) and (**f**) CRP levels ($r = 0.592$; $p = 0.025$) during exacerbation (Spearman correlation).

4. Discussion

The main finding of this study is the altered miRNA expression profile in the airways, but not in blood, during pulmonary exacerbation. We also found that altered miRNAs (miR-223-3p, miR-451a, miR-27b, miR486-5p) correlate with clinical outcomes (bacterial infections, the severity of symptoms, lung function, peripheral inflammation) in sputum and exhaled breath condensate of CF patients.

Previous studies showed that miR-223 is a negative regulator of neutrophil activation and chemotaxis in experimental models of inflammatory diseases. This miRNA mediates intracellular neutrophil action as well as extracellular inflammation responses in the lungs [26,27]. In CF, neutrophilic inflammation in the lung correlated with more severe lung disease [28,29]. Previous data indicated that *Aspergillus* colonization may be associated with reduced lung function and that *Aspergillus* infection increased neutrophil count and elevated the levels of inflammatory cytokines (e.g., IL-8) in BALF [30,31]. In our study, we found increased expression of miR-223 during exacerbation with concurrent *Aspergillus* infection. Thus, miR-223-3p upregulation may be a response to infection and enhanced airway inflammation induced by *Aspergillus*.

Regarding miR-451a, a previous study showed increased expression of this miRNA in BALF from healthy subjects in the lower lung lobes compared to the upper lobes [32]. In silico analysis indicated several targets for miR-451a, e.g., macrophage migration inhibitory factor (MIF) and matrix metalloproteinase-2 (MMP-2), that are innate immunity mediators [33]. MIF is a proinflammatory molecule that enhances Gram-negative inflammatory responses, and its high level accelerates end-organ injury in CF [33]. In our study, we found the highest miR-451a expression in EBC during exacerbation in patients infected with *Hemophilus influenzae*. Infection with these Gram-negative bacteria in cystic fibrosis often co-occurs with PE [34]. An inverse correlation of miR-451a expression with the Brasfield score suggests that increased expression in the upper airways (EBC) may be a marker of disease progression assessed by radiological changes. Interestingly, the expression of miR-451a in CF exacerbation slightly decreased in sputum and did not correlate with *Hemophilus* infection. This observation indicates that miRNA alterations are site-specific within the respiratory tract and differ between body fluids from the upper and lower airways.

The expression of miR-27b-3p decreased during pulmonary exacerbation in both EBC and sputum supernatant, however, this change was not significant. Previous studies indicated this miRNA silences the immune response by reducing cytokine secretion, thus inhibiting local macrophage recruitment. Its expression increased during acute infection, e.g., sepsis preventing the spreading of inflammation [35]. This action was confirmed in an animal model of *Mycobacterium tuberculosis* infection [36]. Infected mice overexpressed in the airways miR-27b that suppressed the production of pro-inflammatory factors and excessive inflammation. Similarly, we observed that *Pseudomonas aeruginosa* infection correlated with overexpression of miR-27b in sputum in a stable period. Thus, its increase seems to suppress the exaggerated inflammatory response. Its significant decrease during exacerbation correlated with enhanced inflammation induced by *Pseudomonas* infection. Increased expression of miR-27b in EBC also associated with better lung function parameters, e.g., FEV_1 or FVC, suggesting that airway inflammation suppressed by miR-27b overexpression may translate into improved lung function in CF.

Previous data regarding mir-486–5p showed its increased plasma expression in CF patients than healthy controls [37]. We confirmed its expression in whole blood and also in sputum and EBC. A recent study showed that mice with induced acute lung injury presented higher miR-486-5p expression, whereas its inhibition with antagomir blocked inflammatory response and apoptosis, thus reducing lung injury [38]. Our results showed an increased expression of exosomal miR-486-5p in the sputum of CF patients infected with *P. aeruginosa*. Its expression inversely correlated with symptoms severity (Shwachman–Kulczycki and Brasfield scores) and lung function indicating a worse course of lung disease. Therefore, the increased local expression of this microRNA may be a marker of worse prognosis in CF patients. However, further studies are needed to confirm this assumption.

One of the main limitations of the study is small sample size of our group and the fact that patients from the exacerbation group were different from patients from the stable group.

Another limitation may be high variability in clinical and miRNA expression data comparisons in the correlation analysis and to address this issue, we used nonparametric tests to minimize the influence of outliers on the results interpretation.

5. Conclusions

In conclusion, we found the altered miRNA expression profile in the airways of CF patients. These changes correlate with the clinical outcomes and suggest the involvement of miRNA regulation in pulmonary exacerbation. Our study also indicates the potential of non-invasively collected material from the airways (exhaled breath condensate) that may be a source of extracellular biomarkers of CF pulmonary exacerbation in children.

Author Contributions: Z.S. participated in the study design, sample collection, molecular analysis and data interpretation and drafting the manuscript; I.W.-B. participated in the study design, recruitment of patients, data analysis and the revision of the manuscript; K.J.-P. participated in the study design, clinical assessment of patients, data analysis and the revision of the manuscript; B.N. participated in sample collection, data analysis and preparation of the manuscript; W.L. participated in the data analysis and curation and preparing the manuscript; Z.K. participated in the clinical supervision and preparing the manuscript, P.S. participated in the clinical supervision and preparing the manuscript, A.B. participated in the study design, clinical supervision and preparing the manuscript; A.S. designed the study, performed molecular analysis, interpreted the data, revised and edited the manuscript, acquired the funding and administered the project. All authors have read and agreed to the published version of the manuscript.

Funding: This research was funded by the Polish National Science Center, grant no. 2016/22/E/NZ5/00383 (A. Szczepankiewicz).

Conflicts of Interest: The authors declare no conflict of interest. The funders had no role in the design of the study; in the collection, analyses or interpretation of data; in the writing of the manuscript or in the decision to publish the results.

References

1. Dos Santos, A.L.M.; de Melo Santos, H.; Nogueira, M.B.; Tavora, H.T.O.; de Lourdes Jaborandy Paim da Cunha, M.; de Melo Seixas, R.B.P.; de Freitas Velloso Monte, L.; de Carvalho, E. Cystic Fibrosis: Clinical Phenotypes in Children and Adolescents. *Pediatric Gastroenterol. Hepatol. Nutr.* **2018**, *21*, 306314. [CrossRef]
2. Belkin, R.A.; Henig, N.R.; Singer, L.G.; Chaparro, C.; Rubenstein, R.C.; Xie, S.X.; Yee, J.Y.; Kotloff, R.M.; Lipson, D.A.; Bunin, G.R. Risk factors for death of patients with cystic fibrosis awaiting lung transplantation. *Am. J. Respir. Crit. Care Med.* **2006**, *173*, 659–666. [CrossRef] [PubMed]
3. Waters, V.; Ratjen, F. Pulmonary Exacerbations in Children with Cystic Fibrosis. *Ann. Am. Thoracic Soc.* **2015**, *12* (Suppl. S2), S200–S206. [CrossRef]
4. Zemanick, E.T.; Hoffman, L.R. Cystic Fibrosis: Microbiology and Host Response. *Pediatric Clin. N. Am.* **2016**, *63*, 617–636. [CrossRef] [PubMed]
5. Stressmann, F.A.; Rogers, G.B.; Marsh, P.; Lilley, A.K.; Daniels, T.W.; Carroll, M.P.; Hoffman, L.R.; Jones, G.; Allen, C.E.; Patel, N.; et al. Does bacterial density in cystic fibrosis sputum increase prior to pulmonary exacerbation? *J. Cyst. Fibros. Off. J. Eur. Cyst. Fibrosis Soc.* **2011**, *10*, 357–365. [CrossRef] [PubMed]
6. Zemanick, E.T.; Wagner, B.D.; Harris, J.K.; Wagener, J.S.; Accurso, F.J.; Sagel, S.D. Pulmonary exacerbations in cystic fibrosis with negative bacterial cultures. *Pediatric Pulmonol.* **2010**, *45*, 569–577. [CrossRef] [PubMed]
7. Bhatt, J.M. Treatment of pulmonary exacerbations in cystic fibrosis. *Eur. Respir. Rev. Off. J. Eur. Respir. Soc.* **2013**, *22*, 205–216. [CrossRef]
8. Jacquot, J.; Tabary, O.; Clement, A. Hyperinflammation in airways of cystic fibrosis patients: What's new? *Ex. Rev. Mol. Diagn.* **2008**, *8*, 359–363. [CrossRef]
9. Gray, R.D.; Imrie, M.; Boyd, A.C.; Porteous, D.; Innes, J.A.; Greening, A.P. Sputum and serum calprotectin are useful biomarkers during CF exacerbation. *J. Cyst. Fibrosis Off. J. Eur. Cyst. Fibros. Soc.* **2010**, *9*, 193–198. [CrossRef] [PubMed]

10. Colombo, C.; Costantini, D.; Rocchi, A.; Cariani, L.; Garlaschi, M.L.; Tirelli, S.; Calori, G.; Copreni, E.; Conese, M. Cytokine levels in sputum of cystic fibrosis patients before and after antibiotic therapy. *Pediatric Pulmonol.* **2005**, *40*, 15–21. [CrossRef] [PubMed]
11. Gray, R.D.; Downey, D.; Taggart, C.C. Biomarkers to monitor exacerbations in cystic fibrosis. *Ex. Rev. Respir. Med.* **2017**, *11*, 255–257. [CrossRef] [PubMed]
12. Maes, T.; Cobos, F.A.; Schleich, F.; Sorbello, V.; Henket, M.; De Preter, K.; Bracke, K.R.; Conickx, G.; Mesnil, C.; Vandesompele, J.; et al. Asthma inflammatory phenotypes show differential microRNA expression in sputum. *J. All. Clin. Immunol.* **2016**, *137*, 1433–1446. [CrossRef] [PubMed]
13. Sagel, S.D.; Wagner, B.D.; Anthony, M.M.; Emmett, P.; Zemanick, E.T. Sputum biomarkers of inflammation and lung function decline in children with cystic fibrosis. *Am. J. Respir. Crit. Care Med.* **2012**, *186*, 857–865. [CrossRef]
14. Mendes, F.C.; Paciencia, I.; Ferreira, A.C.; Martins, C.; Rufo, J.C.; Silva, D.; Cunha, P.; Farraia, M.; Moreira, P.; Delgado, L.; et al. Development and validation of exhaled breath condensate microRNAs to identify and endotype asthma in children. *PLoS ONE* **2019**, *14*, e0224983. [CrossRef] [PubMed]
15. Stolzenburg, L.R.; Harris, A. The role of microRNAs in chronic respiratory disease: Recent insights. *Biol. Chem.* **2018**, *399*, 219–234. [CrossRef]
16. Gon, Y.; Shimizu, T.; Mizumura, K.; Maruoka, S.; Hikichi, M. Molecular techniques for respiratory diseases: MicroRNA and extracellular vesicles. *Respirology* **2020**, *25*, 149–160. [CrossRef]
17. Sonneville, F.; Ruffin, M.; Guillot, L.; Rousselet, N.; Le Rouzic, P.; Corvol, H.; Tabary, O. New insights about miRNAs in cystic fibrosis. *Am. J. Pathol.* **2015**, *185*, 897–908. [CrossRef]
18. Krause, K.; Kopp, B.T.; Tazi, M.F.; Caution, K.; Hamilton, K.; Badr, A.; Shrestha, C.; Tumin, D.; Hayes, D., Jr.; Robledo-Avila, F.; et al. The expression of Mirc1/Mir17-92 cluster in sputum samples correlates with pulmonary exacerbations in cystic fibrosis patients. *J. Cyst. Fibros. Off. J. Eur. Cyst. Fibros. Soc.* **2018**, *17*, 454–461. [CrossRef]
19. Oglesby, I.K.; Bray, I.M.; Chotirmall, S.H.; Stallings, R.L.; O'Neill, S.J.; McElvaney, N.G.; Greene, C.M. miR-126 is downregulated in cystic fibrosis airway epithelial cells and regulates TOM1 expression. *J. Immunol.* **2010**, *184*, 1702–1709. [CrossRef]
20. McKiernan, P.J.; Greene, C.M. MicroRNA Dysregulation in Cystic Fibrosis. *Med. Inflamm.* **2015**, *2015*, 529642. [CrossRef]
21. Mooney, C.; McKiernan, P.J.; Raoof, R.; Henshall, D.C.; Linnane, B.; McNally, P.; Glasgow, A.M.A.; Greene, C.M. Plasma microRNA levels in male and female children with cystic fibrosis. *Sci. Rep.* **2020**, *10*, 1141. [CrossRef] [PubMed]
22. Szentpetery, S.; Flume, P.A. Optimizing outcomes of pulmonary exacerbations in cystic fibrosis. *Curr. Opin. Pulm. Med.* **2018**, *24*, 606–611. [CrossRef] [PubMed]
23. Bilton, D.; Canny, G.; Conway, S.; Dumcius, S.; Hjelte, L.; Proesmans, M.; Tummler, B.; Vavrova, V.; De Boeck, K. Pulmonary exacerbation: Towards a definition for use in clinical trials. Report from the EuroCareCF Working Group on outcome parameters in clinical trials. *J. Cyst. Fibros. Off. J. Eur. Cyst. Fibros. Soc.* **2011**, *10* (Suppl. S2), S79–S81. [CrossRef]
24. Wojsyk-Banaszak, I.; Sobkowiak, P.; Jonczyk-Potoczna, K.; Narozna, B.; Langwinski, W.; Szczepanik, M.; Kycler, Z.; Breborowicz, A.; Szczepankiewicz, A. Evaluation of Copeptin during Pulmonary Exacerbation in Cystic Fibrosis. *Med. Inflamm.* **2019**, *2019*, 1939740. [CrossRef]
25. Horvath, I.; Hunt, J.; Barnes, P.J.; Alving, K.; Antczak, A.; Baraldi, E.; Becher, G.; van Beurden, W.J.; Corradi, M.; Dekhuijzen, R.; et al. Exhaled breath condensate: Methodological recommendations and unresolved questions. *Eur. Respir. J.* **2005**, *26*, 523–548. [CrossRef] [PubMed]
26. Dorhoi, A.; Iannaccone, M.; Farinacci, M.; Fae, K.C.; Schreiber, J.; Moura-Alves, P.; Nouailles, G.; Mollenkopf, H.J.; Oberbeck-Muller, D.; Jorg, S.; et al. MicroRNA-223 controls susceptibility to tuberculosis by regulating lung neutrophil recruitment. *J. Clin. Investig.* **2013**, *123*, 4836–4848. [CrossRef] [PubMed]
27. Hall, C.H.T.; Campbell, E.L.; Colgan, S.P. Neutrophils as Components of Mucosal Homeostasis. *Cell. Mol. Gastroenterol. Hepatol.* **2017**, *4*, 329–337. [CrossRef] [PubMed]
28. Tirouvanziam, R. Neutrophilic inflammation as a major determinant in the progression of cystic fibrosis. *Drug News Perspect.* **2006**, *19*, 609–614. [CrossRef]

29. Pillarisetti, N.; Williamson, E.; Linnane, B.; Skoric, B.; Robertson, C.F.; Robinson, P.; Massie, J.; Hall, G.L.; Sly, P.; Stick, S.; et al. Infection, inflammation, and lung function decline in infants with cystic fibrosis. *Am. J. Respir. Crit. Care Med.* **2011**, *184*, 75–81. [CrossRef]
30. Gangell, C.; Gard, S.; Douglas, T.; Park, J.; de Klerk, N.; Keil, T.; Brennan, S.; Ranganathan, S.; Robins-Browne, R.; Sly, P.D.; et al. Inflammatory responses to individual microorganisms in the lungs of children with cystic fibrosis. *Clin. Infect. Dis. Off. Publ. Infect. Dis. Soc. Am.* **2011**, *53*, 425–432. [CrossRef]
31. Amin, R.; Dupuis, A.; Aaron, S.D.; Ratjen, F. The effect of chronic infection with Aspergillus fumigatus on lung function and hospitalization in patients with cystic fibrosis. *Chest* **2010**, *137*, 171–176. [CrossRef] [PubMed]
32. Armstrong, D.A.; Nymon, A.B.; Ringelberg, C.S.; Lesseur, C.; Hazlett, H.F.; Howard, L.; Marsit, C.J.; Ashare, A. Pulmonary microRNA profiling: Implications in upper lobe predominant lung disease. *Clin. Epigenetics* **2017**, *9*, 56. [CrossRef] [PubMed]
33. Adamali, H.; Armstrong, M.E.; McLaughlin, A.M.; Cooke, G.; McKone, E.; Costello, C.M.; Gallagher, C.G.; Leng, L.; Baugh, J.A.; Fingerle-Rowson, G.; et al. Macrophage migration inhibitory factor enzymatic activity, lung inflammation, and cystic fibrosis. *Am. J. Respir. Crit. Care Med.* **2012**, *186*, 162–169. [CrossRef]
34. Rayner, R.J.; Hiller, E.J.; Ispahani, P.; Baker, M. Haemophilus infection in cystic fibrosis. *Arch. Dis. Child.* **1990**, *65*, 255–258. [CrossRef] [PubMed]
35. Wang, Z.; Ruan, Z.; Mao, Y.; Dong, W.; Zhang, Y.; Yin, N.; Jiang, L. miR-27a is up regulated and promotes inflammatory response in sepsis. *Cell. Immunol.* **2014**, *290*, 190–195. [CrossRef] [PubMed]
36. Liang, S.; Song, Z.; Wu, Y.; Gao, Y.; Gao, M.; Liu, F.; Wang, F.; Zhang, Y. MicroRNA-27b Modulates Inflammatory Response and Apoptosis during Mycobacterium tuberculosis Infection. *J. Immunol.* **2018**, *200*, 3506–3518. [CrossRef] [PubMed]
37. Ideozu, J.E.; Zhang, X.; Rangaraj, V.; McColley, S.; Levy, H. Microarray profiling identifies extracellular circulating miRNAs dysregulated in cystic fibrosis. *Sci. Rep.* **2019**, *9*, 15483. [CrossRef]
38. Luo, Q.; Zhu, J.; Zhang, Q.; Xie, J.; Yi, C.; Li, T. MicroRNA-486-5p Promotes Acute Lung Injury via Inducing Inflammation and Apoptosis by Targeting OTUD7B. *Inflammation* **2020**. [CrossRef]

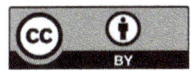

© 2020 by the authors. Licensee MDPI, Basel, Switzerland. This article is an open access article distributed under the terms and conditions of the Creative Commons Attribution (CC BY) license (http://creativecommons.org/licenses/by/4.0/).

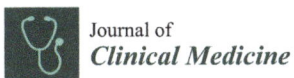
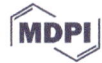

Review

Implications of a Change of Paradigm in Alpha1 Antitrypsin Deficiency Augmentation Therapy: From Biochemical to Clinical Efficacy

José Luis López-Campos [1,2,*], Laura Carrasco Hernandez [1,2] and Candelaria Caballero Eraso [1,2]

1. Unidad Médico-Quirúrgica de Enfermedades Respiratorias, Instituto de Biomedicina de Sevilla (IBiS), Hospital Universitario Virgen del Rocío/Universidad de Sevilla, 41013 Seville, Spain; lauracarrascohdez@gmail.com (L.C.H.); ccaballero-ibis@us.es (C.C.E.)
2. Centro de Investigación Biomédica en Red de Enfermedades Respiratorias (CIBERES), Instituto de Salud Carlos III, 28029 Madrid, Spain
* Correspondence: lcampos@separ.es

Received: 4 July 2020; Accepted: 3 August 2020; Published: 5 August 2020

Abstract: Ever since the first studies, restoring proteinase imbalance in the lung has traditionally been considered as the main goal of alpha1 antitrypsin (AAT) replacement therapy. This strategy was therefore based on ensuring biochemical efficacy, identifying a protection threshold, and evaluating different dosage regimens. Subsequently, the publication of the results of the main clinical trials showing a decrease in the progression of pulmonary emphysema has led to a debate over a possible change in the main objective of treatment, from biochemical efficacy to clinical efficacy in terms of lung densitometry deterioration prevention. This new paradigm has produced a series controversies and unanswered questions which face clinicians managing AAT deficiency. In this review, the concepts that led to the approval of AAT replacement therapy are reviewed and discussed under a new prism of achieving clinical efficacy, with the reduction of lung deterioration as the main objective. Here, we propose the use of current knowledge and clinical experience to face existing challenges in different clinical scenarios, in order to help clinicians in decision-making, increase interest in the disease, and stimulate research in this field.

Keywords: alpha1 antitrypsin deficiency; augmentation therapy; replacement therapy; rare diseases

1. Introduction

Alpha1 antitrypsin deficiency (AATD) is a rare genetic condition that determines the appearance of pulmonary emphysema and liver damage in its severe forms [1]. As a rare condition, the available evidence indicating how to proceed in different clinical situations that may occur is limited and not always clear-cut. Therefore, controversies and doubts may arise about the management of different aspects of this condition in daily clinical practice. This is particularly evident when it comes to considering exogenous alpha1 antitrypsin (AAT) replacement therapy, which is also known as augmentation therapy, for severely deficient patients. Different aspects including indications, the dose regimen for dose intervals, or the differences between the presentations available are still a matter for debate. Interestingly, in recent years, there have been some advances that have clarified, at least in part, some of the previous controversies in relation to this therapy. One major finding is the ability of AAT augmentation therapy to decrease emphysema progression as measured by lung densitometry [2–4]. Consequently, the preservation of pulmonary density with exogenous AAT has sparked a debate over a potential change in the main aims of treatment from biochemical efficacy to clinical efficacy, based on emphysema progression evaluated by lung densitometry. Under this new paradigm, clinicians managing AATD are faced with a number of controversies and unanswered questions. In this work, we propose harnessing current knowledge and clinical experience to find answers to the current debate, with a view to helping clinicians to take key decisions, arouse interest in the disease, and foster research in this field.

2. Initial Assumptions

2.1. Biochemical Efficacy

Plasma AAT normally diffuses through the endothelial barrier into the interstitium. Here, most of the AAT flows out through the lymphatic vessels; however, part of the diffuse AAT passes through the epithelial barrier into the alveolar epithelial lining fluid (Figure 1). Accordingly, the amount of serum AAT is directly proportional to the amount of AAT that migrates to the interstitium and the epithelial lining fluid of the lungs [5]. As a result, the initial trials on AAT replacement therapy were focused on demonstrating that this therapy could restore the AAT levels and anti-elastase activity in the epithelial lining fluid. This aim is referred to as biochemical efficacy.

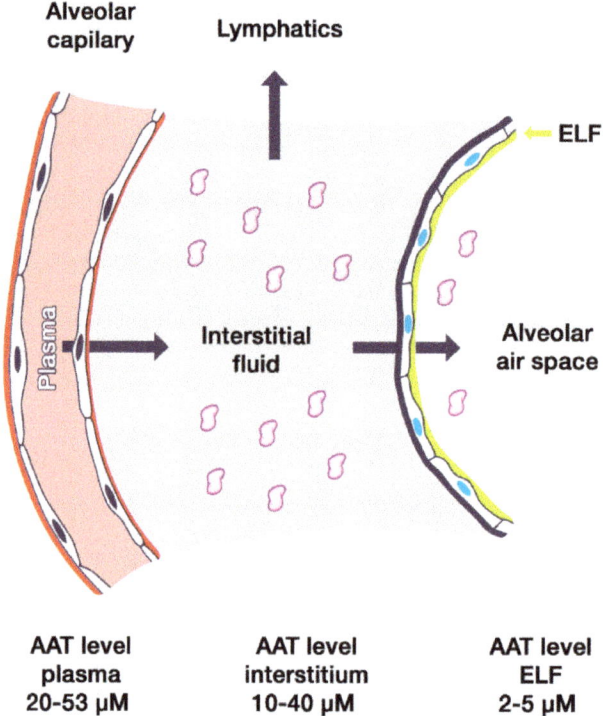

Figure 1. Diagram indicating alpha1 antitrypsin in plasma from normal individuals diffusing across the alveolar capillary endothelial barrier into the interstitium. AAT, Alpha1 antitrypsin; ELF, epithelial lining fluid. The sizes of the vascular, interstitial, and alveolar compartments are not to scale, for educational purposes.

However, four figures obtained from five patients (Figure 2) in 1981 [6] were enough to start a path that would culminate in the approval of the Food and Drug Administration in 1987. This initial study demonstrated that, by administering intravenous exogenous AAT in seven-day infusion periods, exogenous AAT could reach the epithelial lining fluid, increase the protein concentration at this compartment, and improve the anti-elastase activity [7]. A subsequent study in a few patients also confirmed that, by administering AAT infusions every seven days, serum levels of AAT were kept above a level defined as a protective threshold (discussed below) [8].

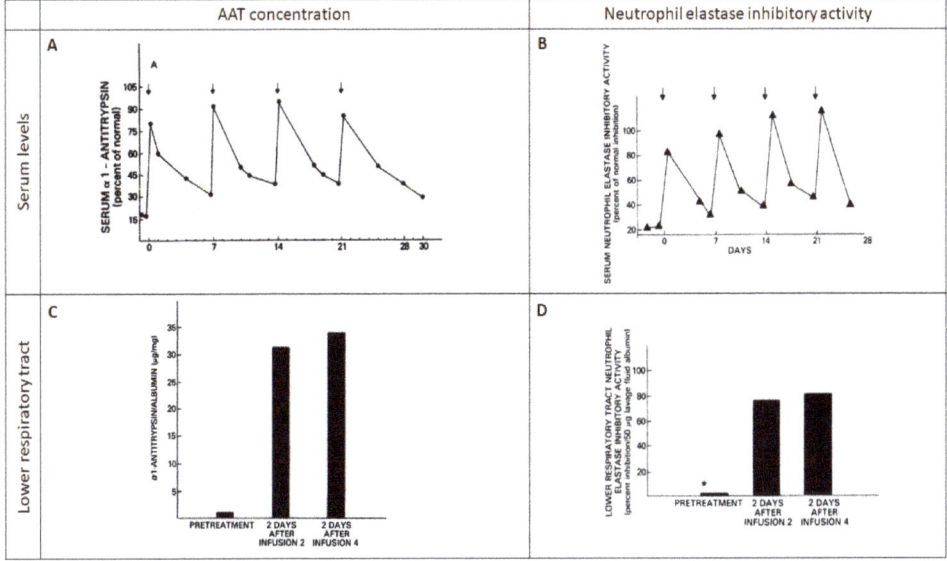

Figure 2. Initial study evaluating the biochemical efficacy of AAT augmentation therapy. Reproduced with permission from Reference [6]. (**A**) The response of serum a1-antitrypsin levels to the infusion of 4.0 g of AAT. (**B**) Serum neutrophil elastase inhibitory activity following weekly intravenous infusions of 4.0 g of AAT. (**C**) Lower respiratory tract a1-antitrypsin levels during intravenous replacement therapy with 4.0 g of AAT. (**D**) Lower respiratory tract neutrophil elastase inhibitory activity following weekly intravenous infusions of 4.0 g of AAT.

Finally, AAT replacement therapy was approved for intravenous infusion based on biochemical efficacy and preliminary safety data. Therefore, it is important to remember that, at those times, augmentation therapy for AATD was an example of a treatment that had been approved for use in patients, without being evaluated for efficacy and safety in cohorts of patients through traditional clinical trials in clinical, functional, or radiological terms.

2.2. Protective Threshold Level

A so-called protective threshold level has been defined as the amount of AAT in serum from which there is no increased risk of developing emphysema. Notably, this limit was not based on specific patient data but on epidemiological data, following the description of the presence of emphysema in the initial cases [8]. Interestingly, this threshold level was first described by radial immunodiffusion, which suggests that that AAT levels ≤50 mg/dL are associated with a high risk for the development of emphysema, levels between 50 and 80 mg/dL confer an uncertain risk, and levels >80 mg/dL confer no increase in risk above the background risk [8]. Therefore, 80 mg/dL by radial immunodiffusion was the initial accepted limit.

However, there is a considerable confusion regarding this level. In those days, commercially available standards yielded values for amounts of AAT that were identified as higher than the true values [8]. Therefore, the result had to be adjusted depending on which standard was used—the commercially available standard or a true laboratory standard. To differentiate the procedures, initial studies expressed values as milligrams per deciliter when based on the commercial standard, and as micromolar units when based on the true laboratory standard. According to these different units,

80 mg/dL with the commercial standard corresponded to 11.2 µM with the true laboratory standard [8]. Later, in another study, 80 mg/dL by radial immunodiffusion corresponded to 10.9 µM [9]. Consequently, in the ATS consensus, it was established that 80 mg/dL by radial immunodiffusion corresponded to 50 mg/dL by nephelometry, using commercially available standards, which in turn corresponded to 11 µM, using the American National Health Lung Blood Institute (NHLBI) standard [10]. Interestingly, 11 µM of the NHLBI standard corresponds to 57.2 mg/dL by nephelometry. Therefore, these two values of 11 µM and 57.2 mg/dL by nephelometry, using the NHBLI standard, have been interchangeably identified as the protective threshold.

Interestingly, what this protective threshold really shows is a level from which emphysema associated with the deficit is more likely to appear, based on epidemiological studies. However, we really have no idea if this is the limit above which the progression of emphysema is slowed down with replacement therapy, as the concept of "protective threshold" would imply. Accordingly, we still do not know the threshold which identifies the optimal therapeutic response in terms of emphysema progression [11], and so, rather than "protective threshold", it would be better to call it "detection threshold" or "severity threshold" or "risk threshold".

2.3. Dose

Since AAT half-life in healthy MM individuals is reported to be from 3.8 to 5.2 days (mean 4.6, standard error of the mean 0.21) [12], the initial trials devised an infusion schedule that would allow once-weekly administrations for PiZ individuals, thus maintaining serum AAT levels above the considered protective level (as discussed above). Weekly infusions containing around 4.0 g of AAT were therefore prepared from 3.5–4.0 L of pooled plasma [6]. This dose corresponds to 57.1 mg/kg for a subject of 70 kg. Accordingly, the subsequent trial used the standard dose of 60 mg/kg in weekly infusions [8], which has been maintained until now.

2.4. Route of Administration

Since the first studies, the administration of AAT has been intravenous [6–8]. This route of administration is the only one available to this day. Inhaled AAT administration has been tried in recent years, but it is still under exploration [13].

2.5. Origin of AAT

From the beginning, the AAT has been obtained from fresh plasma from human donors. Specifically, the first studies reported that between 3 and 4 L of pooled human plasma was necessary to obtain 4 gr of AAT for administration [6]. Alternative ways of obtaining AAT were investigated in the early years, in particular from recombinant DNA in microorganisms [14] or from recombinant AAT associated with virus vectors as a potential tool for the gene therapy [15], cell lines producing AAT [16], silkworm larvae [17], or a plant-made recombinant AAT from Nicotiana benthamiana, a close relative of the tobacco plant which is indigenous to Australia [17]. All of these are exploratory possibilities, but, currently, AAT continues to be obtained from human plasma.

2.6. Final Statement

Starting from the uncertain origins commented above, replacement treatment with exogenous AAT obtained from human plasma, at a dose of 60 mg/kg in weekly intravenous administrations, is the maintenance therapy for severe AATD, with the objective of achieving biochemical efficacy by aiming for serum levels of AAT above 11 µM, using the NHBLI standard.

3. Clinical Efficacy: A Change of Paradigm

It was only from the late 1990s onward when longitudinal data on the impact of AAT replacement therapy started to become available. This information comes mainly from seven major observational studies (Table 1), and mostly from two major cohorts, namely the German scientific working group for the therapy of lung diseases (WALT from the German abbreviation: Wissenschaftliche Arbeitsgemeinschaft zur Therapie von Lungenerkrankungen) [18–20] and the American NHBLI registry for individuals with severe deficiency of AAT [21,22], together with other studies in the USA [23] and Spain [24]. Additionally, three clinical trials plus one pooled analysis of two of these trials explored the clinical impact of AAT augmentation therapy [2–4,25] (Table 1). To cut a long story short, although observational trials reported several significant results favoring augmentation therapy in terms of exacerbations, lung function, or survival, the main finding from the formal clinical trials was a reduction in the loss of lung density by lung densitometry. This finding was relevant since it implied that, by administering intravenous exogenous AAT, not only are we able to regain biochemical efficacy, but the treatment also achieves a change in the natural progression of emphysema, with a potential longer-term prognostic impact [26,27]. Therefore, augmentation therapy has the potential to modify the natural progression of AATD-associated emphysema.

As a main consequence, the objective of exogenous administration of AAT is to be modified from seeking biochemical efficacy to seeking clinical impact in the form of prevention of lung deterioration and emphysema progression. However, this change in therapeutic objective poses a dilemma. If the goal of treatment is no longer to ensure biochemical efficacy but to slow the progression of emphysema, this opens up a number of controversies and unanswered questions as regards when the therapy is indicated and its administration and follow-up, which are discussed hereafter.

Table 1. Description of the population included in the main studies with augmentation therapy.

Study	N	Age		FEV1		Mutations
		Eligibility Criteria	Cohort Results *	Eligibility Criteria	Cohort Result *	Eligibility Criteria	Cohort Result
Observational studies with control							
Seersholm N, et al.; WALT. Eur Respir J, 1997 [18]	295	NR	46 (8)	FEV1 < 65% or decline > 120 mL/year	37 (14)%	Severe AATD (NR)	NR
NHLBI Registry. AJRCCM, 1998 [21]	927	≥18 years	46 (11)	NR	<35%: 43.6% 35–49%: 21.1% 50–79%: 16.2% ≥80%: 19.1%	AAT ≤ 11 µM or ZZ	NR
Wencker M, et al.; WALT. Eur Respir J, 1998 [19]	443	>18 years	45 (7)	FEV1 < 65% or decline > 120 mL/year	Ex-smokers: 35.5 (14.8)% Non-smokers: 42.2 (18.2)%	AAT < 50 mg/dL (nephelometry) AAT < 80 mg/dL (immunodiffusion)	ZZ: 88.9% SZ: 7.1% Other/unknown: 4.0%
Wencker M, et al.; WALT. Chest, 2001 [20]	96	NR	44 (8)	FEV1 < 65% or decline > 120 mL/year	41 (17.3)%	AAT < 35%	ZZ: 85% SZ: 8% Other: 3%
Stoller JK, et al.; NHLBI. Chest, 2003 [22]	747	NR	48 (9)	NR	37 (18)%	AAT ≤ 11 µM or ZZ or null	NR
Tonelli AR, et al. Int J COPD, 2009 [23]	164	NR	61.3 (0.7)	NR	43 (2)%	ZZ	ZZ
Barros-Tizón JC, et al. Ther Adv Respir Dis, 2012 [24]	127	>18 years	51.7 (9.1)	NR	1.25 (0.50) L	AAT ≤ 11 µM (50 mg/dL) and ZZ, rare or null	ZZ: 93.6% SZ: 0.8% Other: 5.6%
Clinical trials							
Dirksen A, et al.; Danish–Dutch study. AJRCCM, 1999 [3]	56	NR	Danish: 50.4 (1.62) Dutch 45.1 (1.17)	FEV1 30–80%	Danish: 1.5 (0.9) L Dutch: 1.6 (0.1) L	ZZ	ZZ
Dirksen A, et al.; EXACTLE. Eur Respir J, 2009 [2]	77	≥18 years	54.7 (8.4)	NR	46.3 (19.6)%	AAT ≤ 11 µM	ZZ or Zn
Chapman KR, et al.; RAPID. Lancet, 2015 [4]	180	18–65	53.8 (6.9)	FEV1 35–70%	47.4 (12.1)%	AAT ≤ 11 µM	ZZ: 93% Other: 7%

* Numerical data expressed as mean (standard deviation). FEV1: forced expiratory volume in 1 s (expressed as absolute values in liters or as percentage of the theoretical value the patient should have according to its age, gender, height, weight, and race). NR, not reported; AAT, alpha1 antitrypsin ; AATD, Alpha1 antitrypsin deficiency; NHLBI, National Health Lung Blood Institute; COPD, chronic obstructive pulmonary disease; WALT, from the German abbreviation: Wissenschaftliche Arbeitsgemeinschaft zur Therapie von Lungenerkrankungen; AJRCCM, American Journal of Respiratory and Critical Care Medicine

4. Controversies over Indication

4.1. Age Limits

The eligibility criteria regarding age are not very explicit in all trials. When available, these are adult studies (>18 years), and the average age is around 45 to 50 years (Table 1). Although there may be extreme values in the distributions, there is little information on very young or very old cases. Although cases in children requiring augmentation therapy have been described anecdotally [28], being young is not normally an issue from a clinical perspective, since by the time emphysema develops, patients are already young adults [29,30]. The issue comes with elderly cases. Currently, there is no information on the impact of AAT augmentation therapy in this cohort. These patients are clearly disease survivors, and the dilemma of initiating a life-long weekly intravenous treatment over the age of 70 or 80 is controversial. In these cases, despite the fact that we could restore AAT anti-elastase activity, achieving the biochemical efficacy, it is not well established how much further the emphysema may progress and what window of opportunity is available to have an impact on long-term lung density deterioration in these elderly patients. Therefore, therapy ought to be individualized and must be agreed with the patient and the caregivers, since many comorbidities and social circumstances may influence this decision. In any case, family screening should be carried out in these cases, to detect severe cases amongst younger relatives. Fortunately, current technologies facilitate these diagnostic procedures in the population [31,32].

4.2. Mutations

AATD is a co-dominant autosomal inherited genetic disease caused by mutations in the SERPINA1 gene on chromosome 14. Mutations are named with a letter from A to Z, according to the migration speed in the isoelectric focusing gel. The normal M allele has an average migration rate. The two most frequent mutated alleles are S and the more severe Z. As shown in Table 1, most studies include ZZ and rare or null allele carriers, with only a minority with SZ or other less frequent mutations. Interestingly, in these trials, the eligibility criteria focused on having a severe AATD (identified by an AAT value below the protective threshold), irrespective of the mutation. Although we can restore the biochemical efficacy of the approved dose for all mutations, the impact on emphysema progression has been shown for those with AAT ≤ 11 µM, which included ZZ, Zn, and other unspecified severe mutations. Accordingly, the drug's technical specifications for augmentation therapy states that the indication is for PiZZ, PiZ (null), Pi (null) (null), and PiSZ. However, in the main study showing a clear impact on lung density, the RAPID trial [4], there were only 12 cases (7%) with severe mutations other than ZZ, which were two SZ, one Z/Null, and nine other non-specified mutations. Unfortunately, these mutations were not evaluated separately and there is no sensitivity analysis evaluating this in the trial. As a result, when aiming at biochemical efficacy, it is reasonable to consider treatment in those with severe deficits (AAT ≤ 11 µM), regardless of the associated mutation. However, the exact impact on the decline of lung densitometry in non-ZZ patients needs to be clarified in the future.

4.3. Lung Function Limits

The evaluation of lung function impairment in chronic obstructive pulmonary disease (COPD) is performed with FEV1. Consequently, the limits of lung function impairment in previous studies was evaluated by this parameter (Table 1). Additionally to the potential relevance of AAT in COPD [33], according to these studies, there were two ways of evaluating FEV1 as the baseline value or as the yearly decline. Although the majority of the cases had an FEV1 below 50%, the included patients presented a wide variability in this spirometric value. Interestingly, the main trial evaluating AAT augmentation therapy on densitometry, the RAPID trial, included patients with FEV1 between 35 and 70% [4]. In fact, the technical specifications for Prolastin include a formal indication of FEV1 limits from 35 to 60%. This has led to the question about whether milder or more severe cases should receive augmentation therapy to impact on emphysema progression. There are two points worth considering about this issue.

First, despite this formal lack of evidence, common sense and clinical experience urge us to indicate or not to stop augmentation therapy below an FEV1 of 35%. The clinical practice guidelines from the Alpha1 Foundation clearly state that intravenous augmentation therapy is recommended for individuals with a predicted FEV1 less than 30%, and, for those with an FEV1 greater than 65%, they recommend discussing with each individual the potential benefits of reducing lung function decline, considering the cost of the therapy and lack of evidence for its benefits [34]. Similarly, the Portuguese guidelines state that augmentation therapy should not be discontinued in case of pulmonary function deterioration, even if it reaches the lowest established limit for its initiation [35].

Second, despite the well-known role of FEV1 in COPD, we know that FEV1 is a poor surrogate measure for emphysema. Notably, gas transfer is reduced much earlier than FEV1 [36,37], and it is therefore a more sensitive marker of disease onset. Additionally, gas transfer keeps worsening in the final stages of the disease, whereas FEV1 decline slows down [38], thus making it also a more sensitive marker of disease deterioration than FEV1 [36]. Finally, during disease progression, gas transfer is a better marker of emphysema progression than FEV1. Altogether, gas transfer may be a more sensitive and specific test of emphysema development than FEV1. However, the indication for augmentation therapy continues to be established according to FEV1 values instead of diffusing capacity. Thus, if emphysema is the goal of treatment rather than biochemical efficacy, it would probably be desirable to use diffusing capacity instead of FEV1 as the basis for indication for therapy and as a monitoring and follow-up parameter. If this is the case, we should consider the FEV1 debate to be over and turn our focus to the functional parameters with a closer relationship to emphysema.

4.4. Indication in Liver Disease

Despite the potential clinical importance of AATD-associated liver failure, the available treatments are still at the very early stages of clinical development. Currently, liver transplantation remains the definitive option for its treatment [39]. However, according to the current records, AATD is a rare cause of liver transplantation [40]. Some treatments are beginning to be evaluated, such as glibenclamide analogs [41], ursodeoxycholic acid homologues [42], or RNA-targeted treatments [43]. In this context, AAT augmentation therapy has not been explored as a potential treatment for AATD-associated liver condition until very recently. Interestingly, a recent collaborative study between Sweden and Germany reported that exogenous AAT lowered SERPINA1 expression in primary human hepatocytes in a dose-dependent manner [44] (Figure 3). Consequently, if the reproducibility and clinical relevance of these findings are confirmed, a possible new indication is opened as a treatment for the prevention of liver involvement that should be prospectively evaluated in trials with patients at risk of developing this complication.

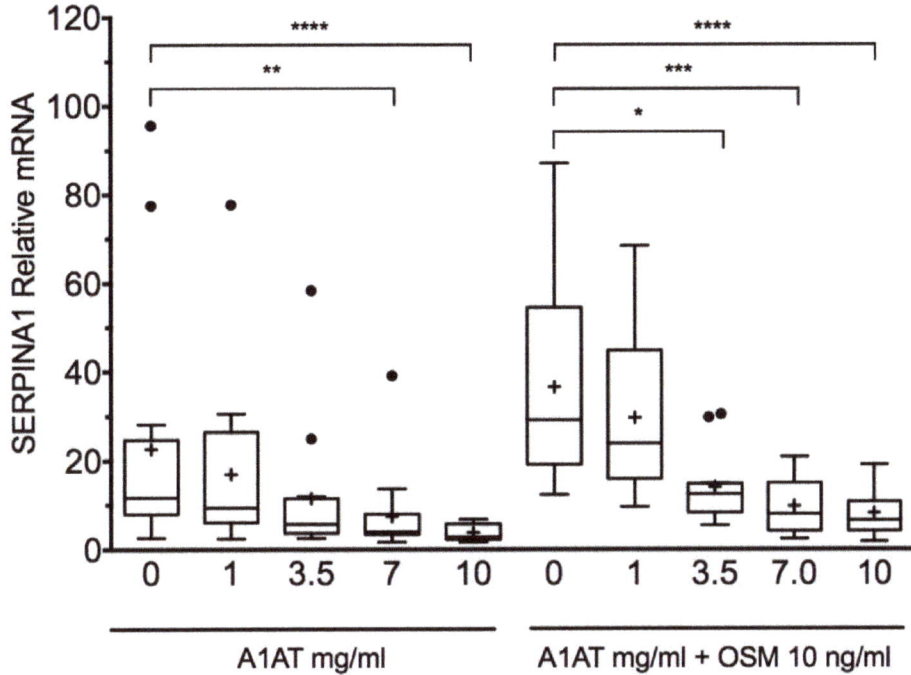

Figure 3. Purified A1AT reduces SERPINA1 expression in a dose-dependent manner in primary human hepatocytes. Exogenously added purified AAT reduced SERPINA1 expression in primary human hepatocytes isolated from both proficient and deficient liver tissue. The reduction was more prominent following Oncostatin M (OSM 10 ng/mL) stimulation, known to increase expression of SERPINA1. *, $P < 0.05$; **, $P < 0.001$; ***, $P < 0.001$; ****, $P < 0.0001$). © 2017 Karadagi, et al. This is an open-access article distributed under the terms of the Creative Commons Attribution License, which permits unrestricted use, distribution, and reproduction in any medium, provided the original author and source are credited. Obtained from Reference [44].

5. Controversies in the Administration

5.1. Infusion Frequency

As discussed above, the weekly frequency of AAT infusions was based on the half-life of this protein and the biochemical efficacy of the first preparations. However, in our search for more comfortable dosages, other alternatives have been tried by doubling, tripling, and even quadrupling the dose and the administration interval to up to 240 mg/kg every four weeks. From the point of view of biochemical efficacy, it seems that administrations every three and every four weeks would be insufficient to keep the trough pre-dose value (C_{min}) above the considered protection threshold (as discussed above) [45]. For this reason, it is recommended to use the usual weekly dose, which, in some cases, can be changed to a biweekly administration with double doses, since this regimen has also been shown to be appropriate [46] and safe [47]. However, if we include in the equation the objective of slowing down the progression of emphysema instead of achieving biochemical efficacy, the scenario changes considerably. Interestingly, the so-called Danish–Dutch study, the first study to evaluate the role of replacement therapy in lung density, used a dose of 250 mg/kg every four weeks, resulting in an improvement in the progression of emphysema [3]. Unfortunately, the study of lung density was an exploratory objective in which the densitometric technique was not standardized. Consequently, it would be desirable to replicate the study with the current lung densitometry methodology. Interestingly, the result of the Danish–Dutch study opens up another question about how it is possible that administration every four weeks does not maintain biochemical efficacy during the four weeks [45] but does have an effect on lung densitometry [3]. This paradox highlights the discrepancy between biochemical and clinical efficacy, which should be explored in future trials. Additionally, it supports the idea mentioned above that the so-called "protective threshold" is a misnomer and should rather be known as "the risk threshold for developing emphysema".

5.2. Correct Dose

As discussed above, the weekly dose of 60 mg/kg was established following the experience of the first researchers, and it has remained to this day, since it ensured biochemical efficacy. However, the RAPID trial identified that lung density decrease rate was related with the median serum AAT concentration, so that the higher the serum concentration, the higher impact on lung density decline prevention. This data also suggested that there was no ceiling effect with the data provided by the RAPID trial [4], implying that achieving higher serum level might have a greater impact on lung density decline. This hypothesis has been recently explored in the SPARK study, which evaluated the safety and pharmacokinetic profile of weekly infusions of a 120 mg/kg dose and showed that this dose is safe and well-tolerated and provides more favorable physiologic AAT serum levels [48]. SPARTA (Study of ProlAstin-C Randomized Therapy with Alpha-1 augmentation), an ongoing randomized, placebo-controlled trial is currently assessing the efficacy and safety of 120 mg/kg administered weekly over three years [11]. The recruitment for this trial is now over, and the results, once available, will have to be evaluated to complete this discussion between the discrepancy between biochemical and clinical efficacy.

5.3. Differences between Preparations

Augmentation therapy with AAT has undergone extensive pharmacological development since the first approval of Prolastin in 1987 (Figure 4). All the preparations can be divided into three types: lyophilized preparations (Prolastin and other country-specific brand names, Trypsone, Alfalastin, and Aralast, originally named Respitin), lyophilized concentrated preparations (Zemaira in the USA—known as Respreeza in Europe—Prolastin C, and Aralast NP), and finally the preparations with a liquid presentation (Prolastin C liquid and Glassia). From a biochemical efficacy perspective, all of these gained approval by comparing their clinical efficacy with either Prolastin, as the first approved presentation, or Prolastin C (pivotal studies showing biochemical efficacy are depicted in Figure 5).

However, if the aim of the treatment is to decrease loss of lung density rather than biochemical efficacy, then only three of these products have been evaluated in clinical trials, namely Alfalastin in the Danish–Dutch study [3], Prolastin in the EXACTLE (EXAcerbations and Computed Tomography scan as Lung End-points) trial [2], and Zemaira/Respreeza in the RAPID trial [4]. Nevertheless, neither the standard methodology of lung densitometry nor the approved explored dose was followed in the Danish–Dutch study. Therefore, it would be of interest to compare the differences between Prolastin and Zemaira/Respreeza in trials.

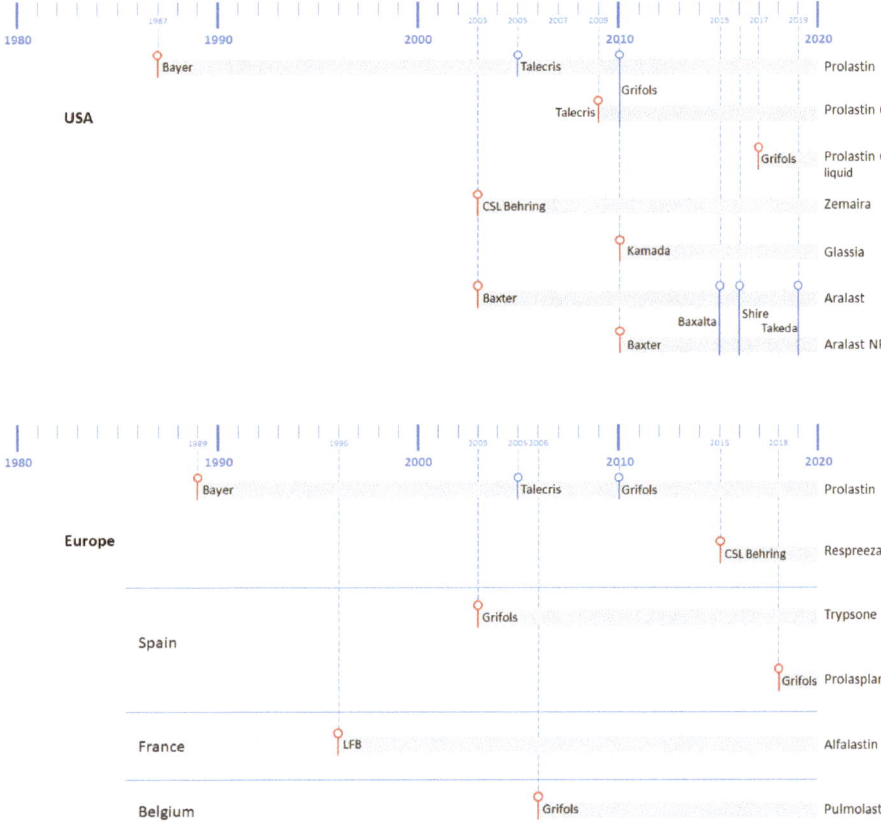

Figure 4. Temporal distribution of the years of approval of augmentative AAT treatments in the USA (upper) and Europe and European countries, with their own presentation (lower). In red: year of initial official approval. In blue: year when company changed. LFB, Laboratoire français du fractionnement et des biotechnologies.

To begin with, there are certain differences between these two presentations [49]. First, it has been reported in biochemical comparisons between both that Zemaira/Respreeza shows a better profile in terms of total protein content, AAT potency, specific AAT activity, and purity [50,51]. Secondly, the concentration of AAT is different in both preparations with Zemaira/Respreeza having a higher concentration (Table 2). Thirdly, the results of the clinical trials are probably not directly comparable due to the different population and study design (Table 2). Therefore, until the possible emergence of new therapeutic options, augmentative treatment with AAT is the only specific treatment for patients with congenital emphysema, and both products have demonstrated their efficacy in slowing the progression of emphysema (Table 2). Accordingly, this treatment should be available for patients who meet internationally established criteria and are controlled and supervised by reference health centers [49]. Unfortunately, we will probably not be able to directly explore these differences further, since future trials are being planned with lyophilized concentrated or liquid preparations.

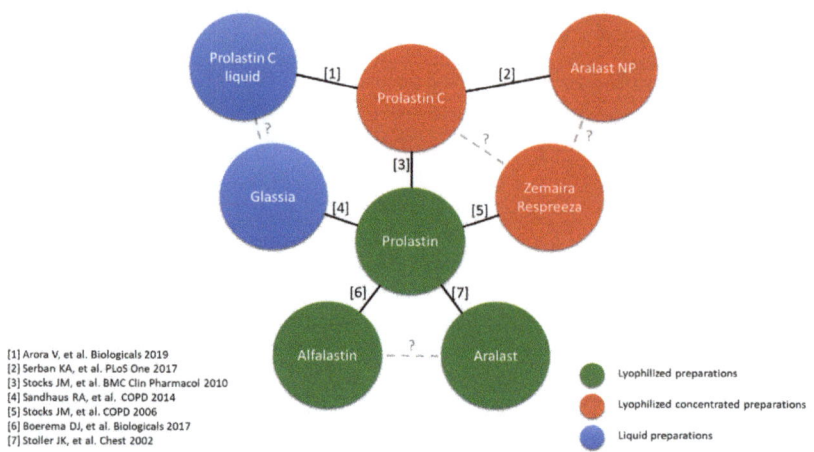

Figure 5. List of studies evaluating biochemical efficacy by type of preparation.

Table 2. Differences between Prolastin and Zemaira/Respreeza.

	Prolastin	Zemaira/Respreeza
Origin *	Human donor plasma	Human donor plasma
Presentations *	1 gr + 40 mL solvent (25 mg/mL)	1 gr + 20 mL solvent (50 mg/mL) 4 gr + 76 mL solvent (50 mg/mL) 5 gr + 95 mL solvent (50 mg/mL)
Excipients *	Powder: Sodium chloride Sodium dihydrogen phosphate Solvent: Water for injections	Powder: Sodium chloride Sodium dihydrogen phosphate monohydrate Mannitol Solvent: Water for injections
Purity (AAT/proteins) [49]	76.9%	97.4%
Specific activity (active AAT/proteins) [49]	64%	86.2%
Infusion velocity *	0.08 mL/kg/min	0.08 mL/kg/min
Time of infusion 60 mg/kg dose †	30 min	15 min
Time of infusion 120 mg/kg dose ‡	60 min	30 min
Lung density decline reduction [4,25]	Versus basal: −1.73 g/L/year Versus placebo: 1.01 g/L/year	Versus basal: −1.45 g/L/year Versus placebo: 0.74 g/L/year

*, Obtained from the technical leaflet; †, At a dose of 60 mg/kg/wk for a 75 kg patient; ‡, At a dose of 120 mg/kg/2 wk for a 75 kg patient.

6. Controversies in the Follow-Up

6.1. Monitoring Control in the First Few Months

Due to the current controversy over dosage therapy and replacement therapy, once indicated, the next question is how to establish the suitable dose. From the perspective of biochemical efficacy, the debate is about the use of C_{min} during the initial administration as a way of identifying which patients can receive biweekly infusions. Here, some authors warn against systematic measurements of C_{min} [52], whereas others suggest there is scope for an individualized dosage regimen for AAT augmentation therapy [53]. Interestingly, if we are aiming for individualized biochemical efficacy, it follows that measuring C_{min} during the first infusions is the only way to identify how patients respond to other regimens than weekly administrations. Once established, there is no further need to evaluate it. However, if we are aiming to achieve clinical efficacy in terms of preventing lung density decline progression, we will have to admit that further information is needed. We have the results of the Danish–Dutch study, which quadrupled the dose and the administration interval and showed a significant impact on the outcome (with the limitations mentioned above) [3], despite biochemical efficacy not being guaranteed [45]. Additionally, the really interesting measure would be the evaluation of the progression of emphysema by lung densitometry. Unfortunately, the methodology used in the RAPID trial for lung density evaluation is not available for clinical practice. Alternatively, other forms of evaluation emphysema progression should be evaluated in the future to identify lung function or radiological parameters that allow us to identify the correct dose for emphysema progression prevention in the follow-up.

6.2. Discontinuation of Augmentation Therapy

The impact of discontinuation of augmentative treatment has not been a major topic of debate in recent years until the recent publication of two letters. McElvaney, et al. [54] recently reported on the consequences of abrupt cessation of AAT replacement therapy, showing an increase in the frequency of exacerbations over a 77-day period, with two deaths due to exacerbation (Figure 6), accompanied by increased circulating levels of inflammatory biomarkers. Recently, another study [55] described post-transplant complications leading to reduced survival only in patients who had discontinued replacement therapy a few weeks before transplant. Interestingly, the effect seemed to have faded by 11 months, suggesting a possible role of the timing of the withdrawal of replacement therapy. These authors [55] hypothesized about a transient inflammatory rebound phenomenon short after withdrawal of therapy. Interestingly, the study by McElvaney, et al. [54] describes this increase in the inflammatory load during the weeks after withdrawal, which seems to peak at three months (Figure 6). The progression of the inflammatory markers and the clinical consequences beyond that point should be explored, to define the window of risk, since two behaviors could potentially be seen thereafter (Figure 6). As a result, these two letters have opened up new questions about the repercussion of abrupt cessation of augmentation therapy that should be further explored. Very recently the role of AAT as a modulator of the neutrophil membrane has been described, providing new data on the role of neutrophil-associated AATD disease [56].

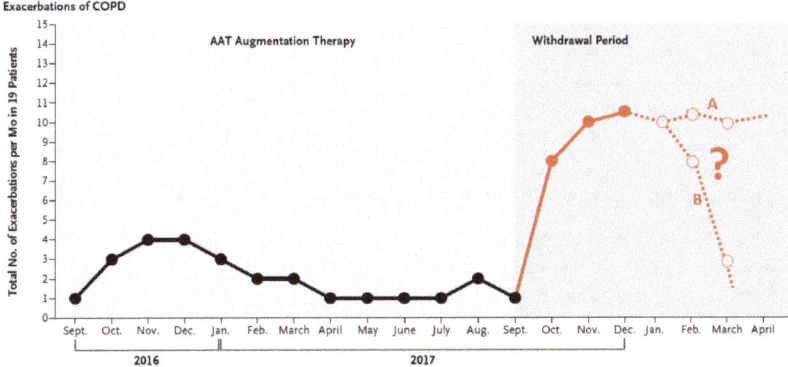

Figure 6. Total number of pulmonary exacerbations per month in the 19 patients in Ireland receiving AAT augmentation therapy for AAT deficiency–associated emphysema during the year before the study (black line) and during the withdrawal period (red line), as reported in the original article. Reproduced with permission from Reference [54]. On the right, we have added (dashed line) two possible hypothetical changes that the curve could have had if the patients had been followed longer, with two possibilities: curve A, with a persistent increase of exacerbations risk, and curve B, with a transient increase in the exacerbation risk. COPD, chronic obstructive pulmonary disease.

6.3. Pulmonary Transplantation

The relationship between augmentation therapy and lung transplantation has sparked another major controversy. Beyond the debate on the survival benefits of lung transplantation in AATD [57–59], the issue at hand now is the role of augmentation therapy in the peritransplantation. At this point, the debate is largely mediated by the decision over whether to continue replacement therapy after transplantation, with two conflicting opinions with their own arguments (Table 3). On the one hand, augmentation therapy has been shown to have several potential benefits. First, intravenous AAT inhibits elastase mediated injury to the transplanted lung in humans [60]. Second, animal models have shown that the administration of human AAT before reperfusion in recipients improved immediate post-transplant lung function [61]. Third, AAT attenuates acute lung allograft injury [62]. On the other hand, as expected, augmentation therapy retains its biochemical efficacy in the recipient, although we do not know about the potential preventive effect of augmentation therapy on newly developed emphysema in the transplanted lung. With the available information, this decision is especially relevant, in the light of the study by Kleinerova, et al. [55] mentioned above, in which the authors suggested that discontinuation of augmentation therapy should be undertaken several months before lung transplantation, to avoid an increased risk of complications. Therefore, either augmentation therapy is stopped just at inclusion in the lung-transplant waiting list or is maintained non-stop during the complete process. Trials are needed to clarify this confusing situation.

Table 3. Arguments for and against maintaining augmentation therapy after lung transplant.

In Favor	Against
The biochemical efficacy is expected to be the same as in non-transplanted AATD patients.	There are no formal trials on its clinical efficacy in lung density deterioration after transplant.
Augmentation therapy is safe and well-tolerated, and patients get used to it as part of their lives. It is not expected to create an additional burden.	Lung transplant patients already have to cope with a considerable amount of medication with potential adverse effects that determine their lives, without adding another treatment of unproven efficacy in this context.
AATD lung-transplant patients are generally younger, with a longer life expectancy, so it is vital to take all the necessary measures to protect the transplanted lung.	Emphysema due to AATD is a slow, progressive disease. It may take decades until clinically relevant emphysema is developed in the new lung.
The number of lung donors is limited, so every transplant has an opportunity cost, since it could have been received by another patient. Therefore, it is unethical not to take all possible steps to preserve the transplanted lung.	It has not been proven that the risk of rejection is increased if recipients do not receive augmentation therapy.

7. The Future: A Second Change of Paradigm Coming

Despite the fact that the diagnostic approach to AATD currently varies between different health institutions and countries [63], diagnosis currently begins with the determination of AAT levels in blood as the main form of screening for the disease. Although this approach is probably the most suitable at the moment, it leaves us with some unknowns. It has been reported a variable disease penetrance of AATD, with different patients with the same mutations suffering different degrees of disease burden. Of note, AAT levels do not clarify why some patients develop severe lung disease, while others do not carry the same mutation [64,65]. In this context, the potential role of evaluating anti-elastase activity could be of help. Anti-elastase activity is one of the main markers in the importance of a specific mutation [66]. Beyond serum AAT levels, anti-elastase activity is also influenced by external and environmental factors like alcohol intake [67] or active smoking [68], as well as by inorganic compounds [69] and inflammatory processes [70]. In human-immunodeficiency virus patients, AAT levels increased in bronchoalveolar lavage fluid and blood. However, anti-elastase activity decreased in bronchoalveolar lavage from human-immunodeficiency virus patients, suggesting impaired AAT function [71]. Accordingly, it has been described that there is a disagreement between protein concentration in peripheral blood with anti-elastase activity [72]. Finally, to complicate things further, a mutation has been described which is secreted at normal levels in cellular models of AATD but with a severe reduction in anti-elastase activity, therefore identifying the first pure functionally deficient AATD mutation [73].

Consequently, we may need to address the debate about the adequacy of basing AATD screening exclusively on the peripheral blood concentration of AAT or if it is possible to determine anti-elastase activity as a complementary marker of lung involvement in AATD [74,75]. Beyond making general recommendations for a healthy lifestyle, which is also necessary, anti-elastase activity should probably be measured to provide a clearer idea of the potential penetration of the disease and enable us to give more thorough patient-based diagnosis and information on the presence and importance of the disease in specific cases in order to evaluate its impact on the long-term deterioration of lung density. Here, multinational clinical research collaboration initiatives [76] will pave the way for acquiring more thorough knowledge on AATD that will result in a more personalized approach for these patients.

Author Contributions: Conceptualization, J.L.L.-C., L.C.H. and C.C.E.; writing—original draft preparation, J.L.L.-C.; writing—review and editing, L.C.H. and C.C.E. All authors have read and agreed to the published version of the manuscript.

Funding: This research received no external funding.

Acknowledgments: The authors are grateful to Simon Armour from Academia Británica for his assistance in the improving the English of the original version.

Conflicts of Interest: J.L.L.-C. has received honoraria during the last three years, for lecturing, scientific advice, participation in clinical studies, or writing for the following publications (in alphabetical order): AstraZeneca, Boehringer Ingelheim, Chiesi, CSL Behring, Esteve, Ferrer, Gebro, GlaxoSmithKline, Grifols, Menarini, Novartis, Rovi, and Teva. The other authors declare no conflicts of interest.

References

1. Strnad, P.; McElvaney, N.G.; Lomas, D.A. Alpha1-Antitrypsin Deficiency. *N. Engl. J. Med.* **2020**, *382*, 1443–1455. [CrossRef] [PubMed]
2. Dirksen, A.; Piitulainen, E.; Parr, D.G.; Deng, C.; Wencker, M.; Shaker, S.B.; Stockley, R.A. Exploring the role of CT densitometry: A randomised study of augmentation therapy in alpha1-antitrypsin deficiency. *Eur. Respir. J. Off. J. Eur. Soc. Clin. Respir. Physiol.* **2009**, *33*, 1345–1353. [CrossRef] [PubMed]
3. Dirksen, A.; Dijkman, J.H.; Madsen, F.; Stoel, B.; Hutchison, D.C.; Ulrik, C.S.; Skovgaard, L.T.; Kok-Jensen, A.; Rudolphus, A.; Seersholm, N.; et al. A randomized clinical trial of alpha(1)-antitrypsin augmentation therapy. *Am. J. Respir. Crit. Care Med.* **1999**, *160*, 1468–1472. [CrossRef] [PubMed]
4. Chapman, K.R.; Burdon, J.G.; Piitulainen, E.; Sandhaus, R.A.; Seersholm, N.; Stocks, J.M.; Stoel, B.C.; Huang, L.; Yao, Z.; Edelman, J.M.; et al. Intravenous augmentation treatment and lung density in severe alpha1 antitrypsin deficiency (RAPID): A randomised, double-blind, placebo-controlled trial. *Lancet* **2015**, *386*, 360–368. [CrossRef]
5. McElvaney, N.G. Alpha-1 Antitrypsin Therapy in Cystic Fibrosis and the Lung Disease Associated with Alpha-1 Antitrypsin Deficiency. *Ann. Am. Thorac. Soc.* **2016**, *13* (Suppl. S2), S191–S196. [CrossRef]
6. Gadek, J.E.; Klein, H.G.; Holland, P.V.; Crystal, R.G. Replacement therapy of alpha 1-antitrypsin deficiency. Reversal of protease-antiprotease imbalance within the alveolar structures of PiZ subjects. *J. Clin. Investig.* **1981**, *68*, 1158–1165. [CrossRef] [PubMed]
7. Gadek, J.E.; Crystal, R.G. Experience with replacement therapy in the destructive lung disease associated with severe alpha-1-antitrypsin deficiency. *Am. Rev. Respir. Dis.* **1983**, *127*, S45–S46. [CrossRef]
8. Wewers, M.D.; Casolaro, M.A.; Sellers, S.E.; Swayze, S.C.; McPhaul, K.M.; Wittes, J.T.; Crystal, R.G. Replacement therapy for alpha 1-antitrypsin deficiency associated with emphysema. *N. Engl. J. Med.* **1987**, *316*, 1055–1062. [CrossRef]
9. Hubbard, R.C.; Sellers, S.; Czerski, D.; Stephens, L.; Crystal, R.G. Biochemical efficacy and safety of monthly augmentation therapy for alpha 1-antitrypsin deficiency. *JAMA J. Am. Med. Assoc.* **1988**, *260*, 1259–1264. [CrossRef]

10. American Thoracic, S.; European Respiratory, S. American Thoracic Society/European Respiratory Society statement: Standards for the diagnosis and management of individuals with alpha-1 antitrypsin deficiency. *Am. J. Respir. Crit. Care Med.* **2003**, *168*, 818–900. [CrossRef]
11. Sorrells, S.; Camprubi, S.; Griffin, R.; Chen, J.; Ayguasanosa, J. SPARTA clinical trial design: Exploring the efficacy and safety of two dose regimens of alpha1-proteinase inhibitor augmentation therapy in alpha1-antitrypsin deficiency. *Respir. Med.* **2015**, *109*, 490–499. [CrossRef] [PubMed]
12. Jones, E.A.; Vergalla, J.; Steer, C.J.; Bradley-Moore, P.R.; Vierling, J.M. Metabolism of intact and desialylated alpha 1-antitrypsin. *Clin. Sci. Mol. Med.* **1978**, *55*, 139–148. [CrossRef] [PubMed]
13. Stolk, J.; Tov, N.; Chapman, K.R.; Fernandez, P.; MacNee, W.; Hopkinson, N.S.; Piitulainen, E.; Seersholm, N.; Vogelmeier, C.F.; Bals, R.; et al. Efficacy and safety of inhaled α1-antitrypsin in patients with severe α1-antitrypsin deficiency and frequent exacerbations of COPD. *Eur. Respir. J. Off. J. Eur. Soc. Clin. Respir. Physiol.* **2019**, *54*. [CrossRef] [PubMed]
14. Straus, S.D.; Fells, G.A.; Wewers, M.D.; Courtney, M.; Tessier, L.H.; Tolstoshev, P.; Lecocq, J.P.; Crystal, R.G. Evaluation of recombinant DNA-directed E. coli produced alpha 1-antitrypsin as an anti-neutrophil elastase for potential use as replacement therapy of alpha 1-antitrypsin deficiency. *Biochem. Biophys. Res. Commun.* **1985**, *130*, 1177–1184. [CrossRef]
15. Flotte, T.R.; Trapnell, B.C.; Humphries, M.; Carey, B.; Calcedo, R.; Rouhani, F.; Campbell-Thompson, M.; Yachnis, A.T.; Sandhaus, R.A.; McElvaney, N.G.; et al. Phase 2 clinical trial of a recombinant adeno-associated viral vector expressing alpha1-antitrypsin: Interim results. *Hum. Gene Ther.* **2011**, *22*, 1239–1247. [CrossRef]
16. Amann, T.; Hansen, A.H.; Kol, S.; Hansen, H.G.; Arnsdorf, J.; Nallapareddy, S.; Voldborg, B.; Lee, G.M.; Andersen, M.R.; Kildegaard, H.F. Glyco-engineered CHO cell lines producing alpha-1-antitrypsin and C1 esterase inhibitor with fully humanized N-glycosylation profiles. *Metab. Eng.* **2019**, *52*, 143–152. [CrossRef]
17. Morifuji, Y.; Xu, J.; Karasaki, N.; Iiyama, K.; Morokuma, D.; Hino, M.; Masuda, A.; Yano, T.; Mon, H.; Kusakabe, T.; et al. Expression, Purification, and Characterization of Recombinant Human alpha1-Antitrypsin Produced Using Silkworm-Baculovirus Expression System. *Mol. Biotechnol.* **2018**, *60*, 924–934. [CrossRef]
18. Seersholm, N.; Wencker, M.; Banik, N.; Viskum, K.; Dirksen, A.; Kok-Jensen, A.; Konietzko, N. Does alpha1-antitrypsin augmentation therapy slow the annual decline in FEV1 in patients with severe hereditary alpha1-antitrypsin deficiency? Wissenschaftliche Arbeitsgemeinschaft zur Therapie von Lungenerkrankungen (WATL) alpha1-AT study group. *Eur. Respir. J. Off. J. Eur. Soc. Clin. Respir. Physiol.* **1997**, *10*, 2260–2263. [CrossRef]
19. Wencker, M.; Banik, N.; Buhl, R.; Seidel, R.; Konietzko, N. Long-term treatment of alpha1-antitrypsin deficiency-related pulmonary emphysema with human alpha1-antitrypsin. Wissenschaftliche Arbeitsgemeinschaft zur Therapie von Lungenerkrankungen (WATL)-alpha1-AT-study group. *Eur. Respir. J. Off. J. Eur. Soc. Clin. Respir. Physiol.* **1998**, *11*, 428–433. [CrossRef]
20. Wencker, M.; Fuhrmann, B.; Banik, N.; Konietzko, N. Longitudinal follow-up of patients with alpha(1)-protease inhibitor deficiency before and during therapy with IV alpha(1)-protease inhibitor. *Chest* **2001**, *119*, 737–744. [CrossRef]
21. The Alpha-1-Antitrypsin Deficiency Registry Study Group. Survival and FEV1 decline in individuals with severe deficiency of alpha1-antitrypsin. *Am. J. Respir. Crit. Care Med.* **1998**, *158*, 49–59. [CrossRef]
22. Stoller, J.K.; Fallat, R.; Schluchter, M.D.; O'Brien, R.G.; Connor, J.T.; Gross, N.; O'Neil, K.; Sandhaus, R.; Crystal, R.G. Augmentation therapy with alpha1-antitrypsin: Patterns of use and adverse events. *Chest* **2003**, *123*, 1425–1434. [CrossRef] [PubMed]
23. Tonelli, A.R.; Rouhani, F.; Li, N.; Schreck, P.; Brantly, M.L. Alpha-1-antitrypsin augmentation therapy in deficient individuals enrolled in the Alpha-1 Foundation DNA and Tissue Bank. *Int. J. Chronic Obstr. Pulm. Dis.* **2009**, *4*, 443–452. [CrossRef] [PubMed]
24. Barros-Tizon, J.C.; Torres, M.L.; Blanco, I.; Martinez, M.T.; Investigators of the rEXA Study Group. Reduction of severe exacerbations and hospitalization-derived costs in alpha-1-antitrypsin-deficient patients treated with alpha-1-antitrypsin augmentation therapy. *Ther. Adv. Respir. Dis.* **2012**, *6*, 67–78. [CrossRef]
25. Stockley, R.A.; Parr, D.G.; Piitulainen, E.; Stolk, J.; Stoel, B.C.; Dirksen, A. Therapeutic efficacy of alpha-1 antitrypsin augmentation therapy on the loss of lung tissue: An integrated analysis of 2 randomised clinical trials using computed tomography densitometry. *Respir. Res.* **2010**, *11*, 136. [CrossRef]

26. McElvaney, N.G.; Burdon, J.; Holmes, M.; Glanville, A.; Wark, P.A.; Thompson, P.J.; Hernandez, P.; Chlumsky, J.; Teschler, H.; Ficker, J.H.; et al. Long-term efficacy and safety of alpha1 proteinase inhibitor treatment for emphysema caused by severe alpha1 antitrypsin deficiency: An open-label extension trial (RAPID-OLE). *Lancet Respir. Med.* **2017**, *5*, 51–60. [CrossRef]
27. Chapman, K.R.; Chorostowska-Wynimko, J.; Koczulla, A.R.; Ferrarotti, I.; McElvaney, N.G. Alpha 1 antitrypsin to treat lung disease in alpha 1 antitrypsin deficiency: Recent developments and clinical implications. *Int. J. Chronic Obstr. Pulm. Dis.* **2018**, *13*, 419–432. [CrossRef]
28. Esteves Brandão, M.; Conde, B.; Seixas, S.; Clotilde Silva, J.; Fernandes, A. Pulmonary Emphysema in a Child With Alpha-1 Antitrypsin Deficiency: Evaluation of 2 Years of Intravenous Augmentation Therapy. *Arch. Bronconeumol.* **2019**, *55*, 502–504. [CrossRef]
29. Menga, G.; Fernandez Acquier, M.; Echazarreta, A.L.; Sorroche, P.B.; Lorenzon, M.V.; Fernandez, M.E.; Saez, M.S.; grupo de estudio, D.A. Prevalence of Alpha-1 Antitrypsin Deficiency in COPD Patients in Argentina. The DAAT.AR Study. *Arch. Bronconeumol.* **2019**. [CrossRef]
30. Janciauskiene, S.; DeLuca, D.S.; Barrecheguren, M.; Welte, T.; Miravitlles, M.; Ancochea, J.; Badiola, C.; Sánchez, G.; Duran, E.; Río, F.G.; et al. Serum Levels of Alpha1-antitrypsin and Their Relationship with COPD in the General Spanish Population. *Arch. Bronconeumol.* **2020**, *56*, 76–83. [CrossRef]
31. Lopez-Campos, J.L.; Casas-Maldonado, F.; Torres-Duran, M.; Medina-Gonzálvez, A.; Rodriguez-Fidalgo, M.L.; Carrascosa, I.; Calle, M.; Osaba, L.; Rapun, N.; Drobnic, E.; et al. Results of a diagnostic procedure based on multiplex technology on dried blood spots and buccal swabs for subjects with suspected alpha1 antitrypsin deficiency. *Arch. Bronconeumol.* **2020**, in press. [CrossRef] [PubMed]
32. Lopez-Campos, J.L.; Carrasco Hernandez, L.; Marquez-Martin, E.; Ortega Ruiz, F.; Martinez Delgado, B. Diagnostic Performance of a Lateral Flow Assay for the Detection of Alpha-1-Antitrypsin Deficiency. *Arch. Bronconeumol.* **2020**, *56*, 124–126. [CrossRef] [PubMed]
33. Ellis, P.; Turner, A. What Do Alpha-1 Antitrypsin Levels Tell Us About Chronic Inflammation in COPD? *Arch. Bronconeumol.* **2020**, *56*, 72–73. [CrossRef] [PubMed]
34. Sandhaus, R.A.; Turino, G.; Brantly, M.L.; Campos, M.; Cross, C.E.; Goodman, K.; Hogarth, D.K.; Knight, S.L.; Stocks, J.M.; Stoller, J.K.; et al. The Diagnosis and Management of Alpha-1 Antitrypsin Deficiency in the Adult. *Chronic Obstr. Pulm. Dis.* **2016**, *3*, 668–682. [CrossRef] [PubMed]
35. Lopes, A.P.; Mineiro, M.A.; Costa, F.; Gomes, J.; Santos, C.; Antunes, C.; Maia, D.; Melo, R.; Canotilho, M.; Magalhaes, E.; et al. Portuguese consensus document for the management of alpha-1-antitrypsin deficiency. *Pulmonology* **2018**, *24* (Suppl. S1), 1–21. [CrossRef]
36. Piitulainen, E.; Montero, L.C.; Nystedt-Duzakin, M.; Stoel, B.C.; Sveger, T.; Wollmer, P.; Tanash, H.A.; Diaz, S. Lung Function and CT Densitometry in Subjects with alpha-1-Antitrypsin Deficiency and Healthy Controls at 35 Years of Age. *COPD* **2015**, *12*, 162–167. [CrossRef]
37. Stockley, R.A.; Edgar, R.G.; Pillai, A.; Turner, A.M. Individualized lung function trends in alpha-1-antitrypsin deficiency: A need for patience in order to provide patient centered management? *Int. J. Chronic Obstr. Pulm. Dis.* **2016**, *11*, 1745–1756. [CrossRef]
38. Dawkins, P.A.; Dawkins, C.L.; Wood, A.M.; Nightingale, P.G.; Stockley, J.A.; Stockley, R.A. Rate of progression of lung function impairment in alpha1-antitrypsin deficiency. *Eur. Respir. J. Off. J. Eur. Soc. Clin. Respir. Physiol.* **2009**, *33*, 1338–1344. [CrossRef]
39. Clark, V.C. Liver Transplantation in Alpha-1 Antitrypsin Deficiency. *Clin. Liver Dis.* **2017**, *21*, 355–365. [CrossRef]
40. Strange, C.; Stoller, J.K.; Sandhaus, R.A.; Dickson, R.; Turino, G. Results of a survey of patients with alpha-1 antitrypsin deficiency. *Respir. Int. Rev. Thorac. Dis.* **2006**, *73*, 185–190. [CrossRef]
41. Wang, Y.; Cobanoglu, M.C.; Li, J.; Hidvegi, T.; Hale, P.; Ewing, M.; Chu, A.S.; Gong, Z.; Muzumdar, R.; Pak, S.C.; et al. An analog of glibenclamide selectively enhances autophagic degradation of misfolded alpha1-antitrypsin Z. *PLoS ONE* **2019**, *14*, e0209748. [CrossRef]
42. Tang, Y.; Blomenkamp, K.S.; Fickert, P.; Trauner, M.; Teckman, J.H. NorUDCA promotes degradation of alpha1-antitrypsin mutant Z protein by inducing autophagy through AMPK/ULK1 pathway. *PLoS ONE* **2018**, *13*, e0200897. [CrossRef] [PubMed]
43. Wooddell, C.I.; Blomenkamp, K.; Peterson, R.M.; Subbotin, V.M.; Schwabe, C.; Hamilton, J.; Chu, Q.; Christianson, D.R.; Hegge, J.O.; Kolbe, J.; et al. Development of an RNAi therapeutic for alpha-1-antitrypsin liver disease. *JCI Insight* **2020**. [CrossRef]

44. Karadagi, A.; Johansson, H.; Zemack, H.; Salipalli, S.; Mork, L.M.; Kannisto, K.; Jorns, C.; Gramignoli, R.; Strom, S.; Stokkeland, K.; et al. Exogenous alpha 1-antitrypsin down-regulates SERPINA1 expression. *PLoS ONE* **2017**, *12*, e0177279. [CrossRef] [PubMed]
45. Soy, D.; de la Roza, C.; Lara, B.; Esquinas, C.; Torres, A.; Miravitlles, M. Alpha-1-antitrypsin deficiency: Optimal therapeutic regimen based on population pharmacokinetics. *Thorax* **2006**, *61*, 1059–1064. [CrossRef]
46. Vidal Pla, R.; Padullés Zamora, N.; Sala Piñol, F.; Jardí Margaleff, R.; Rodríguez Frías, F.; Montoro Ronsano, J.B. Pharmacokinetics of alpha1-antitrypsin replacement therapy in severe congenital emphysema. *Arch. Bronconeumol.* **2006**, *42*, 553–556. [CrossRef]
47. Greulich, T.; Chlumsky, J.; Wencker, M.; Vit, O.; Fries, M.; Chung, T.; Shebl, A.; Vogelmeier, C.; Chapman, K.R.; McElvaney, N.G.; et al. Safety of biweekly alpha1-antitrypsin treatment in the RAPID programme. *Eur. Respir. J. Off. J. Eur. Soc. Clin. Respir. Physiol.* **2018**, *52*. [CrossRef]
48. Campos, M.A.; Kueppers, F.; Stocks, J.M.; Strange, C.; Chen, J.; Griffin, R.; Wang-Smith, L.; Brantly, M.L. Safety and pharmacokinetics of 120 mg/kg versus 60 mg/kg weekly intravenous infusions of alpha-1 proteinase inhibitor in alpha-1 antitrypsin deficiency: A multicenter, randomized, double-blind, crossover study (SPARK). *COPD* **2013**, *10*, 687–695. [CrossRef]
49. Esquinas, C.; Miravitlles, M. Are There Differences Between the Available Treatments for Emphysema Associated with Alpha-1 Antitrypsin Deficiency? *Arch. Bronconeumol.* **2018**, *54*, 451–452. [CrossRef]
50. Boerema, D.J.; An, B.; Gandhi, R.P.; Papineau, R.; Regnier, E.; Wilder, A.; Molitor, A.; Tang, A.P.; Kee, S.M. Biochemical comparison of four commercially available human alpha1-proteinase inhibitors for treatment of alpha1-antitrypsin deficiency. *Biologicals* **2017**, *50*, 63–72. [CrossRef]
51. Cowden, D.I.; Fisher, G.E.; Weeks, R.L. A pilot study comparing the purity, functionality and isoform composition of alpha-1-proteinase inhibitor (human) products. *Curr. Med. Res. Opin.* **2005**, *21*, 877–883. [CrossRef] [PubMed]
52. Tirado-Conde, G.; Lara, B.; Miravitlles, M. Augmentation therapy for emphysema due to alpha-1-antitrypsin deficiency. *Ther. Adv. Respir. Dis.* **2008**, *2*, 13–21. [CrossRef] [PubMed]
53. Ellis, P.; Dirksen, A.; Turner, A.M. Treatment of lung disease. In *Alpha1-Antitrypsin Deficiency*; Strnad, P., Brantly, M.L., Bals, R., Eds.; ERS: Lausanne, Switzerland, 2019; pp. 78–92.
54. McElvaney, O.J.; Carroll, T.P.; Franciosi, A.N.; Sweeney, J.; Hobbs, B.D.; Kowlessar, V.; Gunaratnam, C.; Reeves, E.P.; McElvaney, N.G. Consequences of Abrupt Cessation of Alpha1-Antitrypsin Replacement Therapy. *N. Engl. J. Med.* **2020**, *382*, 1478–1480. [CrossRef] [PubMed]
55. Kleinerova, J.; Ging, P.; Rutherford, C.; Lawrie, I.; Winward, S.; Eaton, D.; Redmond, K.C.; Egan, J.J. The withdrawal of replacement therapy and outcomes in alpha-1 antitrypsin deficiency lung transplant recipients. *Eur. Respir. J. Off. J. Eur. Soc. Clin. Respir. Physiol.* **2019**, *53*. [CrossRef]
56. Murphy, M.P.; McEnery, T.; McQuillan, K.; McElvaney, O.F.; McElvaney, O.J.; Landers, S.; Coleman, O.; Bussayajirapong, A.; Hawkins, P.; Henry, M.; et al. alpha1 Antitrypsin therapy modulates the neutrophil membrane proteome and secretome. *Eur. Respir. J. Off. J. Eur. Soc. Clin. Respir. Physiol.* **2020**, *55*. [CrossRef]
57. Tanash, H.A.; Riise, G.C.; Hansson, L.; Nilsson, P.M.; Piitulainen, E. Survival benefit of lung transplantation in individuals with severe alpha1-anti-trypsin deficiency (PiZZ) and emphysema. *J. Heart Lung Transpl.* **2011**, *30*, 1342–1347. [CrossRef]
58. Stone, H.M.; Edgar, R.G.; Thompson, R.D.; Stockley, R.A. Lung Transplantation in Alpha-1-Antitrypsin Deficiency. *COPD* **2016**, *13*, 146–152. [CrossRef]
59. Thabut, G. Estimating the Survival Benefit of Lung Transplantation: Considering the Disease Course during the Wait. *Ann. Am. Thorac. Soc.* **2017**, *14*, 163–164. [CrossRef]
60. King, M.B.; Campbell, E.J.; Gray, B.H.; Hertz, M.I. The proteinase-antiproteinase balance in alpha-1-proteinase inhibitor-deficient lung transplant recipients. *Am. J. Respir. Crit. Care Med.* **1994**, *149*, 966–971. [CrossRef]
61. Iskender, I.; Sakamoto, J.; Nakajima, D.; Lin, H.; Chen, M.; Kim, H.; Guan, Z.; Del Sorbo, L.; Hwang, D.; Waddell, T.K.; et al. Human alpha1-antitrypsin improves early post-transplant lung function: Pre-clinical studies in a pig lung transplant model. *J. Heart Lung Transpl.* **2016**, *35*, 913–921. [CrossRef]
62. Emtiazjoo, A.M.; Hu, H.; Lu, L.; Brantly, M.L. Alpha-1 Antitrypsin Attenuates Acute Lung Allograft Injury in a Rat Lung Transplant Model. *Transpl. Direct* **2019**, *5*, e458. [CrossRef] [PubMed]

63. Miravitlles, M.; Dirksen, A.; Ferrarotti, I.; Koblizek, V.; Lange, P.; Mahadeva, R.; McElvaney, N.G.; Parr, D.; Piitulainen, E.; Roche, N.; et al. European Respiratory Society statement: Diagnosis and treatment of pulmonary disease in alpha1-antitrypsin deficiency. *Eur. Respir. J. Off. J. Eur. Soc. Clin. Respir. Physiol.* **2017**, *50*, 1700610. [CrossRef] [PubMed]
64. Piras, B.; Ferrarotti, I.; Lara, B.; Martinez, M.T.; Bustamante, A.; Ottaviani, S.; Pirina, P.; Luisetti, M.; Miravitlles, M. Clinical phenotypes of Italian and Spanish patients with alpha1-antitrypsin deficiency. *Eur. Respir. J. Off. J. Eur. Soc. Clin. Respir. Physiol.* **2013**, *42*, 54–64. [CrossRef]
65. Matamala, N.; Lara, B.; Gómez-Mariano, G.; Martínez, S.; Vázquez-Domízquez, I.; Otero-Sobrino, Á.; Muñoz-Callejas, A.; Sánchez, E.; Esquinas, C.; Bustamante, A.; et al. miR-320c Regulates SERPINA1 Expression and Is Induced in Patients With Pulmonary Disease. *Arch. Bronconeumol.* **2020**. [CrossRef]
66. Matamala, N.; Lara, B.; Gomez-Mariano, G.; Martinez, S.; Retana, D.; Fernandez, T.; Silvestre, R.A.; Belmonte, I.; Rodriguez-Frias, F.; Vilar, M.; et al. Characterization of Novel Missense Variants of SERPINA1 Gene Causing Alpha-1 Antitrypsin Deficiency. *Am. J. Respir. Cell Mol. Biol.* **2018**, *58*, 706–716. [CrossRef] [PubMed]
67. Brecher, A.S.; Thevananther, S.; Franco-Saenz, R. Acetaldehyde inhibits the anti-elastase activity of alpha 1-antitrypsin. *Alcohol* **1994**, *11*, 181–185. [CrossRef]
68. Gadek, J.E.; Fells, G.A.; Crystal, R.G. Cigarette smoking induces functional antiprotease deficiency in the lower respiratory tract of humans. *Science* **1979**, *206*, 1315–1316. [CrossRef]
69. Cohen, M.D.; Sisco, M.; Baker, K.; Chen, L.C.; Schlesinger, R.B. Rapid communication: Effect of inhaled chromium on pulmonary A1AT. *Inhal. Toxicol.* **2002**, *14*, 765–771. [CrossRef]
70. Carter, R.I.; Mumford, R.A.; Treonze, K.M.; Finke, P.E.; Davies, P.; Si, Q.; Humes, J.L.; Dirksen, A.; Piitulainen, E.; Ahmad, A.; et al. The fibrinogen cleavage product Aα-Val360, a specific marker of neutrophil elastase activity in vivo. *Thorax* **2011**, *66*, 686–691. [CrossRef]
71. Stephenson, S.E.; Wilson, C.L.; Crothers, K.; Attia, E.F.; Wongtrakool, C.; Petrache, I.; Schnapp, L.M. Impact of HIV infection on α(1)-antitrypsin in the lung. *Am. J. Physiol. Lung Cell. Mol. Physiol.* **2018**, *314*, L583–L592. [CrossRef]
72. Cook, L.; Burdon, J.; Brenton, S.; Janus, E.D.; Knight, K. Alpha-1-antitrypsin PLowell: A normally functioning variant present in low concentration. *Aust. New Zealand J. Med.* **1995**, *25*, 695–697. [CrossRef] [PubMed]
73. Laffranchi, M.; Elliston, E.L.K.; Gangemi, F.; Berardelli, R.; Lomas, D.A.; Irving, J.A.; Fra, A. Characterisation of a type II functionally-deficient variant of alpha-1-antitrypsin discovered in the general population. *PLoS ONE* **2019**, *14*, e0206955. [CrossRef]
74. Fujita, J.; Nelson, N.L.; Daughton, D.M.; Dobry, C.A.; Spurzem, J.R.; Irino, S.; Rennard, S.I. Evaluation of elastase and antielastase balance in patients with chronic bronchitis and pulmonary emphysema. *Am. Rev. Respir. Dis.* **1990**, *142*, 57–62. [CrossRef] [PubMed]
75. Abboud, R.T.; Vimalanathan, S. Pathogenesis of COPD. Part I. The role of protease-antiprotease imbalance in emphysema. *Int. J. Tuberc. Lung Dis. Off. J. Int. Union Tuberc. Lung Dis.* **2008**, *12*, 361–367.
76. Barrecheguren, M.; Torres-Duran, M.; Casas-Maldonado, F.; Miravitlles, M. Spanish Implementation of the New International Alpha-1 Anitrypsin Deficiency International Registry: The European Alpha-1 Research Collaboration (EARCO). *Arch. Bronconeumol.* **2020**. [CrossRef]

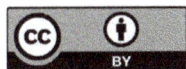

© 2020 by the authors. Licensee MDPI, Basel, Switzerland. This article is an open access article distributed under the terms and conditions of the Creative Commons Attribution (CC BY) license (http://creativecommons.org/licenses/by/4.0/).

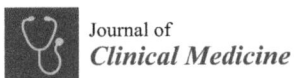
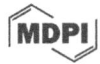

Review

Gene Therapy in Rare Respiratory Diseases: What Have We Learned So Far?

Lucía Bañuls [1,2,†], Daniel Pellicer [1,2,†], Silvia Castillo [2,3], María Mercedes Navarro-García [2], María Magallón [1,2], Cruz González [2,4] and Francisco Dasí [1,2,*]

[1] Research group on Rare Respiratory Diseases (ERR), Department of Physiology, School of Medicine, University of Valencia, Avda. Blasco Ibáñez, 15, 46010 Valencia, Spain; lucia.banyuls.soto@gmail.com (L.B.); dpellicerroig@gmail.com (D.P.); mariamagallon94@gmail.com (M.M.)
[2] Research group on Rare Respiratory Diseases (ERR), Instituto de Investigación Sanitaria INCLIVA, Fundación Investigación Hospital Clínico Valencia, Avda. Menéndez y Pelayo, 4, 46010 Valencia, Spain; sccorullon@gmail.com (S.C.); mer_navarro2002@yahoo.es (M.M.N.-G.); cruz.gonzalez@uv.es (C.G.)
[3] Paediatrics Unit, Hospital Clínico Universitario de Valencia, Avda. Blasco Ibáñez, 17, 46010 Valencia, Spain
[4] Pneumology Unit, Hospital Clínico Universitario de Valencia, Avda. Blasco Ibáñez, 17, 46010 Valencia, Spain
* Correspondence: Francisco.Dasi@uv.es; Tel.: +34-676515598
† These two authors contributed equally to this work.

Received: 3 July 2020; Accepted: 5 August 2020; Published: 8 August 2020

Abstract: Gene therapy is an alternative therapy in many respiratory diseases with genetic origin and currently without curative treatment. After five decades of progress, many different vectors and gene editing tools for genetic engineering are now available. However, we are still a long way from achieving a safe and efficient approach to gene therapy application in clinical practice. Here, we review three of the most common rare respiratory conditions—cystic fibrosis (CF), alpha-1 antitrypsin deficiency (AATD), and primary ciliary dyskinesia (PCD)—alongside attempts to develop genetic treatment for these diseases. Since the 1990s, gene augmentation therapy has been applied in multiple clinical trials targeting CF and AATD, especially using adeno-associated viral vectors, resulting in a good safety profile but with low efficacy in protein expression. Other strategies, such as non-viral vectors and more recently gene editing tools, have also been used to address these diseases in pre-clinical studies. The first gene therapy approach in PCD was in 2009 when a lentiviral transduction was performed to restore gene expression in vitro; since then, transcription activator-like effector nucleases (TALEN) technology has also been applied in primary cell culture. Gene therapy is an encouraging alternative treatment for these respiratory diseases; however, more research is needed to ensure treatment safety and efficacy.

Keywords: gene therapy; rare respiratory diseases; alpha-1-antitrypsin deficit; cystic fibrosis; primary ciliary dyskinesia

1. Introduction

1.1. Why Gene Therapy?

Since the discovery of the way DNA transmits information from parents to progeny, medical research has focused on finding a way to reverse malfunctions to improve the quality of life in people suffering genetic-related conditions. Advances in the understanding of gene interactions and their physiological consequences have put gene therapy in the spotlight as the key for creating personalized medicine.

Gene therapy can be described as a disease treatment that introduces exogenous genetic material such as plasmid DNA, antisense oligonucleotides, mRNA or peptide nucleic acids into cells or tissues with the aim of treating hereditary or acquired genetic disorders. In essence, it is the use of nucleic acids as a drug to obtain therapeutic benefits for the patient [1].

1.2. A Brief History of Gene Therapy

When Theodore Friedmann introduced the idea that gene therapy could treat monogenic diseases in 1972 [2], the novel gene therapists started facing the barriers that the body has to protect us from foreign DNA. We are currently on the race to treatments that promise a one-dose administration and a stable expression of a protein of interest. Thus, through the last 50 years, gene therapy development has been facing countless challenges and feeding back on itself until it has reached the first glimpses of clinical uses. At the beginning of the 1990s, clinical assays using viral vectors started with high optimism, but a series of catastrophic events ended up with the death of the first volunteer during gene therapy clinical trials, Jesse Gelsinger [3]. That particular event reached far beyond the scientific community and severely damaged the already controversial studies on human research. Lack of support from the institutions during the beginning of the millennia revived the debate on the concerns of gene editing. Thus, in order to improve the safety of the possible treatments, basic science continued studying the mechanisms of the viral vectors used and developed synthetic particles that could mimic the process of delivering genetic material without the risk of letting a virus get out of control. The deeper knowledge on the metabolic routes allowed more and more clinical trials, and after exhaustive tests, the FDA approved the first gene therapy in 2017, Luxturna from Novartis [4]. To date, 17 cellular and gene therapy drugs have been FDA-approved and listed in the Office of Tissues and Advanced Therapies (OTAT), and there are hundreds of clinical trials on the way due to the broad range of available viral and non-viral vectors and techniques to modify genetic information. At the same time, we have gained a greater understanding of molecular bases and genetic causes of many diseases, which encourages gene therapy applications targeting key cells and organs for almost any genetic disease.

One of the most promising branches of gene therapy uses avant garde gene-editing techniques such as CRISPR Cas9. The appearance of these techniques in scientific papers saw exponential growth from 2012 on, and clinical trials have started to appear during the recent years. In 2018, the first human in vivo test using CRISPR technology was performed by Editas with the drug EDIT-101 [5], which used associated adenoviruses to introduce the genetic material for editing a mutation causing Leber congenital amaurosis 10. Results from the clinical trial were satisfactory, and the first patient has received treatment in 2020 during the clinical trial phase II [6]. The events are promising; nevertheless, especially concerning are the possible off-target effects, mutations that appear in erratic locations, and the transmission of those mutations to the germ cells, which could end up in the progeny and cause several problems. History has shown that further tests are needed to prove the safety of these therapies in the long term.

1.3. Gene Therapy Challenges in Rare Respiratory Diseases

Many respiratory conditions have a genetic origin that can be addressed by gene therapy techniques. Lungs are an attractive organ for gene therapy as vector delivery can be performed directly into the lungs via the air with nebulization, bronchoscopy, pleural administration, or through the blood via intravenous administration [7–9]. Nevertheless, the complexity of the lung structure places certain physical and chemical barriers to vector delivery, especially for viral vectors. The airway epithelium is covered by a mucus layer whose function is to trap and clear exogenous material, including gene therapy vectors. Moreover, most of the vector's cell receptors are located in the basolateral surface of the cells. Epithelial cells form tight junctions between them, making it very difficult for vectors aiming at the basolateral side to reach their destination [10,11]. Given the exposure of airways to the external environment, lungs have natural protection from the immune system against viruses and other exogenous agents, which increases the possibility of adverse effects due to inflammatory response [12]. In addition, in many respiratory diseases, these barriers are often exacerbated: mucus production is increased, and there is a proinflammatory basal state. The constant renewal of epithelial cells is also challenging, provoking the need for repeated administration, which increases the possibility of activating the immune system [13]. One possible solution could be to target stem cells with integrating vectors, but there are some associated concerns such as integrational mutagenesis and the low efficiency of stem cell transduction in vivo due to their location in the basal surface of the tissue. Preclinical studies are also challenging, due to the difficulty of finding an animal model that mimics human lung cell biology and function, with the result that therapies successful in animals are complicated to translate to humans [14]. Despite all these obstacles, there have been many attempts to develop both in vitro and in vivo gene therapy, using all kinds of vectors and strategies to treat different respiratory diseases [14].

In this review, we aim to provide a general overview of the state of the art of gene therapy applied to three of the most common rare respiratory diseases such as cystic fibrosis (CF), alpha-1 antitrypsin deficiency (AATD), and primary ciliary dyskinesia (PCD). We summarize the vectors used and developed to treat these diseases, the administration routes implemented, and the outcomes obtained, successful or otherwise. Among the approaches used to address these respiratory conditions are augmentation therapy introducing a wild-type copy of the gene, silencing defective gene expression, directly removing the mutation, and trying to edit and correct the nucleotide sequence. Finally, we shed some light on future perspectives for gene therapy and lung disease.

2. Gene Therapy Strategies

2.1. Transfection Vectors

The effective delivery of genetic material inside cells of interest can be achieved by a myriad of methods. Focusing on gene editing, the vectors have to be capable of inserting Cas9, the associated tracrRNA (trans-activated Clustered Regularly Interspaced Short Palindromic Repeats (CRISPR) RNA) and gRNA (guide RNA). Some approaches are more suitable for in vitro and others for in vivo therapies. However, the key aspect for selecting between different methods is undoubtedly the kind of project carried out [15].

2.2. Viral Vectors

Viral methods exploit the innate abilities of viruses to insert the desired genetic material, although their generally high efficiency in delivering and expressing genetic material has a major drawback: they require at least a level II biosafety laboratory and safety procedures to ensure no major complications arise when manipulating the virus. Viral methods are generally divided into genome-integrative and non-genome integrative, and their advantages and disadvantages are shown in the table below (Table 1) [16]. The last column indicates the existence of studies using the virus for CF, AATD, or PCD. Strict regulations and safety concerns only allow few viral vectors to reach the clinical trial phase. In CF and AATD, there are several studies and clinical trials explained in their corresponding sections. In PCD, there is no information about clinical trials using viral vectors.

2.3. Non Viral Vectors

Non-viral methods take advantage of different chemical and physical properties to pierce the membrane and insert the genetic material or proteins. The optimal method depends on the cell or tissue to be transfected. Naked DNA may be inserted directly in the cells, using a physical method; however, its lack of stability and low permeability through the membrane due to its negative charges cause a very low expression of the gene of interest and can cause inflammatory responses [24]. For these reasons, chemical coating systems are highly recommended or necessary in some cases. This issue has been overcome using different creative solutions such as physical methods, inorganic molecules, and other biocomponents. Combining different methods best optimizes the transfection process [25].

Table 1. Viral vectors used in gene therapy reporting genome integration capability and summary of main advantages and drawbacks. The "studies in CF, AATD, PCD" column shows if there are any in vitro or in vivo studies using the viral method. * Herpes simplex virus is used as a complementation method for the adeno-associated virus. CF (Cystic fibrosis), AATD (Alpha 1 antitrypsin deficiency), PCD (Primary ciliary dyskinesia).

Viral Vector	Genome Integration	Advantages	Disadvantages	Studies in CF, AATD, PCD
Lentivirus	Yes	Long-term expression	Mutagenesis potential	Yes [17], yes [18], yes [19]
Retrovirus	Yes	Long-term expression in dividing cells	Mutagenesis potential	Yes [20], yes [18], no
Adenovirus	No	Transduction is efficient in many cells	Strong antiviral immune response	Yes [21], yes [22], no
Adeno-associated virus	No	Non-inflammatory and non-pathogenic	Requires helper virus Small packaging capacity	Yes [21], yes [18], no
Herpes simplex virus	No	Large capacity	No expression when the infection is latent Tropism to neurons	No, yes [23] *, no

2.4. Physical Methods

Physical methods (Table 2) are mainly used to penetrate the cell membrane barrier. This can be done by briefly creating holes and making it permeable for a sufficient amount of time to allow the material of interest to enter the cytoplasm [26].

Table 2. Physical methods used for DNA insertion into cells with a summary of the main advantages, disadvantages, and the physical principle underlying the method.

Physical Methods	Advantages	Disadvantages	Principle
Microinjection	Specific delivery Safe, Simple	Low efficiency	Uses a needle to inject the material [27]
Ballistic DNA	Precise delivery	Limited applications	Application of a pressurized gas to introduce nanoparticles in the cell [28]
Electroporation	Good efficiency Reproducible results	Low viability	Uses a high-voltage electric current to destabilize membrane polarity [29]
Sonoporation	Safe, Flexible	Cell damage	Ultrasounds create pores in the membrane [28]
Photoporation	Theoretically very efficient	Expensive Complex	Use of highly concentrated light beams that perforate the membrane [28]
Magnetofection	Specific delivery Used for difficult to transfect cells	Expensive Complex	Uses magnetic fields to move magnetic-sensitive particles to the cells of interest [30]
Hydroporation	Safe, Simple	Low efficiency Complex in large animals	Exerting osmotic pressure in the tissue environment Promotes particle movement to the interior of the cells [28]
Mechanical Massage	Safe, Simple	Low efficiency	Mechanical movement of the liver makes it permeable to DNA and nanoparticles [31]

Some of these methods of mammal cell modification can only be performed in cell culture and they are useful in understanding the mechanisms of the disease, while others are used to modify animal models and have the potential to be used in medical trials. Decisions about their use are made depending on the size of the plasmid, the cell type and organization, or the aim of the project.

The use of the techniques used in rare respiratory diseases is expanded in each of the sections of the diseases of the article.

There are different approaches for improving the efficiency of the physical methods; binding the DNA to different structures increases the stability and reproducibility of results. Conventionally, they are stratified into inorganic particles and biocomponents.

2.5. Inorganic Particles

Inorganic particles (Table 3) bind to DNA due to their chemical properties and allow better insertion control than naked DNA; they are also generally cheap to produce and easy to store [32].

Table 3. Inorganic particles used to stimulate DNA insertion into the cells with a summary of the main advantages, disadvantages, and the chemical principle underlying the method.

Inorganic Particles	Advantages	Disadvantages	Principle
Calcium Phosphate	Biocompatible Biodegradable	Might crystalize when stored	Calcium is naturally absorbed by the cell [33]
Silica	Low toxicity Easy to store Very versatile	Interacts with serum proteins	Silica-functionalized nanoparticles are recognized and engulfed by cells [34]
Gold	Inert High transfection efficiency	Accumulation Long-term effects have not been studied	Its small size allows it to permeate the cell, the near infrared light absorption can be used for selective delivery [35]

2.6. Biocomponents

Biocomponents (Table 4) are biodegradable structures enclosing DNA or biopolymers that interact with their negative charges. Their versatility and chemical properties are highly attractive for gene therapy use. Their main benefit against inorganic particles is that their degradation products are organic and normally enter the citric acid cycle after use, lowering toxicity and increasing biosafety.

Table 4. Biocomponents used to stimulate DNA insertion into the cells with a summary of the main advantages, disadvantages, and the chemical principle relying on the method.

Biocomponents	Advantages	Disadvantages	Principle
Cationic lipids	Flexible	Can become toxic at certain concentrations	Positive charges interact with the negative charged proteoglycans and glycoproteins in the membrane, helping the particles of interest enter the interior of the cells [36]
Lipid Nano Emulsions	Stable Very low toxicity	Less toxic than cationic lipids	
Solid lipid particles	Increased protection for the delivery material	Complex to produce	
Peptide based	Multifunctional Specific Safe	Complex to produce	Peptides can be added to lipoparticles for specific recognition or delivery [37]
Polyethylenimine	Widely used	Difficult to use in in vivo models	Increases osmotic pressure in the cell, creating pores in the membrane [38]
Chitosan	Non-toxic Mucoadhesive	Low efficiency	Increases osmotic pressure in the cell [39]
PLA/PLGA	Small, Phagocyted	Can induce immune reaction	Biodegradable polyesters that deliver their content by hydrolysis [40]
Dendrimers	Flexible, Good interaction	Toxicity	Small size allows them to interact with cell membranes, favoring DNA uptake in cells [41]
Polymethacrylate	Small	Poor membrane interaction	Small size allows them to reach the whole organism and deliver the content [42]

2.7. Gene Editing Techniques

Gene editing techniques allow researchers to manipulate genes according to their interests. These tools are based on a domain that specifically binds to a DNA sequence associated with an endonuclease domain that produces a double-strand break (DSB). Then, the damage on the genome is repaired by the cell mechanisms. During the process, a small insertion or deletion can be produced or a single nucleotide can be precisely changed due to the presence of two alternative pathways to repair the DSB: non-homologous end joining (NHEJ) or homology-directed repair (HDR). The first, NHEJ, generates random insertions or deletions to repair the DSB, which results in disruption of the gene function useful for gene knockout experiments, while the HDR pathway repairs the DNA damage by copying a homologous template. By delivering a DNA donor encoding the sequence of interest into the cell, the genome can be precisely edited [43] (Figure 1).

2.8. Zinc Fingers and Transcription Activator-Like Effector Nucleases

The first gene editing tool to be developed was zinc finger nucleases (ZFN). Cys2His2 zinc fingers proteins are DNA-binding proteins with a particular structure that interact with a specific triplet on the DNA. By varying the amino acid sequence of the finger, different DNA triplets can be recognized. Due to the modular nature of zinc fingers, different fingers can be linked together to recognize a specific DNA sequence. In addition, zinc fingers are fused to the proteolytic domain of nuclease FokI to obtain the ZFN editing tool [44] (Figure 1).

Another approach in gene editing is transcription activator-like effector nucleases (TALEN), based on the transcription activator-like (TAL) effectors from plant pathogenic Xanthomonas spp. The bacteria use TAL effectors to bind the host DNA and activate the expression of certain genes. They consist of modules of 33–35 amino acids that recognize one specific nucleotide. Through creating a modular protein by fusing different TAL effectors, virtually any sequence on the genome can be targeted. These proteins have been fused to the endonuclease activity of FokI, just as in ZFN, to develop the TALENs gene editing tool (Figure 1). The only requirement of TALENs is that the target sequence must start with a thymine. Since two domains of FokI are needed to produce a DSB, both ZFN and TALENs must be designed in pairs, binding the two complementary DNA strands while leaving enough space for FokI to dimerize [45].

2.9. CRISPR/Cas9

The most recently emerged gene editing tool is the CRISPR/Cas9 system (Clustered Regularly Interspaced Short Palindromic Repeats). It is an adaptation of an adaptive immune system against viruses from bacteria and archaea. In 2012, two independent publications pointed to the CRISPR/Cas9 system as a potential gene editing tool, describing it as a two-RNA structure targeting a specific DNA sequence and the Cas9 nuclease that cuts it [46,47]. It is this simplicity that has boosted the spread of CRISPR/Cas9 among thousands of laboratories worldwide. Basically, it consists of (1) a single guide RNA (sgRNA), formed by two RNA molecules: a crRNA with approximately 20 nucleotides complementary to the target sequence, fused to an invariable trans-activating crRNA (tracRNA), and (2) the Cas9 protein that contains two nuclease domains, an endonuclease domain named HNH for having characteristic histidine and asparagine residuesand another domain named Ruv-C, producing a DSB. The main drawback of the CRISPR/Cas9 system is that a protospacer adjacent motif (PAM) with an NGG sequence is required at the end of the target site. After binding, the Cas9 protein cuts three bases upstream of the PAM sequence [48] (Figure 1).

In addition to knock-in and knockout experiments such as ZFN and TALENs, different applications have been developed by modifying the Cas9 protein function. Endogenous genes can be activated or repressed using CRISPR activation (CRISPRa) [49] or CRISPR interference (CRISPRi) [50]. By fusing a dead Cas9 with other deaminase enzymes, one nitrogenous base can be transformed into another in a specific way without producing a DBS. These tools are called CRISPR base editors [51,52]. One of the main concerns regarding the CRISPR/Cas9 system is off-target activity. In order to reduce it, the widely used Streptococcus pyogenes Cas9 nuclease (SpCas9) has been engineered to improve its specificity, such as for instance the D10A Cas9, which only cuts one DNA strand, thus necessitating two proteins binding in the same locus to produce a DSB [53]. Other examples are modified Cas9 proteins such as enhanced specificity Cas9 (eSpCas) [54] or SpCas9-HF [55]. Aiming to expand the limits of the Cas9 protein, other nucleases have been reported as efficient and specific when editing human cells. Among examples are the smaller but also efficient Staphylococcus aureus Cas9 (SaCas9), which recognizes NNG(A/G)(A/G)T PAM sequence, and its variant KKH SaCas9 [56], which recognizes the NNN(A/G)(A/G)T PAM sequence, but it also nucleases different from Cas9 proteins, such as Cpf1 nucleases: AsCpf1 (from Acidaminococcus sp. BV3L6) and LbCpf1 (from Lachnospiraceae bacterium ND2006). Cpf1 nucleases are guided by a 42-nt crRNA, without tracRNA, and recognizes the TTTN PAM sequence, which is located at the 5′ end of the target sequence [57]. AsCpf1 nuclease has also been engineered to obtain new variants associated with new PAM sequences [58].

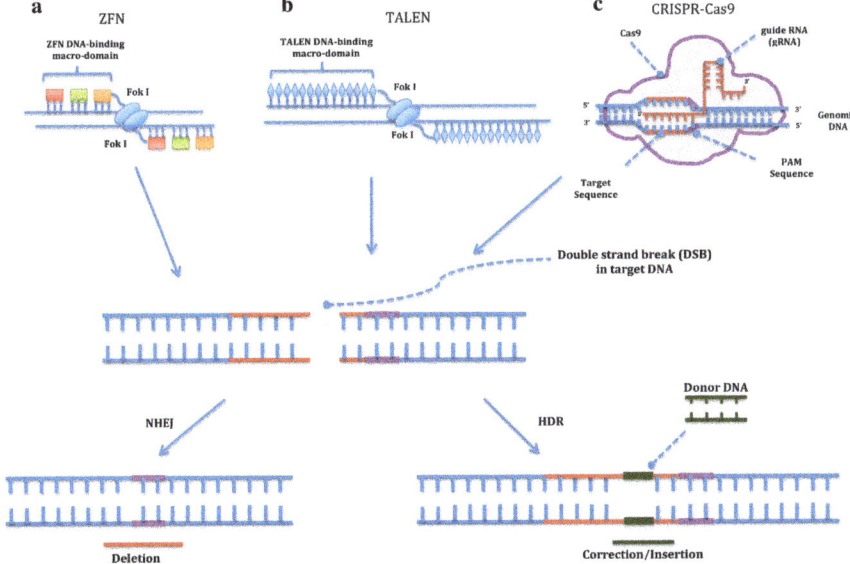

Figure 1. Genome editing with zinc finger nucleases (ZFN) (**a**), transcription activator-like effector nucleases (TALEN) (**b**) and CRISPR/Cas9 (Clustered Regularly Interspaced Short Palindromic Repeats). (**c**) First, a double-strand break (DSB) is produced in the target sequence, and then, it is repaired by non-homologous end joining (NHEJ) or homology-directed repair (HDR). NHEJ produces random insertions and deletions useful for knockout experiments, while HDR results in a precise modification of the target sequence. Reproduced with permission from Torres-Durán et al. [59] under the terms of the Creative Commons Attribution 4.0 International License (http://creativecommons.org/licenses/by/4.0/).

2.10. Cellular and Animal Models

Animal models are key to understanding the physiopathology of a disease. Rare diseases are generally caused by one or a cluster of genes that are conserved among species, so finding the orthologue of the gene of interest in an animal allows detailed studies on malfunction and unravels different approaches on how to find a therapy. Each animal model has its pros and cons, and using one or the other depends on the nature of the study to be conducted.

Murine models are the classical example of an animal model, and they are useful for their fast reproduction, relatively easy maintenance, well-studied genomes, and highly reproducible results.

Focusing on respiratory diseases, mice, guinea pigs, rats, and pigs are the most frequently used models, noting that inflammatory processes are mimicked in mice. Pigs have the most similar lungs to humans due to the presence of the connective tissue, the size, and the arrangement of the lymphoid tissues in the nasopharynx [60].

2.11. Animal Models in CF

The most important trait for CF animal models is CFTR gene homology, so listing the animals most commonly used as CF models in this order, pigs have a homology percentage of 93% [61], while ferrets have 92% [62], sheep have 91% [63], mice have 78% [64], rats have 75.5% [65], and zebrafish have 55% [66]. CF models should also ideally have spontaneous lung disease and/or infection by the common pathogens that appear in CF patients.

Each animal has its advantages and drawbacks, and research is focused on finding a model that reproduces the physiopathology of the disease [67].

2.12. Animal Models in AATD

AAT is a multi-functional molecule that requires complex organisms for understanding its different roles. Murine models used in the studies provide excellent information on how AAT is created and transported, but hepatopathies, lung emphysema, and anomalous inflammatory responses do not affect mice as much as humans [68]. First, human Protein inhibitor Z mutacion (PiZ) AAT murine models were developed in 1987 and were used to measure the expression of PiZ in different tissues, mainly liver and kidneys [69]. Liver accumulation and damage was reported similar to that in humans, but pulmonary disease was not reported due to the presence of other antiproteases [70]. Due to the complexity of the murine *Serpina1*-gene locus, that presents up to six *Serpina1* paralogs, it was not until 2018 that Borel et al. created a *Serpina1*(a–e) knockout mouse to mimic AATD lung physiopathology. This mouse could be used not only for a better understanding of the formation of panlobular emphysema in AATD, but also for the genetics pathways of the disease [71]. So far, there is no murine model with concurrent lung and liver disease [72]. In silico approaches for the creation of humanized AAT mice might help to create better models for testing gene editing techniques in living organisms. Nevertheless, some of the techniques applied in mice genetic modifications, such as hydroporation, which is further explained later on the article, are not scalable to bigger animals such as pigs because the stress exerted causes fatal organ damage. New techniques developed to overcome these issues make it a better approach to find a human therapy [73].

Besides murine models, a transgenic zebrafish model has recently been developed which expresse the Z mutant form of the human AAT(Z-hAAT) and shows liver stress and decrease in AAT circulating levels. This new animal model may help explore AATD physiological bases and treatment [74].

2.13. Animal Models in PCD

Murine models are adequate to study the function of the cilia in an organism because of their left-right asymmetry, lungs, mucociliary clearance, and similar genetic disposition to humans. However, many mutant alleles have proven lethal due to hydrocephalus, cardiac, or kidney defects caused in neonatal or early live stages [75]. Due to the nature of the disease, which consists of a defect in an organelle, different approaches may be taken according to the nature of the malfunction to study. Unicellular organisms are useful for understanding cilia biology, among which *Chlamydomonas reinhardtii* is the most commonly used, particularly due to its wide spectrum of mutants, which exhibit different mutations. Studies using this model have furthered understanding of the basics of the cilia structure [76]. Other unicellular organisms such as *Trypanosoma brucei* and *Paramecium tetraurelia* provide different insights into motility mechanisms [77] and genetics [78]. However, complex organisms are required to understand the pathophysiology of the disease. *Drosophila melanogaster* has two types of cilia, with 9 + 0 (in cells involved in hearing and coordination) and 9 + 2 (in sperm cells) structures, and it shares transcription factors with humans [79]. However, cilia assembly mechanisms are different, and mucociliary clearance is absent.

Xenopus laevis and *tropicalis* are very useful to study these traits because of their ciliated epidermis, which creates a flow from the head to the tail [80], and additionally, left–right asymmetry developmental studies can be performed due to their short developmental cycle [81]. Meanwhile, zebrafish (*Danio rerio*) is a well-known model for left–right asymmetry [82] and is suitable for gene editing techniques such as the ones previously mentioned; however, it has no lungs, and some of the cilia-related genes are duplicated, which can create confusion due to genetic redundancy.

3. Gene Therapy in Rare Respiratory Diseases

3.1. Cystic Fibrosis

Cystic fibrosis (CF) is an autosomal recessive disease caused by mutations in the cystic fibrosis transmembrane conductance regulator (CFTR) gene, with pediatric onset and a median life expectancy of 36.8 years. Over 70,000 people are affected by CF in Europe and the United States, and around 2000 different mutations in CFTR gene have been described. Unfortunately, it is found in a wide range of phenotypes, and affected organs that are not always explained by the genotype–phenotype relation, leading experts to postulate whether CF could be the result of multiple combining effects such as modifier genes or epigenetics [21,83].

The CFTR protein is a chloride and bicarbonate channel expressed in epithelial cells located in different organs. Dysfunctional CFTR provokes abnormalities in epithelial electrolyte transport leading to complications in the lungs, intestine, colon, liver, reproductive system, salivary, and sweat glands. In general, CF is characterized by increased salt concentration in sweat and thickened secretions in affected systems (Figure 2). However, specific symptoms can vary from chronic respiratory tract infections due to thick mucus immobility, chronic sinusitis, nasal polyps, bronchiectasis, and abnormal chest computed tomography to pancreatitis, failure to thrive or fat malabsorption, and many others. Among all these affected organs and symptoms, it is respiratory disease that provokes the most severe effects and is the main cause of CF-related death. Historically, CF diagnosis was based on sweat chloride levels and clinical symptoms. Today, it is confirmed by the presence of characteristic symptoms and evidence of dysfunctional CFTR. Over time, a tendency has emerged toward molecular diagnosis that can detect both symptomatic and pre-symptomatic patients [83].

Mutations described for CF have been organized into five groups. Class I mutations provoked the partial or complete absence of CFTR protein due to nonsense or frameshift mutations or mRNA splicing defects. Class II mutations are defects in protein processing causing the partial or complete absence of CFTR. The most common CF mutation, ΔF508, belongs to this group and results in complete absence of the protein. Class III mutations are called gating mutations because the resulting channels are resistant to normal activation and gating. Cass IV mutations affect transmembrane domains; the protein is functional but has a reduced capacity to conduct anions through the pore. Finally, class V mutations are found on the gene introns, so the protein is functional but the expression level is low or zero. This wide variety of mutations complicates finding a single drug to treat all CF patients. However, in 2012, the US Food and Drug Administration (FDA) approved ivacaftor, a CFTR potentiator, to treat patients with class III G551D mutation. In combination with lumacaftor (trade name Orkambi), this can treat ΔF508 homozygous patients. Although promising, these treatments are not indicated for all CF patients [84].

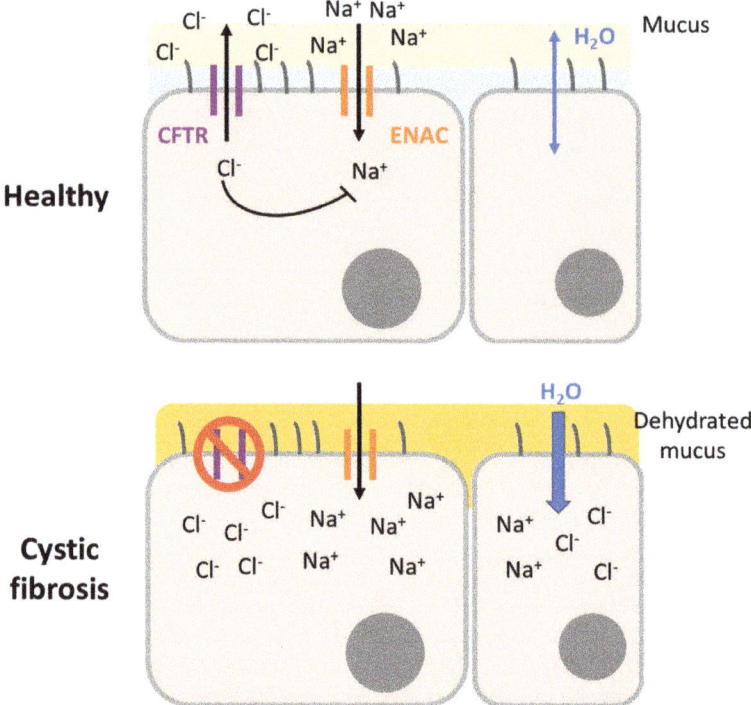

Figure 2. Pathophysiology of CF. Comparison between airway surface from a healthy (top) individual and a CF patient (bottom). In a normal situation, the cystic fibrosis transmembrane conductance regulator (CFTR) channel secretes chloride ions and inhibits sodium ions' entrance, allowing water to hydrate the mucus by osmosis. When CFTR is mutated, ions are kept inside the cell and water moves inside the cell by osmosis, dehydrating the mucus and impeding mucus clearance from the airways.

3.1.1. Adenoviral Vectors

In the last few decades since the discovery of the CFTR gene in 1989 [85], many different strategies have been attempted to develop a gene therapy for CF. The first approaches arrived in the early 1990s, with adenovirus expressing CFTR cDNA. The partial restoration of chloride transport was detected, but patients reported nasal epithelium damage and immune response against the viral vector [86–88]. Recently, using a helper-dependent adenoviral (HD-Ad) vector expressing CFTR, in vivo mouse and pig airway basal cells and airway basal cells from CF patients in air–liquid interface (ALI) culture were transduced, and CFTR activity was restored [89].

3.1.2. Lentiviral Vectors

Sendai virus (SeV) vectors efficiently transduce the apical surface of airway epithelial cells and achieve high gene expression levels. Both characteristics are very useful in CF gene therapy. Meanwhile, lentiviruses such as simian immunodeficiency virus (SIV) are able to transduce non-dividing cells, including airway epithelial cells. The SIV vector has been pseudotyped with key proteins of the Sev envelope: hemagglutinin-neuraminidase (HN) and fusion (F) protein. In addition, F/HN-pseudotyped SIV was optimized with the central popypurine tract (cPPT) and the Woodchuz hepatitis virus post-transcriptional regulatory element (WPRE) to drive CFTR gene expression. The respiratory mouse epithelium was transduced in vivo using a single formulation and without preconditioning, achieving beneficial expression levels. Long-term expression was detected, and readministration was also shown to be feasible. In addition, the F/HN-pseudotyped SIV vector was able to efficiently transduce human ALI cultures, where CFTR channel activity was restored [90]. Assessment of in vitro and in vivo models of toxicity, transduction efficiency, CFTR gene expression, protein functionality, genome integration sites, immune response, and optimization of the enhancer and promoter indicated that this vector could progress to human clinical trials to treat CF [91]. Other lentiviral vectors have been shown to be efficient in restoring CFTR function in animal models. For instance, three newborn pigs received aerosolized feline immunodeficiency virus vector pseudotyped with GP64 envelope encoding CFTR (FIV-CFTR). Two weeks after, functional CFTR, increased airway surface liquid pH and an increase also in bacterial killing was detected [92].

3.1.3. Recombinant Adeno-Associated Viral Vectors

Outcomes of pre-clinical studies in animal models with recombinant adeno-associated virus serotype 2 encoding CFTR (AAV2-CFTR) resulted in a long sequence of clinical trials (Table 5).

Table 5. Summary of clinical trials performed in CF with tgAAVCG viral vector and pGM169/GL67A non-viral vector. FEV1: Forced Expiratory Volume in the first second, IL: interleukin.

Clinical Trial	Vector	Administration Route	Outcome	References
Phase I		Nasal epithelium	Low gene transfer efficiency Safety profile	Flotte et al. (1996)
Phase I/II		Maxillary sinus	Dose-dependent effect Safety profile	Wagner et al. (1998)
Phase II		Maxillary sinus	No significant differences Safety profile	Wagner et al. (2002)
Phase I	rAAV2-CFTR (tgAAVCG)	One-dose nebulization	Safety profile	Aitken et al. (2001)
Phase II		Repeated-dose nebulization	Decrease of IL-8 Improvement of FEV1	Moss et al. (2004)
Phase IIb NCT00073463		Repeated-dose nebulization	No improvement of lung function	Moss et al. (2007)
Phase I NCT00004533			Adverse effects Minimal vector shedding PCR positive only in highest dose	Flotte et al. (2003)
Phase I/IIa NCT00789867	pGM169/GL67A	One-dose nebulization	Safe and efficient	Alton et al. (2015)
Phase IIb NCT01621867		Repeated-dose nebulization each 28 days for one year	Modest improvement in FEV1 value No adverse effects	Alton et al. (2015)

The first one applied in humans consisted of AAV2-CFTR or placebo administration to the nasal epithelium of 12 CF patients. Even though gene transfer efficiency was very low, this study demonstrated that viral therapy was safe [92]. A phase I/II clinical trial concluded that AAV2-CFTR applied on the maxillary sinus was safe and has a dose-dependent effect on chloride secretion without immune response after 10 weeks [93]. Based on these results, a phase II trial was performed in patients who had undergone antrostomy. In one maxillary sinus, AAV2-CFTR was administered and in the other sinus, placebo was administered. Nevertheless, after 90 days, no significant differences were detected. Only anti-inflammatory interleukin-10 (IL-10) was increased in treated sinus. Gene therapy with AAV2 proved again to be safe but not efficient [94]. After a phase I trial to prove the safety of one-dose nebulization of the vector [7], a phase II trial assessed the safety of repeated aerosolized doses in CF patients, showing a decrease in interleukin-8 (IL-8) and an improvement of Forced Expiratory Volume in the first second (FEV1) measurement [95]. However, a phase IIb of this study with a higher number of participants did not prove any amelioration in CF patients, indicating that AAV2-CFTR did not improve lung function in the study conditions [96]. Other administration routes were tested, such as bronchoscopic procedures to reach the lower lobe of the lung, but this resulted in adverse effects related to bronchoscopy, minimal vector shedding, and PCR was only positive in the highest doses [8].

Due to the good safety profile but low expression level of transgene achieved by AAV2-CFTR, new adeno-associated virus serotypes have been investigated. A pseudotyped AAV5 was designed with chicken β-actin (CBA) promoter encoding a CFTR minigene (rAAV5-Δ264CFTR), given that the whole CFTR gene is bigger than the insert capacity of AAV5 vector. Either rAAV5-Δ264CFTR or rAAV5-GFP was aerosolized to macaques. Transfection efficiency, transgene expression, and CFTR protein detection were positive for both Δ264CFTR and GFP in all lung regions of the treated macaques in the absence of inflammatory response [97]. AAV1 has also shown to be more efficient in transducing cells and less immunogenic in chimpanzees and primary human airway cells.

AAV1 has also shown to be more efficient than AAV5 in transducing respiratory cells and less immunogenic when tested in chimpanzees. Both events are independent from one another, since AAV1 transfection efficiency is also higher than AAV5 in ALI culture [98]. Another study proved that AAV6 may be more efficient than AAV2 in mice for gene therapy targeting lung diseases [99]. In a different approach, Excoffon et al. [100] used PCR-based mutagenesis combined with a high-throughput in vitro recombination to create a library of chimeric capsid genes from AAV2 and AAV5. These variants were used to infect the human airway epithelial in ALI culture in order to select the most infectious form: AAV2.5T. This novel chimera vector encoding a shortened CFTR gene was able to restore chloride transport in CF airway epithelia [100]. Similarly, after in vivo selection of successful AAV2 evolved forms in pigs, the AAV2H22 high-efficient capsid was created. AAV2H22 expressing CFTR cDNA transduced to pig airways was able to restore chloride transport, but also to improve bacterial killing capacity [101].

Another possibility to tackle CFTR transduction is pre-mRNA segmental trans-splicing, where two halves of CFTR cDNA are encoded in two AAV6.2 vectors. After infection, the two pre-mRNAs form a full CFTR mRNA. CFTR function was restored in FRT-YFP cells (CFTR negative) and in IB3-1 cells, an airway epithelial cell line derived from an individual with CF [102].

3.1.4. Non-Viral Vectors

Studies have also explored the option of non-viral therapies. For example, the plasmid called pGM169 expresses the CFTR gene under the control of human cytomegalovirus enhancer/elongation factor 1α sequence promoter. This plasmid was treated with cationic lipid GL67A to obtain pGM169/GL67A preparation (Table 5). A first preliminary clinical trial (NCT00789867) assessed the safety and efficacy of a single-dose nebulized administration of pGM169/GL67A [102]. Based on this study, a phase IIb trial performed repeated nebulization each 28 days for a year with 5 mL of pGM169/GL67A in CF patients (NCT01621867). At the end of the trial, a modest improvement in lung function, measured by Forced Expiratory Volume in the first second (FEV1) value, was observed in pGM169/GL67A group compared with the placebo group, and no serious adverse effects were reported [103].

A different non-viral approach was to combine a plasmid carrying CFTR gene with polyethylene glycol (PEG)-substituted 30-mer lysine polymers to form DNA nanoparticles that were administered to CF patient's nostrils. After 14 days, there were no serious adverse effects. The measurement of nasal potential difference evidenced a partial completion of CFTR channel reconstitution in some patients, and PCR analysis demonstrated a mean of 0.58 vector copies/cell [104]. Although initial data are encouraging, more research is needed before development of a non-viral gene therapy that can be efficiently applied to CF patients.

3.1.5. CFTR Gene Correction

Since viral and non-viral vectors failed to reach desirable efficacy outcomes as gene therapy, novel strategies for treating CF were developed as new editing tools appeared. ZFN have been applied to human bronchial epithelial (HBE) and CF tracheal epithelial (CFTE) cell lines, demonstrating that CFTR ΔF508 mutation, the most frequent among CF patients, was a suitable target and can be edited by both NHEJ and HDR [105]. ΔF508 and ΔI507 mutations were corrected with ZFN in iPSC from CF patients; after gene correction, the edited iPSC were derived to epithelial monolayer cells, where CFTR function was restored [106].

Two independent studies showed that ΔF508 mutation can also be corrected by iPSC electroporation from CF patients to introduce TALENs pairs and donor DNA. In one of them, iPSC were differentiated to airway epithelial submucosal gland cells that expressed a wild-type form of CFTR [107,108]. Given the many mutations that are described for CF, Xia et al. opted to use a HD-Ad vector to deliver TALENs in the IB3-1 cell line to introduce CFTR minigene cDNA on the AAVS1 locus. CFRT mRNA expression and protein function correction was detected on transfected cells [109].

Finally, promising results can also be found relative to CRISPR/Cas9 and CF gene therapy. CFTR ΔF508 mutation was corrected by the CRISPR/Cas9 system in intestinal stem cell organoids from CF patients transfected with lipofectamine. Clonally expanded organoids showed corrected allele of the target gene and a functional protein [110]. The same mutation was also corrected in iPSC cells. A 20% correction rate was achieved using electroporation for transfection and introducing the CRISPR/Cas9 system as a ribonucleoprotein complex [111]. Following a different approach, three mutations found in 1.5% of CF patients that provoke alternative strong splice sites were assessed. Two gRNA targeting either side of each mutation were designed to produce two DSBs that resulted in the mutation excision in the region; thus, normal splicing was restored via NHEJ [112].

3.1.6. Conclusion

In summary, CF is a monogenic but complex disease for which definitive treatment has not yet been established. As a consequence, since the CFTR gene was discovered as the cause of CF, there has been considerable interest in developing gene therapy, as exemplified by viral and non-viral vectors, aerosolized and intratracheal administration, single-dose and multiple-dose, wild-type gene integration, and gene editing tools. Although there are promising and hopeful breakthroughs in CF gene therapy, drawbacks such as the renewal of epithelial cells, difficult-to-transduce airway cells, and thick mucus in CF patients together with concerns about immune activity against delivery vectors must be resolved before gene therapy can be brought to clinical practice.

3.2. Alpha-1 Antitrypsin Deficiency, the Genetic COPD

Alpha-1 antitrypsin deficiency (AATD) is a rare genetic condition caused by mutations on the SERPINA1 gene, which is responsible for expression of the protein alpha-1 antitrypsin (AAT). Over 100 mutations have been reported to provoke AATD, but the most frequent defective alleles are called PiZ and PiS (the S mutant form of human AAT), while the wild-type form is called M.

AAT is a glycoprotein whose main function is the inhibition of serine proteases such as neutrophil elastase. Around 80% of AAT is produced and secreted by the hepatocytes. Through systemic circulation, AAT diffuses to the lung, where it protects the tissue from the proteolytic activity of neutrophil elastase. In AATD patients with the PiZZ phenotype, mutated protein forms polymers inside the hepatocyte, which not only leads to a decrease in AAT circulating levels but also produces a chronic liver inflammation state that may result in cirrhosis. In the case of PiS mutation, the misfolded protein is degraded before being secreted and does not reach the bloodstream. Therefore, both PiZ and PiS precipitate a decrease in AAT concentration in the pulmonary tissue. As a result, the lungs are left unprotected from neutrophil elastase, creating a protease–antiprotease activity imbalance and thus facilitating the destruction of parenchymal lung. Consequently, patients often develop chronic obstructive pulmonary disease (COPD); in fact, AATD is known as the genetic COPD, because it is the main genetic cause of this highly common disease (Figure 3).

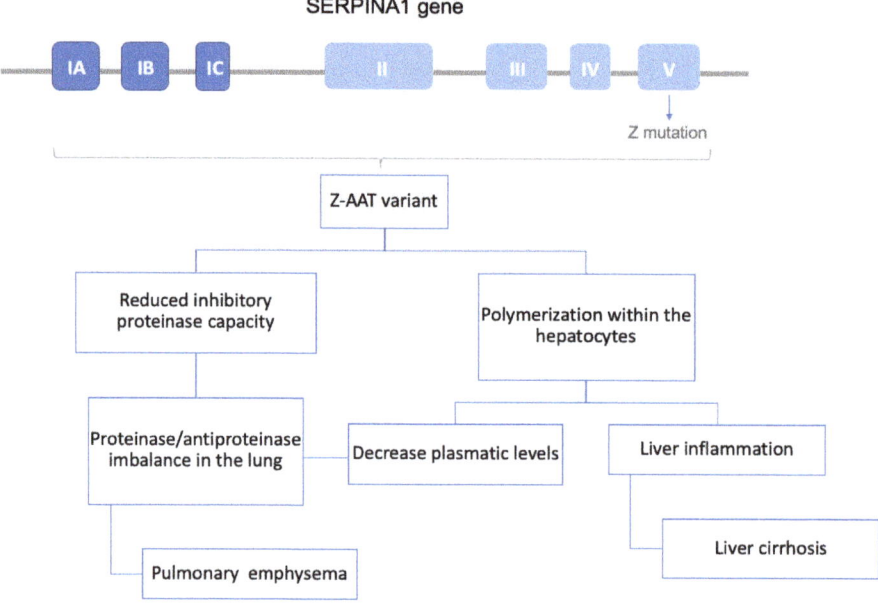

Figure 3. Schematic view of AATD associated with the Z mutant form of human AAT (PiZ) allele pathophysiology. At the top, the SERPINA1 gene scheme with the seven introns and the PiZ mutation in the V exon, where the active site is found. Z-AAT variant, codified by the PiZ allele, polymerized in the hepatocytes leading to a proinflammatory state in the liver that can produce cirrhosis and decrease AAT plasma secretion levels. In addition, the proteinase inhibitory capacity of Z-AAT variant is reduced, facilitating pulmonary emphysema development.

The only approved treatment for AATD is called augmentation therapy. Based on intravenous infusions of purified AAT, it is only able to slow the progression of emphysema and is expensive and time-consuming for the patient [59].

AATD is a complex disorder presenting a wide range of symptoms and severity. The most severe condition is associated with the PiZ allele. Ninety-six percent of diagnosed AATD cases have the PiZZ phenotype, and the remaining 4% are mostly PiSZ [113]. These data can be explained by the fact that it is a highly underdiagnosed disorder, above all in patients with mild symptoms, similar to other prevalent diseases, that usually have PiMS or PiSS phenotypes.

The fact that it is a monogenic disease and that PiZ, the most frequent allele, is a well-characterized point mutation produced by a G > A substitution at codon 342 (Glu342Lys) in exon 5 of SERPINA1 gene make AATD a suitable target for gene therapy [114]. Overall, two different approaches have been performed: gene augmentation therapy by introducing the M allele sequence in the organism and correction of the PiZ allele by gene editing.

3.2.1. Viral Gene Augmentation Therapy

The first gene augmentation therapy attempts used retroviral vectors to deliver AAT into cell lines. Results were promising, but when performed in vivo in animal models, retroviral therapy produced severe adverse effects due to insertional mutagenesis. To avoid these problems, research focus then turned to adenoviral vectors, which do not integrate in the genome. Some in vivo applications in animal models were reported, but they showed two major drawbacks: high immunogenicity and transient protein expression [9].

In the late 1990s, adeno-associated viral (AAV) vectors began to be used in AATD gene therapy. AAV vectors were first tested in different mouse strains with two different promoters via intramuscular injection. It was found that in vivo, cytomegalovirus (CMV) promoter achieved therapeutic and long-term serum levels of human AAT in C57BL6 mice, which were even higher in severe combined immunodeficiency (SCID) mice [115]. These promising data lead to a phase I clinical trial where an rAAV serotype 2 expressing AAT (rAAV2-AAT) vector was administered via intramuscular injection in 12 adults with AATD with at least one PiZ allele. Only low levels of wild-type AAT were achieved, but high safety levels were proven, and although antibodies against rAAV2 were detected, there were no associated adverse effects [116]. In order to improve the efficiency of transgene expression but maintain the safety profile, another phase I clinical trial was launched switching to a rAAV1-AAT vector. One year after administration, M-AAT levels were sustained in two subjects, although 200-fold below the therapeutic level. Although T cell response against rAAV1 capsid was developed within the first 14 days after treatment, no elevation of creatine kinase was detected, so it was concluded that immune response did not completely eliminate transduced myofibers, which allowed the sustained expression of M-AAT over time [117]. In a phase II clinical trial, the same vector was produced by a herpes simplex virus complementation system and administered by intramuscular injection to nine adults with AATD. As in the previous trial, an immune response to AAV capsids was detected, but not against M-AAT. M-AAT levels were dose dependent, peaked at day 30, and then decreased to 3–5% of target concentration for at least 90 days [118]. Five years after the single administration, similar results were obtained. Patients continue to show a persistent but low expression of M form of AAT and a regulatory T cell response that did not provoke adverse effects. Beneficial effects on neutrophil activity such as elastase inhibition and degranulation were also reported [119].

Aiming to circumvent human immune response against rAAV2 and to optimize cell transduction and AAT expression efficiency, alternative administration methods and new AAV serotypes have been explored. The intrapleural administration of rAAV2-hAAT and rAAV5-hAAT in C57BL/6 mice showed that this method generated higher lung and serum levels of hAAT than intramuscular administration and that rAAV5-hAAT was 10-fold more efficient than rAAV2-hAAT in both pleural and intramuscular administration [120]. As a consequence, another study screened 25 AAV vectors derived from human and non-human primates [121]. After intrapleural administration in mice, analysis of AAT serum levels showed that AAV rhesus macaque-derived serotype 10 (AAVrh.10-AAT) was the most efficient vector, and as humans are not exposed to it, there are presumably no problems of previous sensibilization. These results led to an ongoing phase I/II clinical trial called ADVANCE, which assessed two different doses of AAVrh.10-AAT intrapleural administration in individuals with AATD to evaluate the safety and changes in AAT expression in serum and liver (ClinicalTrials.gov Identifier: NCT02168686) [9].

Other approaches for gene augmentation therapy have been applied to in vitro and in vivo mouse models reporting potential strategies to increase serum protein concentration. Stoll et al. [122] created a fusion plasmid vector that contains the Epstein–Barr virus nuclear antigen 1 (EBNA1) gene sequences and the full length *SERPINA1* genomic sequence encoding hAAT. This plasmid showed high expression efficiency when transfected in vitro human and mouse cell lines and also when applied in vivo by hydrodynamic tail-vein injection in mice. Invasive methods such as intratracheal administration of lentivirus or rAAV8 expressing the M allele of hAAT have shown to produce high levels of hAAT in mice lung cells and to ameliorate pulmonary emphysema [123,124]. Recently, in vivo intravenous injection in mice tails with an adenoviral delivery of CRISPR/Cas9 achieved hAAT integration into the ROSA26 safe harbor. Gene integration led to the long-term detection of hAAT in mice serum and liver cells [125]. The autologous transplantation of ex vivo transduced cells with lentiviral or AAV vectors encoding hAAT resulted in sustained hAAT circulating levels in mice [126,127]. Hepatocyte-like cells derived from human mesenchymal stem cells were successfully transduced with a lentiviral vector encoding AAT as a potential source of cells for possible future autologous transplant in the clinical management of AATD [128].

3.2.2. Dual Therapy Approach: Addressing Hepatic and Respiratory Disease with MiRNA

Up to now, our review has focused on various attempts to increase AAT circulating levels; however, AATD is also characterized by the harmful polymerization of Z-AAT forms in hepatocytes, and a complete cure for this syndrome should therefore tackle both hepatic and respiratory symptoms. To assess this dual therapy strategy, Mueller et al. have developed several rAAV vectors containing microRNA (miRNA) targeting the mutant AAT gene and also expressing a miRNA-resistant M-AAT allele. Transgenic mice expressing human Z-AAT were treated with a dual-function rAAV9 vector. Z-AAT aggregates were reduced in hepatocytes at the same time that Z-AAT levels in serum decreased by 80% and M-AAT levels were increased. In addition, the miRNA profile was not altered, suggesting that this miRNA-based dual approach could be safe and efficient to treat AATD, in contrast to small interfering RNA (siRNA) and short hairpin RNA (shRNA) based-therapies that have previously reported side effects [129].

3.2.3. Non-Viral Therapy

Safety concerns about viral vectors have encouraged many researchers to develop other non-viral gene delivery methods for gene therapy. One example is the hydrodynamic procedure, which is based on the rapid intravenous injection of a large volume of a naked DNA solution to transfect mainly liver cells in small animals [28]. Long-term therapeutic levels of hAAT were achieved in mice via the hydrodynamic procedure by transfecting liver cells through the tail vein with the pTG7101 plasmid. This plasmid encodes the full length of the hAAT gene under the control of its natural promoter. The AAT plasma concentration reached therapeutic levels and remained stable for at least 20 days. Furthermore, liver cells showed hAAT expression four months after treatment [130]. However, hydrodynamic transfection has some hemodynamic adverse effects that must be circumvented for this method to be considered in clinical practice. To do that, larger animal models such as pigs have been used to set up a new hydrodynamic approach whereby the liver was surgically sealed and pTG7101 delivery was subsequently performed through the infrahepatic inferior vena cava directly to the liver. The hepatic expression of hAAT was achieved, but at lower levels than in mice, and AAT plasma presence could unfortunately not be detected, which is possibly due to a species-related issue (Figure 4) [131].

Hydrodynamic gene delivery is a promising tool for liver genetic modification to treat AATD and other hepatic pathologies, especially since ex vivo human liver segments have been efficiently transfected with the IL-10 gene [132].

3.3. SERPINA1 Gene Correction

The gene correction of *SERPINA1* mutations in hepatocytes is another option that could provide a definitive therapy to cure AATD. It still needs more in-depth research, but some steps toward gene correction therapy have already been taken. Yusa et al. [133] were able to correct PiZ mutation in both alleles of iPSC from patients with AATD. iPSCs were cotransfected with ZFN targeting PiZ mutation and a puromycin resistance cassette flanked by piggyBac repeats, which after the selection of modified colonies is removed using piggyBac transposase transient expression. This method proved capable of correcting both alleles in 4% of colonies and had little off-target activity. Edited iPSCs were transformed in vitro to hepatocyte-like cells. These hepatocyte-like cells maintain their biological functions, did not form polymers of mutant AAT, and secreted functional AAT. They were successfully transplanted via intrasplenic injection to mice liver, where they integrated into the mouse liver parenchyma, did not form tumors, and expressed M form of hAAT.

Some years later, a similar study was published, also transfecting iPSC with the same integrating vector, but in this case with TALEN constructs, in which the results obtained were successful. All selected clones after gene correction and the excision of selection cassette showed that both PiZ alleles changed to the M sequence. When differentiating iPSC to hepatocyte-like cells, they showed no alteration of growth pattern nor metabolic capabilities. The aggregation of mutant AAT was not detected; instead, levels of wild-type AAT as measured by ELISA assay were normal [114].

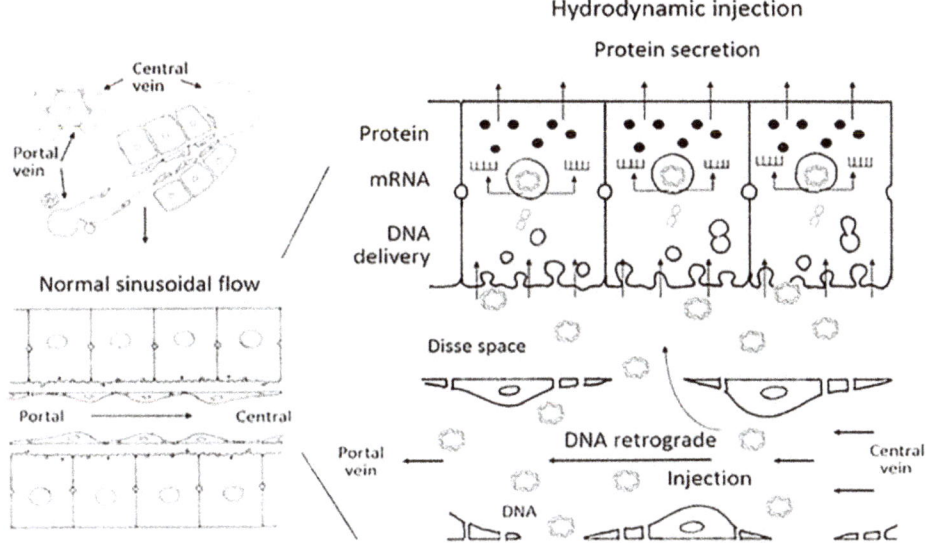

Figure 4. Schema of hydrodynamic transfection within liver tissue in pigs. Retrograde injection of DNA through the infrahepatic inferior vena cava produces a separation between endothelial cells and their fenestration and the formation of endocytic vesicles, allowing DNA molecules to enter the hepatic cells. Modified with permission from Sendra et al. [131] under the terms of the Creative Commons Attribution License (https://creativecommons.org/licenses/by/4.0/).

CRISPR/Cas9 have also been applied to iPSC lines to correct PiZ mutation of the SERPINA1 gene. In the study discussed below, Smith et al. investigated the relative efficiency of CRISPR/Cas9 and TALENs for inducing NHEJ and HDR. Most relevant for this review is the fact that PiZ point mutation was chosen to perform the experiments. iPSC cells were transfected by electroporation with 4D-Nucleofector equipment (Lonza) with the designed TALENs constructs or with two plasmids: one expressing Cas9 protein and the other expressing the sgRNA. The percentage of indel produced was around 2% for CRISPR/Cas9 but was undetectable for TALENs. Curiously, HDR efficiency was very similar across both systems. TALENs showed a relative preference for HDR over NHEJ, while CRISPR/Cas9 was prone to NHEJ. In addition, sgRNA proved to be allele-specific. In heterozygous PiMZ iPSC lines, the CRISPR/Cas9 system was able to discriminate and specifically target PiZ allele [134].

With regard to animal models, the CRISPR/Cas9 system has been delivered with an adenoviral vector to a mouse model of human AATD which expresses the PiZ allele of hAAT. In this study, PiZ expression was disrupted via the NHEJ reparation pathway after the DSB produced by Cas9. Circulating hAAT levels were reduced by 94% at nine weeks after treatment. Liver biopsies showed a significant decrease in AAT aggregates and a decrease in liver fibrosis and inflammation. Obviously, this study does not address the reversal of AATD pathology, but it nonetheless opens a door to research in CRISPR/Cas9 gene editing in vivo treatment to reduce mutant protein, although potential risks must be carefully investigated [135].

Conclusions

In conclusion, gene therapy is a promising substitute to the existing and controversial augmentation therapy, as evidenced by the encouraging results in both pre-clinical and clinical phases. Research is centered mainly on AAV vectors. Despite the safety of these vectors, AAT expression remained far below the minimum therapeutic level. Some projects in animal models are working on optimizing this therapy. Furthermore, new gene editing tools used to correct mutations are trying to find a definitive cure for AATD, but for the moment, testing remains at the animal and in vitro model stage, as there still are many concerns about safety and off-target activity.

4. Primary Ciliary Dyskinesia

Primary ciliary dyskinesia (PCD) is a rare genetically heterogeneous disease that causes the disrupted movement of motile cilia in the organism. This disruption is generally related to poor mucociliary clearance and long-term lung function distress. The main cause of the PCD is inherent to the cilia. Over 600 proteins form its ultrastructure, and the malfunction of any of the genes related to forming or docking the structure could impair movement (Figure 5).

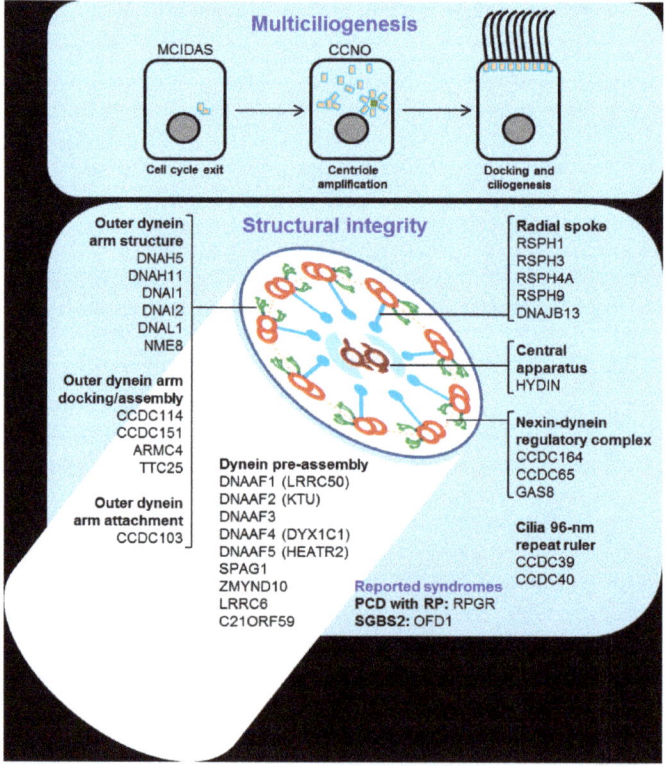

Figure 5. Structure of motile cilia and role of mutant proteins. Motile ciliopathies are caused by mutations in the (top panel) components of the ciliogenesis pathway or (bottom panel) structural and attachment proteins of the axoneme dynein 'arm' motors (green), the dynein arm docking complex, the nexin–dynein regulatory complex (dotted lines), the central apparatus (brown), the radial spokes (blue), as well as molecular ruler proteins and cytoplasmic dynein arm assembly factors. Reported syndromes are: primary ciliary dyskinesia (PCD) associated with retinitis pigmentosa (RP), and Simpson–Golabi–Behmel syndrome, type 2 (SGBS2). Reproduced with permission from [136].

Thus, over 40 genes are known to be related to PCD. Of the total diagnosed patients, around 70% have a mutation in one of those 40 genes, while in the remaining 30%, the origin is unknown [137]. The most common mutations found in patients are located in the outer dynein arm (ODA) docking proteins, with DNAH5 mutations being the cause of around 25% to 30% of all PCD cases [138–140]. Other ODA-related genes are also commonly mutated in PCD such as DNAI1 (approximately 10%), DNAH11 (approximately 6%) and DNAI2, which are genes related to radial spokes (RSPH4A, RSPH9) and other genes involved in ciliary assembly (KTU, LRRC50) [141].

The complexity and heterogeneity of this disease is a major concern when testing new approaches to find a suitable gene therapy. Due to the multigenic nature of the disease, finding a single drug that can treat the whole patient pool is highly unlikely, so personalized medicine will play a key role in PCD.

Restoring cilia motility in PCD using genetic tools started back in 2009 with studies in the ODA gene DNAI1. DNAI1 is a PCD-related gene whose deficiency has been observed to cause a loss of ODA structures and thus impair cilia motility. Incidence is estimated to be 10% of PCD cases. Dnaic1 is the murine DNAI1 orthologue, so Dnaic1-deficient cells show a lack of ODA in ALI culture. In order to mimic PCD, Dnaic1$^{-/-}$ mice were created using tamoxifen-inducible Cre-Lox technology to overcome embryo development complications. When tamoxifen is applied, Dnaic1$^{-/-}$ mice show reduced mucociliary clearance and chronic rhinosinusitis [142].

The transduction of Dnaic1$^{-/-}$ undifferentiated ALI culture with a full-length Dnaic1 cDNA encoded in a lentiviral vector showed a visible increase in ciliary activity, from approximately 0.4% to 10%, and the CBF remained roughly the same. On the other hand, the transduction of a differentiated ALI culture also showed a surface area increase from approximately 1.0% to a maximum of 8.8% and a 10-fold increase in ciliary activity. On differentiated cultures, active ciliated cell appearance showed a 5–6 day delay after treatment.

The tamoxifen-induced deletion of Dnaic1 in a murine model showed that less than 20% of normal gene expression could restore a significant mucociliary clearance and reduce the severity of the disease. To observe gene transfer in the airway epithelium, a luciferase and β-gal lentiviral vector was administered by nasal inhalation. Vector infection rates in PCD mice showed an 8-fold drop compared to control. This inhibited gene transfer was afterwards attributed to the chronic rhinosinusitis [19].

In 2016, new gene therapy approaches using TALENs were used for the ex vivo restoration of the DNAH11 gene. Ciliated cells were collected via nasal brushing from PCD patients heterozygous for a known mutation (p.R2250*/p.Q3604*). Left and right TALENs were designed to target p.R2250*, and after successful design, they were cloned into LAW34 lentivirus, which is a feline immunodeficiency virus (FIV) vector.

Nasal brushings from the patients were cultivated in spheroids containing the ciliated cells inside. Six to eight days after obtaining the spheroids, the lentiviral vector containing the TALEN sequences was added to the media and successfully corrected the mutated sequence to the wild-type one, as proven by molecular analysis, evaluation of ciliary beat phenotype, and visual examination of cells treated for immunohistochemistry (Figure 6) [143].

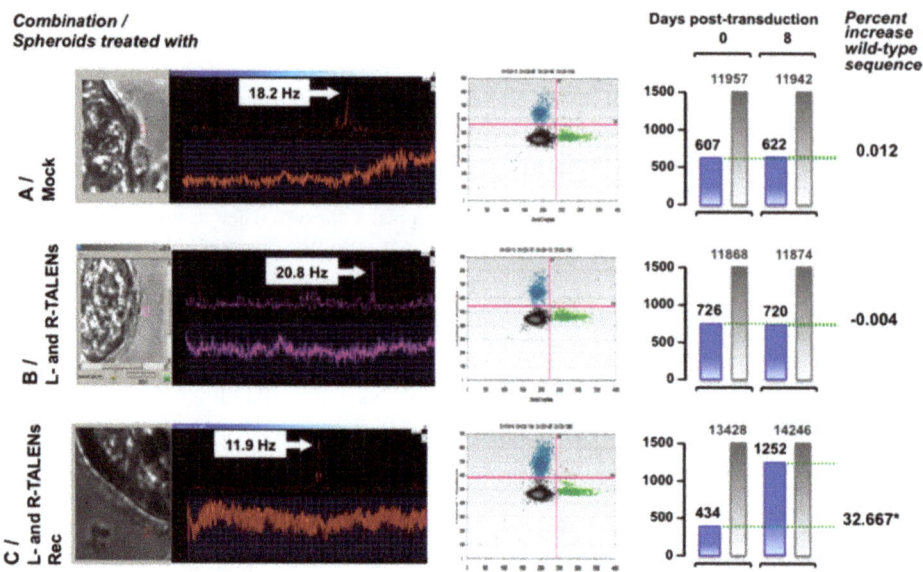

Figure 6. Analysis of ciliary motility and number of wild-type alleles at day 0 and 8 post-transduction. Spheroids from patient A were transduced with the vectors indicated on the left and monitored every 2 days for ciliary beating pattern and frequency. Panels show the ciliary beat frequency measured at day 5 post-transduction for untreated cells (upper panel), cells treated with L-and R-transcription activator-like effector nucleases (TALENs) (middle panel), and L-and R-TALENs and Rec (lower panel). The latter treatment reduced beating frequency to normal levels (12–14 Hz). Normalization lasted throughout the observation treatment. At day 0 and 8 post-treatment, spheroids were collected in part and processed to extract the genomic DNA. Extracted nucleic acids were analyzed by droplet digital PCR (ddPCR) to count the number of molecules containing the wild-type sequence at nucleotide position 172 381. The center gray panels show, spatially separated, the wild-type sequence molecules in the top left quadrant (blue dots), mutated sequence molecules in the lower right quadrant (green dots), and irrelevant molecules in the lower left quadrant (gray dots) counted by ddPCR. The histograms on the right show the number of wild-type sequence molecules counted in spheroids at day 0 and 8 post-transduction and the percentage increment increase in wild-type molecules between the time points. Spheroids treated with L- and R-TALENs and Rec show >30% increase in wild-type molecules. This increase reached statistical significance (*) as determined by the sequential probability ratio test (α value 0.01). Reproduced with permission from [143].

In conclusion, there is still a long road ahead to find a suitable treatment for PCD, but by deepening our insight into cilia biology, its role in molecule trafficking and its assembly, we have created new approaches for restoring motility.

5. Discussion

Nowadays, there are numerous tools available to conduct a gene therapy experiment. Endogenous genes can be modified, edited, disrupted, inhibited, and enhanced; likewise, exogenous genetic material can be introduced into the cell as an episome or integrated in the genome. Many different organs can be targeted via different administration routes; theoretically, cells can even be modified ex vivo and then implanted back in the same individual. Extensive research effort has gone into bringing gene therapy from bench to bedside and hundreds of clinical trials have been performed; however, only a few gene or cell therapies are approved at the moment. Yet during the last few decades, especially since the development of CRISPR/Cas9 technology, there is renewed hope in gene therapy as a treatment for genetic conditions.

As regards respiratory diseases, many of them are chronic and caused by genetic defects. The lung is an organ accessible to gene therapy, but it also presents physical and immunological barriers that impair gene delivery, especially for viral transduction. Aside from physiological barriers, symptomatology such as a thick mucus layer in CF or rhinosinusitis in PCD complicate the process. In addition, to achieve the long-term expression needed in chronic conditions, repeated administrations are needed because of the constant cell renewal in the lung, thus potentially stimulating the immune response. As observed in CF and AATD clinical trials with rAAV vectors, efficacy in gene delivery is very low, and although there are no related adverse effects, there is an immune response to the viral capsid. To circumvent this problem and obtain permanent effects with a unique administration therapy, respiratory stem cells should be targeted, requiring integrative vectors that can produced insertional mutagenesis. Furthermore, gene delivery into these cells in vivo is an important limitation, as they are located in the basal surface of distal airways, and available vectors are not able to reach them efficiently. Undoubtedly, lung stem cell gene delivery is one of the main future challenges for gene therapy development.

In the case of CF and AATD, rAAV vectors have turned out to be the most efficient and safe for therapy, and many clinical trials have been run using them as drugs. However, research is focused on optimizing transfection efficiency by pseudotyping and optimizing promoters and enhancers, such as F/HN-pseudotyped SIV, or looking for new serotypes, such as the AAVrh.10. Conversely, the most frequently used vector for PCD is the lentiviral type. Target cells for PCD therapy are ciliated epithelial cells, which are non-dividing cells that only can be infected with lentivirus or retrovirus.

Alternatively, non-viral vectors can also be used for gene therapy. They are safer but also less efficient than viral vectors. A handful of non-viral vector clinical trials can be found using plasmids encoding CFTR gene combined with cationic lipids and PEG, with modest results. The hydrodynamic procedure has shown encouraging outcomes to treat AATD in pre-clinical studies in vivo, but there are many concerns about the hemodynamic effects if applied to humans. In contrast, non-viral vectors are very useful for in vitro or ex vivo applications.

Gene augmentation therapy is the most widely used approach to treat CF, AATD, and PCD. However, the development of gene editing tools has opened up a new range of possibilities in gene therapy, one of the most promising of which involves editing iPSC ex vivo and then inducing differentiation in the target cell of interest, and finally, autotransplantation with corrected cells. Recently, a number of clinical trials using CRISPR/Cas9 have been approved for oncologic conditions. Pending the results of these trials, the successful application of gene editing tools in CF, AATD, and PCD might be the first step toward definitive and personalized treatment.

In conclusion, the three conditions considered in this review are rare genetic respiratory diseases with complex clinical expression and without definitive treatment. For all three, gene therapy is an encouraging alternative treatment to conventional drugs that have been inefficient up to now. As discussed in this review, recent decades have seen great strides in applying gene therapy in these respiratory conditions; however, researchers are still working toward new breakthroughs due to ongoing concerns about safety, specificity, and efficacy.

Author Contributions: Conceptualization, F.D.; S.C.; and C.G.; Methodology, L.B.; D.P.; F.D.; Writing—original draft preparation, L.B., D.P., M.M.; Writing—Figure drawing and preparation, M.M.N.-G.; Writing—review and editing, F.D.; Project administration, M.M.N.-G.; Funding acquisition, F.D., S.C., C.G. All authors have read and agreed to the published version of the manuscript.

Funding: This research was funded by 2016 Sociedad Valenciana de Neumología grant, SEPAR grant number 112/2016" and European Regional Development Funds (FEDER). Part of the equipment employed in this work has been funded by Generalitat Valenciana and co-financed with ERDF funds (OP ERDF of Comunitat Valenciana 2014–2020). Lucía Bañuls is funded by GVA grant number ACIF/2019/231".

Acknowledgments: We would like to thank the Spanish association of patients with alpha-1 antitrypsin deficiency for donations of research funds to our research group on rare respiratory diseases at IIS INCLIVA/UVEG.

Conflicts of Interest: The authors declare no conflict of interest.

References

1. Xiong, F.; Mi, Z.; Gu, N.; Gu, N. Cationic liposomes as gene delivery system: Transfection efficiency and new application. *Pharmazie* **2011**, *66*, 158–164. [CrossRef]
2. Friedmann, T.; Roblin, R. Gene therapy for human genetic disease? *Science* **1972**, *175*, 949–955. [CrossRef] [PubMed]
3. Wilson, J.M. Lessons learned from the gene therapy trial for ornithine transcarbamylase deficiency. *Mol. Genet. Metab.* **2009**, *96*, 151–157. [CrossRef] [PubMed]
4. Russell, S.; Bennett, J.; Wellman, J.A.; Chung, D.C.; Yu, Z.-F.; Tillman, A.; Wittes, J.; Pappas, J.; Elci, O.; McCague, S.; et al. Efficacy and safety of voretigene neparvovec (AAV2-hRPE65v2) in patients with RPE65-mediated inherited retinal dystrophy: A randomised, controlled, open-label, phase 3 trial. *Lancet Lond. Engl.* **2017**, *390*, 849–860. [CrossRef]
5. Sheridan, C. Go-ahead for first in-body CRISPR medicine testing. *Nat. Biotechnol.* **2018**. [CrossRef]
6. Single Ascending Dose Study in Participants with LCA10-Full Text View-ClinicalTrials.gov. Available online: https://clinicaltrials.gov/ct2/show/NCT03872479 (accessed on 18 June 2020).
7. Aitken, M.L.; Moss, R.B.; Waltz, D.A.; Dovey, M.E.; Tonelli, M.R.; McNamara, S.C.; Gibson, R.L.; Ramsey, B.W.; Carter, B.J.; Reynolds, T.C. A phase I study of aerosolized administration of tgAAVCF to cystic fibrosis subjects with mild lung disease. *Hum. Gene Ther.* **2001**, *12*, 1907–1916. [CrossRef] [PubMed]
8. Flotte, T.R.; Sullivan, K.; Wetzel, R.; Taylor, G.; Carter, B.J.; Guggino, W.B.; Zeitlin, P.L.; Reynolds, T.C.; Heald, A.E.; Pedersen, P.; et al. Phase I trial of intranasal and endobronchial administration of a recombinant adeno-associated virus serotype 2 (raav2)-cftr vector in adult cystic fibrosis patients: A two-part clinical study. *Hum. Gene Ther.* **2003**, *14*, 1079–1088. [CrossRef]
9. Stiles, K.M.; Sondhi, D.; Kaminsky, S.M.; De, B.P.; Rosenberg, J.B.; Crystal, R.G. Intrapleural Gene Therapy for Alpha-1 Antitrypsin Deficiency-Related Lung Disease. *Chronic Obstr. Pulm. Dis. Miami Fla* **2018**, *5*, 244–257. [CrossRef]
10. Pickles, R.J. Physical and biological barriers to viral vector-mediated delivery of genes to the airway epithelium. *Proc. Am. Thorac. Soc.* **2004**, *1*, 302–308. [CrossRef]
11. Kolb, M.; Martin, G.; Medina, M.; Ask, K.; Gauldie, J. Gene therapy for pulmonary diseases. *Chest* **2006**, *130*, 879–884. [CrossRef]
12. Ferrari, S.; Griesenbach, U.; Geddes, D.M.; Alton, E. Immunological hurdles to lung gene therapy. *Clin. Exp. Immunol.* **2003**, *132*, 1–8. [CrossRef] [PubMed]
13. Crystal, R.G.; Randell, S.H.; Engelhardt, J.F.; Voynow, J.; Sunday, M.E. Airway epithelial cells: Current concepts and challenges. *Proc. Am. Thorac. Soc.* **2008**, *5*, 772–777. [CrossRef] [PubMed]
14. Sondhi, D.; Stiles, K.M.; De, B.P.; Crystal, R.G. Genetic modification of the lung directed toward treatment of human disease. *Hum. Gene Ther.* **2017**, *28*, 3–84. [CrossRef] [PubMed]
15. Baliou, S.; Adamaki, M.; Kyriakopoulos, A.M.; Spandidos, D.A.; Panayiotidis, M.; Christodoulou, I.; Zoumpourlis, V. CRISPR therapeutic tools for complex genetic disorders and cancer (Review). *Int. J. Oncol.* **2018**, *53*, 443–468. [CrossRef]
16. Lundstrom, K. Viral Vectors in Gene Therapy. *Diseases* **2018**, *6*, 42. [CrossRef]
17. Marquez Loza, L.I.; Yuen, E.C.; McCray, P.B. Lentiviral Vectors for the Treatment and Prevention of Cystic Fibrosis Lung Disease. *Genes* **2019**, *10*, 218. [CrossRef]
18. Wozniak, J.; Wandtke, T.; Kopinski, P.; Chorostowska-Wynimko, J. Challenges and Prospects for Alpha-1 Antitrypsin Deficiency Gene Therapy. *Hum. Gene Ther.* **2015**, *26*, 709–718. [CrossRef]
19. Ostrowski, L.E.; Yin, W.; Patel, M.; Sechelski, J.; Rogers, T.; Burns, K.; Grubb, B.R.; Olsen, J.C. Restoring ciliary function to differentiated primary ciliary dyskinesia cells with a lentiviral vector. *Gene Ther.* **2014**, *21*, 253–261. [CrossRef]
20. Cooney, A.L.; McCray, P.B.; Sinn, P.L. Cystic Fibrosis Gene Therapy: Looking Back, Looking Forward. *Genes* **2018**, *9*, 538. [CrossRef]
21. Yan, Z.; McCray Jr, P.B.; Engelhardt, J.F. Advances in gene therapy for cystic fibrosis lung disease. *Hum. Mol. Genet.* **2019**, *28*, R88–R94. [CrossRef]

22. Rosenfeld, M.A.; Siegfried, W.; Yoshimura, K.; Yoneyama, K.; Fukayama, M.; Stier, L.E.; Pääkkö, P.K.; Gilardi, P.; Stratford-Perricaudet, L.D.; Perricaudet, M. Adenovirus-mediated transfer of a recombinant alpha 1-antitrypsin gene to the lung epithelium in vivo. *Science* **1991**, *252*, 431–434. [CrossRef] [PubMed]
23. Chulay, J.D.; Ye, G.-J.; Thomas, D.L.; Knop, D.R.; Benson, J.M.; Hutt, J.A.; Wang, G.; Humphries, M.; Flotte, T.R. Preclinical Evaluation of a Recombinant Adeno-Associated Virus Vector Expressing Human Alpha-1 Antitrypsin Made Using a Recombinant Herpes Simplex Virus Production Method. *Hum. Gene Ther.* **2011**, *22*, 155–165. [CrossRef] [PubMed]
24. McMahon, J.M.; Wells, K.E.; Bamfo, J.E.; Cartwright, M.A.; Wells, D.J. Inflammatory responses following direct injection of plasmid DNA into skeletal muscle. *Gene Ther.* **1998**, *5*, 1283–1290. [CrossRef] [PubMed]
25. Wang, W.; Li, W.; Ma, N.; Steinhoff, G. Non-Viral Gene Delivery Methods. *Curr. Pharm. Biotechnol.* **2013**, *14*, 46–60. [CrossRef] [PubMed]
26. Kim, T.K.; Eberwine, J.H. Mammalian cell transfection: The present and the future. *Anal. Bioanal. Chem.* **2010**, *397*, 3173–3178. [CrossRef]
27. DeMayo, J.L.; Wang, J.; Liang, D.; Zhang, R.; DeMayo, F.J. Genetically Engineered Mice by Pronuclear DNA microinjection. *Curr. Protoc. Mouse Biol.* **2012**, *2*, 245–262. [CrossRef]
28. Herrero, M.J.; Sendra, L.; Miguel, A.; Aliño, S.F. Physical Methods of Gene Delivery. In *Safety and Efficacy of Gene-Based Therapeutics for Inherited Disorders*; Brunetti-Pierri, N., Ed.; Springer International Publishing: Cham, Switzerland, 2017; pp. 113–115. ISBN 978-3-319-53457-2.
29. Sherba, J.J.; Hogquist, S.; Lin, H.; Shan, J.W.; Shreiber, D.I.; Zahn, J.D. The effects of electroporation buffer composition on cell viability and electro-transfection efficiency. *Sci. Rep.* **2020**, *10*, 1–9. [CrossRef]
30. Mellott, A.J.; Forrest, M.L.; Detamore, M.S. Physical non-viral gene delivery methods for tissue engineering. *Ann. Biomed. Eng.* **2013**, *41*, 446–468. [CrossRef]
31. Liu, F.; Lei, J.; Vollmer, R.; Huang, L. Mechanism of Liver Gene Transfer by Mechanical Massage. *Mol. Ther.* **2004**, *9*, 452–457. [CrossRef]
32. Giner-Casares, J.J.; Henriksen-Lacey, M.; Coronado-Puchau, M.; Liz-Marzán, L.M. Inorganic nanoparticles for biomedicine: Where materials scientists meet medical research. *Mater. Today* **2016**, *19*, 19–28. [CrossRef]
33. Guo, L.; Wang, L.; Yang, R.; Feng, R.; Li, Z.; Zhou, X.; Dong, Z.; Ghartey-Kwansah, G.; Xu, M.; Nishi, M.; et al. Optimizing conditions for calcium phosphate mediated transient transfection. *Saudi J. Biol. Sci.* **2017**, *24*, 622–629. [CrossRef] [PubMed]
34. Liu, Y.; Lou, C.; Yang, H.; Shi, M.; Miyoshi, H. Silica nanoparticles as promising drug/gene delivery carriers and fluorescent nano-probes: Recent advances. *Curr. Cancer Drug Targets* **2011**, *11*, 156–163. [CrossRef] [PubMed]
35. Huefner, A.; Septiadi, D.; Wilts, B.D.; Patel, I.I.; Kuan, W.L.; Fragniere, A.; Barker, R.A.; Mahajan, S. Gold nanoparticles explore cells: Cellular uptake and their use as intracellular probes. *Methods* **2014**, *68*, 354–363. [CrossRef] [PubMed]
36. Friedman, A.; Claypool, S.; Liu, R. The Smart Targeting of Nanoparticles. *Curr. Pharm. Des.* **2013**, *19*, 6315–6329. [CrossRef]
37. Kang, Z.; Meng, Q.; Liu, K. Peptide-based gene delivery vectors. *J. Mater. Chem. B* **2019**, *7*, 1824–1841. [CrossRef]
38. Baker, A.; Saltik, M.; Lehrmann, H.; Killisch, I.; Mautner, V.; Lamm, G.; Christofori, G.; Cotten, M. Polyethylenimine (PEI) is a simple, inexpensive and effective reagent for condensing and linking plasmid DNA to adenovirus for gene delivery. *Gene Ther.* **1997**, *4*, 773–782. [CrossRef]
39. Santos-Carballal, B.; Fernández, E.F.; Goycoolea, F.M. Chitosan in non-viral gene delivery: Role of structure, characterization methods, and insights in cancer and rare diseases therapies. *Polymers* **2018**, *10*, 444. [CrossRef]
40. Figueiredo, M.; Esenaliev, R. PLGA Nanoparticles for Ultrasound-Mediated Gene Delivery to Solid Tumors. *J. Drug Deliv.* **2012**, *2012*. [CrossRef]
41. Palmerston Mendes, L.; Pan, J.; Torchilin, V.P. Dendrimers as Nanocarriers for Nucleic Acid and Drug Delivery in Cancer Therapy. *Mol. J. Synth. Chem. Nat. Prod. Chem.* **2017**, *22*. [CrossRef]
42. Christiaens, B.; Dubruel, P.; Grooten, J.; Goethals, M.; Vandekerckhove, J.; Schacht, E.; Rosseneu, M. Enhancement of polymethacrylate-mediated gene delivery by Penetratin. *Eur. J. Pharm. Sci.* **2005**, *24*, 525–537. [CrossRef]

43. Miyaoka, Y.; Mayerl, S.J.; Chan, A.H.; Conklin, B.R. Detection and Quantification of HDR and NHEJ Induced by Genome Editing at Endogenous Gene Loci Using Droplet Digital PCR. *Methods Mol. Biol. Clifton NJ* **2018**, *1768*, 349–362. [CrossRef]
44. Kim, Y.-G.; Cha, J.; Chandrasegaran, S. Hybrid restriction enzymes: Zinc finger fusions to Fok I cleavage domain. *Proc. Natl. Acad. Sci. USA* **1996**, *93*, 1156–1160. [CrossRef] [PubMed]
45. Cermak, T.; Doyle, E.L.; Christian, M.; Wang, L.; Zhang, Y.; Schmidt, C.; Baller, J.A.; Somia, N.V.; Bogdanove, A.J.; Voytas, D.F. Efficient design and assembly of custom TALEN and other TAL effector-based constructs for DNA targeting. *Nucleic Acids Res.* **2011**, *39*, e82. [CrossRef] [PubMed]
46. Jinek, M.; Chylinski, K.; Fonfara, I.; Hauer, M.; Doudna, J.A.; Charpentier, E. A programmable dual RNA-guided DNA endonuclease in adaptive bacterial immunity. *Science* **2012**, *337*, 816–821. [CrossRef] [PubMed]
47. Gasiunas, G.; Barrangou, R.; Horvath, P.; Siksnys, V. Cas9–crRNA ribonucleoprotein complex mediates specific DNA cleavage for adaptive immunity in bacteria. *Proc. Natl. Acad. Sci. USA* **2012**, *109*, E2579–E2586. [CrossRef]
48. Zhang, F.; Wen, Y.; Guo, X. CRISPR/Cas9 for genome editing: Progress, implications and challenges. *Hum. Mol. Genet.* **2014**, *23*, R40–R46. [CrossRef]
49. Maeder, M.L.; Linder, S.J.; Cascio, V.M.; Fu, Y.; Ho, Q.H.; Keith Joung, J. CRISPR RNA–guided activation of endogenous human genes. *Nat. Methods* **2013**, *10*, 977–979. [CrossRef]
50. Qi, L.S.; Larson, M.H.; Gilbert, L.A.; Doudna, J.A.; Weissman, J.S.; Arkin, A.P.; Lim, W.A. Repurposing CRISPR as an RNA-γuided platform for sequence-specific control of gene expression. *Cell* **2013**, *152*, 1173–1183. [CrossRef]
51. Gajula, K.S. Designing an Elusive C•G→G•C CRISPR Base Editor. *Trends Biochem. Sci.* **2019**, *44*, 91–94. [CrossRef]
52. Gaudelli, N.M.; Komor, A.C.; Rees, H.A.; Packer, M.S.; Badran, A.H.; Bryson, D.I.; Liu, D.R. Programmable base editing of T to G C in genomic DNA without DNA cleavage. *Nature* **2017**, *551*, 464–471. [CrossRef]
53. Gopalappa, R.; Suresh, B.; Ramakrishna, S.; Kim, H. Paired D10A Cas9 nickases are sometimes more efficient than individual nucleases for gene disruption. *Nucleic Acids Res.* **2018**, *46*, 71. [CrossRef] [PubMed]
54. Slaymaker, I.M.; Gao, L.; Zetsche, B.; Scott, D.A.; Yan, W.X.; Zhang, F. Rationally engineered Cas9 nucleases with improved specificity. *Science* **2016**, *351*, 84–88. [CrossRef] [PubMed]
55. Kleinstiver, B.P.; Pattanayak, V.; Prew, M.S.; Tsai, S.Q.; Nguyen, N.T.; Zheng, Z.; Joung, J.K. High-fidelity CRISPR-Cas9 nucleases with no detectable genome-wide off-target effects. *Nature* **2016**, *529*, 490–495. [CrossRef] [PubMed]
56. Ran, F.A.; Cong, L.; Yan, W.X.; Scott, D.A.; Gootenberg, J.S.; Kriz, A.J.; Zetsche, B.; Shalem, O.; Wu, X.; Makarova, K.S.; et al. In vivo genome editing using Staphylococcus aureus Cas9. *Nature* **2015**, *520*, 186–191. [CrossRef] [PubMed]
57. Kleinstiver, B.P.; Tsai, S.Q.; Prew, M.S.; Nguyen, N.T.; Welch, M.M.; Lopez, J.M.; McCaw, Z.R.; Aryee, M.J.; Joung, J.K. Genome-wide specificities of CRISPR-Cas Cpf1 nucleases in human cells. *Nat. Biotechnol.* **2016**, *34*, 869–874. [CrossRef] [PubMed]
58. Gao, L.; Cox, D.B.T.; Yan, W.; Manteiga, J.; Schneider, M.; Yamano, T.; Nishimasu, H.; Nureki, O.; Zhang, F. Engineered Cpf1 Enzymes with Altered PAM Specificities. *bioRxiv* **2016**, 091611–091611. [CrossRef]
59. Torres-Durán, M.; Lopez-Campos, J.L.; Barrecheguren, M.; Miravitlles, M.; Martinez-Delgado, B.; Castillo, S.; Escribano, A.; Baloira, A.; Navarro-Garcia, M.M.; Pellicer, D.; et al. Alpha-1 antitrypsin deficiency: Outstanding questions and future directions. *Orphanet J. Rare Dis.* **2018**, *13*, 114. [CrossRef]
60. Meurens, F.; Summerfield, A.; Nauwynck, H.; Saif, L.; Gerdts, V. The pig: A model for human infectious diseases. *Trends Microbiol.* **2012**, *20*, 50–57. [CrossRef]
61. Ostedgaard, L.S.; Rogers, C.S.; Dong, Q.; Randak, C.O.; Vermeer, D.W.; Rokhlina, T.; Karp, P.H.; Welsh, M.J. Processing and function of CFTR-DeltaF508 are species-dependent. *Proc. Natl. Acad. Sci. USA* **2007**, *104*, 15370–15375. [CrossRef]
62. Fisher, J.T.; Liu, X.; Yan, Z.; Luo, M.; Zhang, Y.; Zhou, W.; Lee, B.J.; Song, Y.; Guo, C.; Wang, Y.; et al. Comparative Processing and Function of Human and Ferret Cystic Fibrosis Transmembrane Conductance Regulator. *J. Biol. Chem.* **2012**, *287*, 21673–21685. [CrossRef]
63. Harris, A. Towards an ovine model of cystic fibrosis. *Hum. Mol. Genet.* **1997**, *6*, 2191–2194. [CrossRef] [PubMed]

64. Tata, F.; Stanier, P.; Wicking, C.; Halford, S.; Kruyer, H.; Lench, N.J.; Scambler, P.J.; Hansen, C.; Braman, J.C.; Williamson, R. Cloning the mouse homolog of the human cystic fibrosis transmembrane conductance regulator gene. *Genomics* **1991**, *10*, 301–307. [CrossRef]
65. Trezise, A.E.; Szpirer, C.; Buchwald, M. Localization of the gene encoding the cystic fibrosis transmembrane conductance regulator (CFTR) in the rat to chromosome 4 and implications for the evolution of mammalian chromosomes. *Genomics* **1992**, *14*, 869–874. [CrossRef]
66. Liu, F.; Zhang, Z.; Csanády, L.; Gadsby, D.C.; Chen, J. Molecular Structure of the Human CFTR Ion Channel. *Cell* **2017**, *169*, 85–95.e8. [CrossRef]
67. Semaniakou, A.; Croll, R.P.; Chappe, V. Animal Models in the Pathophysiology of Cystic Fibrosis. *Front. Pharmacol.* **2018**, *9*, 1475. [CrossRef]
68. Ghorani, V.; Boskabady, M.H.; Khazdair, M.R.; Kianmeher, M. Experimental animal models for COPD: A methodological review. *Tob. Induc. Dis.* **2017**, *15*. [CrossRef]
69. Sifers, R.N.; Carlson, J.A.; Clift, S.M.; DeMayo, F.J.; Bullock, D.W.; Woo, S.L.C. Tissue specific expression of the human alpha-1-antitrypsin gene in transgenic mice. *Nucleic Acids Res.* **1987**, *15*, 1459–1475. [CrossRef]
70. Carlson, J.A.; Rogers, B.B.; Sifers, R.N.; Finegold, M.J.; Clift, S.M.; DeMayo, F.J.; Bullock, D.W.; Woo, S.L. Accumulation of PiZ alpha 1-antitrypsin causes liver damage in transgenic mice. *J. Clin. Investig.* **1989**, *83*, 1183–1190. [CrossRef]
71. Borel, F.; Sun, H.; Zieger, M.; Cox, A.; Cardozo, B.; Li, W.; Oliveira, G.; Davis, A.; Gruntman, A.; Flotte, T.R.; et al. Editing out five Serpina1 paralogs to create a mouse model of genetic emphysema. *Proc. Natl. Acad. Sci. USA* **2018**, *115*, 2788–2793. [CrossRef]
72. Ni, K.; Serban, K.A.; Batra, C.; Petrache, I. Alpha-1 Antitrypsin Investigations Using Animal Models of Emphysema. *Ann. Am. Thorac. Soc.* **2016**, *13*, S311–S316. [CrossRef]
73. Eggenschwiler, R.; Patronov, A.; Hegermann, J.; Fráguas-Eggenschwiler, M.; Wu, G.; Cortnumme, L.; Ochs, M.; Antes, I.; Cantz, T. A combined in silico and in vitro study on mouse Serpina1a antitrypsin-deficiency mutants. *Sci. Rep.* **2019**, *9*, 1–10. [CrossRef] [PubMed]
74. Yip, E.; Giousoh, A.; Fung, C.; Wilding, B.; Prakash, M.D.; Williams, C.; Verkade, H.; Bryson-Richardson, R.J.; Bird, P.I. A transgenic zebrafish model of hepatocyte function in human Z α1-antitrypsin deficiency. *Biol. Chem.* **2019**, *400*, 1603–1616. [CrossRef] [PubMed]
75. Norris, D.P.; Grimes, D.T. Mouse models of ciliopathies: The state of the art. *Dis. Model. Mech.* **2012**, *5*, 299–312. [CrossRef] [PubMed]
76. Wirschell, M.; Yamamoto, R.; Alford, L.; Gokhale, A.; Gaillard, A.; Sale, W.S. Regulation of ciliary motility: Conserved protein kinases and phosphatases are targeted and anchored in the ciliary axoneme. *Arch. Biochem. Biophys.* **2011**, *510*, 93–100. [CrossRef]
77. Schmid, A.; Salathe, M. Ciliary beat co-ordination by calcium. *Biol. Cell* **2011**, *103*, 159–169. [CrossRef]
78. Dean, S.; Sunter, J.D.; Wheeler, R.J. TrypTag.org: A Trypanosome Genome-wide Protein Localisation Resource. *Trends Parasitol.* **2017**, *33*, 80–82. [CrossRef]
79. Dubruille, R.; Laurençon, A.; Vandaele, C.; Shishido, E.; Coulon-Bublex, M.; Swoboda, P.; Couble, P.; Kernan, M.; Durand, B. Drosophila regulatory factor X is necessary for ciliated sensory neuron differentiation. *Development* **2002**, *129*, 5487–5498. [CrossRef]
80. Marshall, W.F.; Kintner, C. Cilia orientation and the fluid mechanics of development. *Curr. Opin. Cell Biol.* **2008**, *20*, 48–52. [CrossRef]
81. Blum, M.; Schweickert, A.; Vick, P.; Wright, C.V.E.; Danilchik, M.V. Symmetry breakage in the vertebrate embryo: When does it happen and how does it work? *Dev. Biol.* **2014**, *393*, 109–123. [CrossRef]
82. Yuan, S.; Zhao, L.; Brueckner, M.; Sun, Z. Intraciliary calcium oscillations initiate vertebrate left-right asymmetry. *Curr. Biol.* **2015**, *25*, 556–567. [CrossRef]
83. Brennan, M.-L.; Schrijver, I. Cystic Fibrosis: A Review of Associated Phenotypes, Use of Molecular Diagnostic Approaches, Genetic Characteristics, Progress, and Dilemmas. *J. Mol. Diagn. JMD* **2016**, *18*, 3–14. [CrossRef] [PubMed]
84. Bradbury, N.A. CFTR and Cystic Fibrosis: A Need for Personalized Medicine. In *Ion Channels and Transporters of Epithelia in Health and Disease*; Springer New York: New York, NY, USA, 2016; pp. 773–802.
85. Riordan, J.R.; Rommens, J.M.; Kerem, B.S.; Alon, N.O.A.; Rozmahel, R.; Grzelczak, Z.; Zielenski, J.; Lok, S.I.; Plavsic, N.; Chou, J.L.; et al. Identification of the cystic fibrosis gene: Cloning and characterization of complementary DNA. *Science* **1989**, *245*, 1066–1073. [CrossRef] [PubMed]

86. Zabner, J.; Couture, L.A.; Gregory, R.J.; Graham, S.M.; Smith, A.E.; Welsh, M.J. Adenovirus-mediated gene transfer transiently corrects the chloride transport defect in nasal epithelia of patients with cystic fibrosis. *Cell* **1993**, *75*, 207–216. [CrossRef]
87. Crystal, R.G.; McElvaney, N.G.; Rosenfeld, M.A.; Chu, C.S.; Mastrangeli, A.; Hay, J.G.; Brody, S.L.; Jaffe, H.A.; Eissa, N.T.; Danel, C. Administration of an adenovirus containing the human CFTR cDNA to the respiratory tract of individuals with cystic fibrosis. *Nat. Genet.* **1994**, *8*, 42–51. [CrossRef] [PubMed]
88. Zabner, J.; Ramsey, B.W.; Meeker, D.P.; Aitken, M.L.; Balfour, R.P.; Gibson, R.L.; Launspach, J.; Moscicki, R.A.; Richards, S.M.; Standaert, T.A.; et al. Repeat administration of an adenovirus vector encoding cystic fibrosis transmembrane conductance regulator to the nasal epithelium of patients with cystic fibrosis. *J. Clin. Investig.* **1996**, *97*, 1504–1511. [CrossRef] [PubMed]
89. Cao, H.; Ouyang, H.; Grasemann, H.; Bartlett, C.; Du, K.; Duan, R.; Shi, F.; Estrada, M.; Seigel, K.E.; Coates, A.L.; et al. Transducing Airway Basal Cells with a Helper-Dependent Adenoviral Vector for Lung Gene Therapy. *Hum. Gene Ther.* **2018**, *29*, 643–652. [CrossRef]
90. Mitomo, K.; Griesenbach, U.; Inoue, M.; Somerton, L.; Meng, C.; Akiba, E.; Tabata, T.; Ueda, Y.; Frankel, G.M.; Farley, R.; et al. Toward gene therapy for cystic fibrosis using a lentivirus pseudotyped with sendai virus envelopes. *Mol. Ther.* **2010**, *18*, 1173–1182. [CrossRef]
91. Alton, E.W.F.W.; Beekman, J.M.; Boyd, A.C.; Brand, J.; Carlon, M.S.; Connolly, M.M.; Chan, M.; Conlon, S.; Davidson, H.E.; Davies, J.C.; et al. Preparation for a first-in-man lentivirus trial in patients with cystic fibrosis. *Thorax* **2017**, *72*, 137–147. [CrossRef]
92. Flotte, T.; Carter, B.; Conrad, C.; Guggino, W.; Reynolds, T.; Rosenstein, B.; Taylor, G.; Walden, S.; Wetzel, R. A phase I study of an adeno-associated virus-CFTR gene vector in adult CF patients with mild lung disease. *Hum. Gene Ther.* **1996**, *7*, 1145–1159. [CrossRef]
93. Wagner, J.A.; Reynolds, T.; Moran, M.L.; Moss, R.B.; Wine, J.J.; Flotte, T.R.; Gardner, P. Efficient and persistent gene transfer of AAV-CFTR in maxillary sinus. *Lancet* **1998**, *351*, 1702–1703. [CrossRef]
94. Wagner, J.A.; Nepomuceno, I.B.; Messner, A.H.; Moran, M.L.; Batson, E.P.; Dimiceli, S.; Brown, B.W.; Desch, J.K.; Norbash, A.M.; Conrad, C.K.; et al. A Phase II, double-blind, randomized, placebo-controlled clinical trial of tgAAVCF using maxillary sinus delivery in patients with cystic fibrosis with antrostomies. *Hum. Gene Ther.* **2002**, *13*, 1349–1359. [CrossRef] [PubMed]
95. Moss, R.B.; Rodman, D.; Spencer, L.T.; Aitken, M.L.; Zeitlin, P.L.; Waltz, D.; Milla, C.; Brody, A.S.; Clancy, J.P.; Ramsey, B.; et al. Repeated Adeno-Associated Virus Serotype 2 Aerosol-Mediated Cystic Fibrosis Transmembrane Regulator Gene Transfer to the Lungs of Patients with Cystic Fibrosis: A Multicenter, Double-Blind, Placebo-Controlled Trial. *Chest* **2004**, *125*, 509–521. [CrossRef] [PubMed]
96. Moss, R.B.; Milla, C.; Colombo, J.; Accurso, F.; Zeitlin, P.L.; Clancy, J.P.; Spencer, L.T.; Pilewski, J.; Waltz, D.A.; Dorkin, H.L.; et al. Repeated aerosolized AAV-CFTR for treatment of cystic fibrosis: A randomized placebo-controlled phase 2B trial. *Hum. Gene Ther.* **2007**, *18*, 726–732. [CrossRef] [PubMed]
97. Fischer, A.C.; Smith, C.I.; Cebotaru, L.; Zhang, X.; Askin, F.B.; Wright, J.; Guggino, S.E.; Adams, R.J.; Flotte, T.; Guggino, W.B. Expression of a truncated cystic Fibrosis transmembrane conductance regulator with an AAV5-pseudotyped vector in primates. *Mol. Ther.* **2007**, *15*, 756–763. [CrossRef]
98. Flotte, T.R.; Fischer, A.C.; Goetzmann, J.; Mueller, C.; Cebotaru, L.; Yan, Z.; Wang, L.; Wilson, J.M.; Guggino, W.B.; Engelhardt, J.F. Dual reporter comparative indexing of rAAV pseudotyped vectors in chimpanzee airway. *Mol. Ther.* **2010**, *18*, 594–600. [CrossRef]
99. Halbert, C.L.; Allen, J.M.; Miller, A.D. Adeno-Associated Virus Type 6 (AAV6) Vectors Mediate Efficient Transduction of Airway Epithelial Cells in Mouse Lungs Compared to That of AAV2 Vectors. *J. Virol.* **2001**, *75*, 6615–6624. [CrossRef]
100. Excoffon, K.J.D.A.; Koerber, J.T.; Dickey, D.D.; Murtha, M.; Keshavjee, S.; Kaspar, B.K.; Zabner, J.; Schaffer, D.V. Directed evolution of adeno-associated virus to an infectious respiratory virus. *Proc. Natl. Acad. Sci. USA* **2009**, *106*, 3865–3870. [CrossRef]
101. Steines, B.; Dickey, D.D.; Bergen, J.; Excoffon, K.J.D.A.; Weinstein, J.R.; Li, X.; Yan, Z.; Alaiwa, M.H.A.; Shah, V.S.; Bouzek, D.C.; et al. CFTR gene transfer with AAV improves early cystic fibrosis pig phenotypes. *JCI Insight* **2016**, *1*, e88728–e88728. [CrossRef]

102. Alton, E.W.F.W.; Boyd, A.C.; Porteous, D.J.; Davies, G.; Davies, J.C.; Griesenbach, U.; Higgins, T.E.; Gill, D.R.; Hyde, S.C.; Innes, J.A.; et al. A Phase I/IIa Safety and Efficacy Study of Nebulized Liposome-mediated Gene Therapy for Cystic Fibrosis Supports a Multidose Trial. *Am. J. Respir. Crit. Care Med.* **2015**, *192*, 1389–1392. [CrossRef]
103. Alton, E.W.F.W.; Armstrong, D.K.; Ashby, D.; Bayfield, K.J.; Bilton, D.; Bloomfield, E.V.; Boyd, A.C.; Brand, J.; Buchan, R.; Calcedo, R.; et al. Repeated nebulisation of non-viral CFTR gene therapy in patients with cystic fibrosis: A randomised, double-blind, placebo-controlled, phase 2b trial. *Lancet Respir. Med.* **2015**, *3*, 684–691. [CrossRef]
104. Konstan, M.W.; Davis, P.B.; Wagener, J.S.; Hilliard, K.A.; Stern, R.C.; Milgram, L.J.H.; Kowalczyk, T.H.; Hyatt, S.L.; Fink, T.L.; Gedeon, C.R.; et al. Compacted DNA nanoparticles administered to the nasal mucosa of cystic fibrosis subjects are safe and demonstrate partial to complete cystic fibrosis transmembrane regulator reconstitution. *Hum. Gene Ther.* **2004**, *15*, 1255–1269. [CrossRef] [PubMed]
105. Lee, C.M.; Flynn, R.; Hollywood, J.A.; Scallan, M.F.; Harrison, P.T. Correction of the Δf508 mutation in the cystic fibrosis transmembrane conductance regulator gene by zinc-finger nuclease homology-directed repair. *BioResearch Open Access* **2012**, *1*, 99–103. [CrossRef] [PubMed]
106. Crane, A.M.; Kramer, P.; Bui, J.H.; Chung, W.J.; Li, X.S.; Gonzalez-Garay, M.L.; Hawkins, F.; Liao, W.; Mora, D.; Choi, S.; et al. Targeted correction and restored function of the CFTR gene in cystic fibrosis induced pluripotent stem cells. *Stem Cell Rep.* **2015**, *4*, 569–577. [CrossRef] [PubMed]
107. Suzuki, S.; Sargent, R.G.; Illek, B.; Fischer, H.; Esmaeili-Shandiz, A.; Yezzi, M.J.; Lee, A.; Yang, Y.; Kim, S.; Renz, P.; et al. TALENs facilitate single-step seamless SDF correction of F508del CFTR in airway epithelial submucosal gland cell-derived CF-iPSCs. *Mol. Ther. Nucleic Acids* **2016**, *5*, e273. [CrossRef] [PubMed]
108. Merkert, S.; Bednarski, C.; Göhring, G.; Cathomen, T.; Martin, U. Generation of a gene-corrected isogenic control iPSC line from cystic fibrosis patient-specific iPSCs homozygous for p.Phe508del mutation mediated by TALENs and ssODN. *Stem Cell Res.* **2017**, *23*, 95–97. [CrossRef] [PubMed]
109. Xia, E.; Zhang, Y.; Cao, H.; Li, J.; Duan, R.; Hu, J. TALEN-Mediated Gene Targeting for Cystic Fibrosis-Gene Therapy. *Genes* **2019**, *10*, 39. [CrossRef]
110. Schwank, G.; Koo, B.K.; Sasselli, V.; Dekkers, J.F.; Heo, I.; Demircan, T.; Sasaki, N.; Boymans, S.; Cuppen, E.; Van Der Ent, C.K.; et al. Functional repair of CFTR by CRISPR/Cas9 in intestinal stem cell organoids of cystic fibrosis patients. *Cell Stem Cell* **2013**, *13*, 653–658. [CrossRef]
111. Ruan, J.; Hirai, H.; Yang, D.; Ma, L.; Hou, X.; Jiang, H.; Wei, H.; Rajagopalan, C.; Mou, H.; Wang, G.; et al. Efficient Gene Editing at Major CFTR Mutation Loci. *Mol. Ther. Nucleic Acids* **2019**, *16*, 73–81. [CrossRef]
112. Sanz, D.J.; Hollywood, J.A.; Scallan, M.F.; Harrison, P.T. Cas9/gRNA targeted excision of cystic fibrosis-causing deep-intronic splicing mutations restores normal splicing of CFTR mRNA. *PLoS ONE* **2017**, *12*, e0184009. [CrossRef]
113. De Serres, F.J.; Blanco, I. Prevalence of α1-antitrypsin deficiency alleles PI*S and PI*Z worldwide and effective screening for each of the five phenotypic classes PI*MS, PI*MZ, PI*SS, PI*SZ, and PI*ZZ: A comprehensive review. *Ther. Adv. Respir. Dis.* **2012**, *6*, 277–295. [CrossRef]
114. Choi, S.M.; Kim, Y.; Shim, J.S.; Park, J.T.; Wang, R.H.; Leach, S.D.; Liu, J.O.; Deng, C.; Ye, Z.; Jang, Y.Y. Efficient drug screening and gene correction for treating liver disease using patient-specific stem cells. *Hepatology* **2013**, *57*, 2458–2468. [CrossRef] [PubMed]
115. Song, S.; Morgan, M.; Ellis, T.; Poirier, A.; Chesnut, K.; Wang, J.; Brantly, M.; Muzyczka, N.; Byrne, B.J.; Atkinson, M.; et al. Sustained secretion of human alpha-1-antitrypsin from murine muscle transduced with adeno-associated virus vectors. *Proc. Natl. Acad. Sci. USA* **1998**, *95*, 14384–14388. [CrossRef] [PubMed]
116. Brantly, M.L.; Spencer, L.T.; Humphries, M.; Conlon, T.J.; Spencer, C.T.; Poirier, A.; Garlington, W.; Baker, D.; Song, S.; Berns, K.I.; et al. Phase I trial of intramuscular injection of a recombinant adeno-associated virus serotype 2 α1-antitrypsin (AAT) vector in AAT-deficient adults. *Hum. Gene Ther.* **2006**, *17*, 1177–1186. [CrossRef] [PubMed]
117. Brantly, M.L.; Chulay, J.D.; Wang, L.; Mueller, C.; Humphries, M.; Spencer, L.T.; Rouhani, F.; Conlon, T.J.; Calcedo, R.; Betts, M.R.; et al. Sustained transgene expression despite T lymphocyte responses in a clinical trial of rAAV1-AAT gene therapy. *Proc. Natl. Acad. Sci. USA* **2009**, *106*, 16363–16368. [CrossRef]
118. Flotte, T.R.; Trapnell, B.C.; Humphries, M.; Carey, B.; Calcedo, R.; Rouhani, F.; Campbell-Thompson, M.; Yachnis, A.T.; Sandhaus, R.A.; McElvaney, N.G.; et al. Phase 2 clinical trial of a recombinant adeno-associated viral vector expressing α 1-antitrypsin: Interim results. *Hum. Gene Ther.* **2011**, *22*, 1239–1247. [CrossRef]

119. Mueller, C.; Gernoux, G.; Gruntman, A.M.; Borel, F.; Reeves, E.P.; Calcedo, R.; Rouhani, F.N.; Yachnis, A.; Humphries, M.; Campbell-Thompson, M.; et al. 5 Year Expression and Neutrophil Defect Repair after Gene Therapy in Alpha-1 Antitrypsin Deficiency. *Mol. Ther.* **2017**, *25*, 1387–1394. [CrossRef]
120. De, B.; Heguy, A.; Leopold, P.L.; Wasif, N.; Korst, R.J.; Hackett, N.R.; Crystal, R.G. Intrapleural administration of a serotype 5 adeno-associated virus coding for α1-antitrypsin mediates persistent, high lung and serum levels of α1-antitrypsin. *Mol. Ther.* **2004**, *10*, 1003–1010. [CrossRef]
121. De, B.P.; Heguy, A.; Hackett, N.R.; Ferris, B.; Leopold, P.L.; Lee, J.; Pierre, L.; Gao, G.; Wilson, J.M.; Crystal, R.G. High levels of persistent expression of α1-Antitrypsin mediated by the nonhuman primate serotype rh.10 adeno-associated virus despite preexisting immunity to common human adeno-associated viruses. *Mol. Ther.* **2006**, *13*, 67–76. [CrossRef]
122. Stoll, S.M.; Sclimenti, C.R.; Baba, E.J.; Meuse, L.; Kay, M.A.; Calos, M.P. Epstein-Barr virus/human vector provides high-level, long-term expression of α1-antitrypsin in mice. *Mol. Ther.* **2001**, *4*, 122–129. [CrossRef]
123. Wilson, A.A.; Murphy, G.J.; Hamakawa, H.; Kwok, L.W.; Srinivasan, S.; Hovav, A.H.; Mulligan, R.C.; Amar, S.; Suki, B.; Kotton, D.N. Amelioration of emphysema in mice through lentiviral transduction of long-lived pulmonary alveolar macrophages. *J. Clin. Investig.* **2010**, *120*, 379–389. [CrossRef]
124. Liqun Wang, R.; McLaughlin, T.; Cossette, T.; Tang, Q.; Foust, K.; Campbell-Thompson, M.; Martino, A.; Cruz, P.; Loiler, S.; Mueller, C.; et al. Recombinant AAV serotype and capsid mutant comparison for pulmonary gene transfer of α-1-antitrypsin using invasive and noninvasive delivery. *Mol. Ther.* **2009**, *17*, 81–87. [CrossRef] [PubMed]
125. Stephens, C.J.; Kashentseva, E.; Everett, W.; Kaliberova, L.; Curiel, D.T. Targeted in vivo knock-in of human alpha-1-antitrypsin cDNA using adenoviral delivery of CRISPR/Cas9. *Gene Ther.* **2018**, *25*, 139–156. [CrossRef] [PubMed]
126. Li, H.; Lu, Y.; Witek, R.P.; Chang, L.J.; Campbell-Thompson, M.; Jorgensen, M.; Petersen, B.; Song, S. Ex vivo transduction and transplantation of bone marrow cells for liver gene delivery of α1-antitrypsin. *Mol. Ther.* **2010**, *18*, 1553–1558. [CrossRef] [PubMed]
127. Wilson, A.A.; Kwok, L.W.; Hovav, A.H.; Ohle, S.J.; Little, F.F.; Fine, A.; Kotton, D.N. Sustained expression of α1-antitrypsin after transplantation of manipulated hematopoietic stem cells. *Am. J. Respir. Cell Mol. Biol.* **2008**, *39*, 133–141. [CrossRef] [PubMed]
128. Ghaedi, M.; Lotfi, A.S.; Soleimani, M. Establishment of lentiviral-vector-mediated model of human alpha-1 antitrypsin delivery into hepatocyte-like cells differentiated from mesenchymal stem cells. *Tissue Cell* **2010**, *42*, 181–189. [CrossRef] [PubMed]
129. Mueller, C.; Tang, Q.; Gruntman, A.; Blomenkamp, K.; Teckman, J.; Song, L.; Zamore, P.D.; Flotte, T.R. Sustained miRNA-mediated knockdown of mutant AAT with simultaneous augmentation of wild-type AAT has minimal effect on global liver miRNA profiles. *Mol. Ther.* **2012**, *20*, 590–600. [CrossRef]
130. Aliño, S.F.; Crespo, A.; Dasí, F. Long-term therapeutic levels of human alpha-1 antitrypsin in plasma after hydrodynamic injection of nonviral DNA. *Gene Ther.* **2003**, *10*, 1672–1679. [CrossRef]
131. Sendra, L.; Miguel, A.; Pérez-Enguix, D.; Herrero, M.J.; Montalvá, E.; García-Gimeno, M.A.; Noguera, I.; Díaz, A.; Pérez, J.; Sanz, P.; et al. Studying closed hydrodynamic models of "in vivo" DNA perfusion in pig liver for gene therapy translation to humans. *PLoS ONE* **2016**, *11*, e0163898. [CrossRef]
132. Sendra Gisbert, L.; Miguel Matas, A.; Sabater Ortí, L.; Herrero, M.J.; Sabater Olivas, L.; Montalvá Orón, E.M.; Frasson, M.; Abargues López, R.; López-Andújar, R.; García-Granero Ximénez, E.; et al. Efficacy of hydrodynamic interleukin 10 gene transfer in human liver segments with interest in transplantation. *Liver Transpl.* **2017**, *23*, 50–62. [CrossRef]
133. Yusa, K.; Rashid, S.T.; Strick-Marchand, H.; Varela, I.; Liu, P.Q.; Paschon, D.E.; Miranda, E.; Ordóñez, A.; Hannan, N.R.F.; Rouhani, F.J.; et al. Targeted gene correction of α1-antitrypsin deficiency in induced pluripotent stem cells. *Nature* **2011**, *478*, 391–394. [CrossRef]
134. Smith, C.; Abalde-Atristain, L.; He, C.; Brodsky, B.R.; Braunstein, E.M.; Chaudhari, P.; Jang, Y.Y.; Cheng, L.; Ye, Z. Efficient and allele-specific genome editing of disease loci in human iPSCs. *Mol. Ther.* **2015**, *23*, 570–577. [CrossRef] [PubMed]
135. Bjursell, M.; Porritt, M.J.; Ericson, E.; Taheri-Ghahfarokhi, A.; Clausen, M.; Magnusson, L.; Admyre, T.; Nitsch, R.; Mayr, L.; Aasehaug, L.; et al. Therapeutic Genome Editing With CRISPR/Cas9 in a Humanized Mouse Model Ameliorates α1-antitrypsin Deficiency Phenotype. *EBioMedicine* **2018**, *29*, 104–111. [CrossRef] [PubMed]

136. Mitchison, H.M.; Valente, E.M. Motile and non-motile cilia in human pathology: From function to phenotypes. *J. Pathol.* **2017**, *241*, 294–309. [CrossRef] [PubMed]
137. Horani, A.; Ferkol, T.W.; Dutcher, S.K.; Brody, S.L. Genetics and Biology of Primary Ciliary Dyskinesia. *Paediatr. Respir. Rev.* **2016**, *18*, 18–24. [CrossRef] [PubMed]
138. Boaretto, F.; Snijders, D.; Salvoro, C.; Spalletta, A.; Mostacciuolo, M.L.; Collura, M.; Cazzato, S.; Girosi, D.; Silvestri, M.; Rossi, G.A.; et al. Diagnosis of Primary Ciliary Dyskinesia by a Targeted Next-Generation Sequencing Panel: Molecular and Clinical Findings in Italian Patients. *J. Mol. Diagn.* **2016**, *18*, 912–922. [CrossRef] [PubMed]
139. Hornef, N.; Olbrich, H.; Horvath, J.; Zariwala, M.A.; Fliegauf, M.; Loges, N.T.; Wildhaber, J.; Noone, P.G.; Kennedy, M.; Antonarakis, S.E.; et al. DNAH5 Mutations Are a Common Cause of Primary Ciliary Dyskinesia with Outer Dynein Arm Defects. *Am. J. Respir. Crit. Care Med.* **2006**, *174*, 120–126. [CrossRef]
140. Loges, N.T.; Omran, H. 14-Dynein dysfunction as a cause of primary ciliary dyskinesia and other ciliopathies. In *Dyneins: Structure, Biology and Disease (Second Edition)*; King, S.M., Ed.; Academic Press: Cambridge, MA, USA, 2018; pp. 316–355. ISBN 978-0-12-809470-9.
141. Zietkiewicz, E.; Bukowy-Bieryłło, Z.; Voelkel, K.; Klimek, B.; Dmeńska, H.; Pogorzelski, A.; Sulikowska-Rowińska, A.; Rutkiewicz, E.; Witt, M. Mutations in radial spoke head genes and ultrastructural cilia defects in east-european cohort of primary ciliary dyskinesia patients. *PLoS ONE* **2012**, *7*, e33667. [CrossRef]
142. Ostrowski, L.E.; Yin, W.; Rogers, T.D.; Busalacchi, K.B.; Chua, M.; O'Neal, W.K.; Grubb, B.R. Conditional deletion of Dnaic1 in a murine model of primary ciliary dyskinesia causes chronic rhinosinusitis. *Am. J. Respir. Cell Mol. Biol.* **2010**, *43*, 55–63. [CrossRef]
143. Lai, M.; Pifferi, M.; Bush, A.; Piras, M.; Michelucci, A.; Di Cicco, M.; Del Grosso, A.; Quaranta, P.; Cursi, C.; Tantillo, E.; et al. Gene editing of DNAH11 restores normal cilia motility in primary ciliary dyskinesia. *J. Med. Genet.* **2016**, *53*, 242–249. [CrossRef]

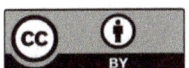

© 2020 by the authors. Licensee MDPI, Basel, Switzerland. This article is an open access article distributed under the terms and conditions of the Creative Commons Attribution (CC BY) license (http://creativecommons.org/licenses/by/4.0/).

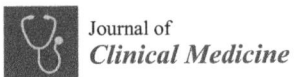

Article

Late Diagnosis of Infants with PCD and Neonatal Respiratory Distress

Myrofora Goutaki [1,2], Florian S. Halbeisen [1], Angelo Barbato [3,†], Suzanne Crowley [4], Amanda Harris [5], Robert A. Hirst [6], Bülent Karadag [7], Vendula Martinu [8], Lucy Morgan [9], Christopher O'Callaghan [6,10], Ugur Ozçelik [11], Sergio Scigliano [12], Santiago Ucros [13], Panayiotis Yiallouros [14], Sven M. Schulzke [15] and Claudia E. Kuehni [1,2,*]

1. Institute of Social and Preventive Medicine, University of Bern, 3012 Bern, Switzerland; myrofora.goutaki@ispm.unibe.ch (M.G.); florian.halbeisen@ispm.unibe.ch (F.S.H.)
2. Paediatric Respiratory Medicine, Children's University Hospital of Bern, University of Bern, 3010 Bern, Switzerland
3. Primary Ciliary Dyskinesia Centre, Department of Women's and Children's Health (SDB), University of Padova, 1848 Padova, Italy; angelo.barbato45@gmail.com
4. Paediatric Department of Allergy and Lung Diseases, Oslo University Hospital, 0372 Oslo, Norway; suzcro@ous-hf.no
5. Primary Ciliary Dyskinesia Centre, NIHR Respiratory Biomedical Research Centre, University of Southampton, Southampton SO 16 6YD, UK; Amanda-Lea.Harris@uhs.nhs.uk
6. Department of Respiratory Sciences, College of Life Sciences, University of Leicester, Leicester LE1 7RH, UK; rah9@leicester.ac.uk (R.A.H.); c.ocallaghan@ucl.ac.uk (C.O.)
7. Department of Pediatric Pulmonology, Marmara University, School of Medicine, Istanbul 34854, Turkey; bkaradag@hotmail.com
8. Department of Paediatrics, 2nd Faculty of Medicine, Charles University and University Hospital Motol, 38FQ+FX Prague, Czech Republic; vendy.martinu@gmail.com
9. Department of Respiratory Medicine, Concord Hospital Clinical School, University of Sydney, Sydney, NSW 2138, Australia; Lucy.Morgan@health.nsw.gov.au
10. Respiratory Critical Care & Anaesthesia, UCL Great Ormond Street Institute of Child Health, London WC1N 1EH, UK
11. Department of Pediatric Pulmonology, Hacettepe University Faculty of Medicine, 06230 Ankara, Turkey; uozcelik@hacettepe.edu.tr
12. Centro Respiratorio, Hospital de Niños Ricardo Gutierrez, Buenos Aires C1425EFD, Argentina; sergioscigliano@gmail.com
13. Departamento de Pediatría, Fundación Santa Fe, Clínica de Neumología Pediátrica Compensar, Bogotá 12390, Colombia; santiago_ucros@yahoo.com
14. Medical School, University of Cyprus, 596G+R2 Nicosia, Cyprus; yiallouros.panayiotis@ucy.ac.cy
15. Department of Neonatology, University Children's Hospital Basel UKBB, 4056 Basel, Switzerland; sven.schulzke@unibas.ch
* Correspondence: Claudia.kuehni@ispm.unibe.ch; Tel.: +41-31-631-35-07
† on behalf of the Italian PCD Consortium.

Received: 27 July 2020; Accepted: 3 September 2020; Published: 4 September 2020

Abstract: Neonatal respiratory distress (NRD) is common among infants with primary ciliary dyskinesia (PCD), but we do not know whether affected neonates receive a timely diagnosis. We used data from the international PCD cohort and assessed the proportion of patients with PCD who had a history of NRD and their age at diagnosis, stratifying by presence of laterality defects. First we analyzed data from all participants diagnosed after 2000, followed by individuals from a subgroup diagnosed using stricter criteria. Among the 1375 patients in the study, 45% had a history of NRD and 42% had laterality defects. Out of the 476 children with definite PCD diagnosis, 55% had a history of NRD and 50% had laterality defects. Overall, 30% of children with PCD were diagnosed during the first 12 months of life. This varied from 13% in those with situs solitus and no NRD, to 21% in those with situs solitus and NRD, 33% in those with situs anomalies but no NRD, and 52% in those with both situs anomalies and NRD. Our results suggest that we need to improve our knowledge of the neonatal presentation of infants with PCD and apply it so that these patients will receive appropriate care sooner.

Keywords: primary ciliary dyskinesia; neonatal respiratory distress; laterality defect; orphan diseases

1. Introduction

Primary ciliary dyskinesia (PCD) is a multiorgan genetic disease that affects approximately 1 in 10,000 people [1,2], or as many as 1 in 400 in highly consanguineous populations [3,4]. The clinical phenotype is variable, but most patients have chronic upper and lower airway disease with rhinitis and cough resulting in recurrent infections of ears, sinuses, and lungs [5,6]. About half of patients with PCD have situs inversus, and an additional 10–12% have other laterality defects, which may be associated with congenital heart disease [7,8]. Already in childhood, lung function is comparable to patients with cystic fibrosis (CF), and as the disease progresses most patients develop progressive lung disease with bronchiectasis and chronic pseudomonas infection [9–13]. At advanced disease stages, many adults become oxygen dependent and undergo a lobectomy, with some eventually requiring lung transplantation [14,15]. It is believed that, as in other genetic respiratory diseases such as CF, early diagnosis followed by initiation of regular physiotherapy and prompt antibiotic treatment may reduce lung function decline and improve long-term outcomes [16].

Patients with PCD are usually born at term, and typically present with chronic respiratory symptoms from birth such as rhinitis and a wet-sounding cough. A large proportion present with neonatal respiratory distress (NRD) [17–19]. The frequency of these symptoms in neonates with PCD is unclear; in a systematic review, the proportion of PCD patients reported to have NRD varied widely between studies, from 15% to 91%. However, these data were generally of poor quality [20]. In a single-center case-control study from Canada, detailed neonatal data were extracted from health records to identify characteristics that distinguish PCD from other causes of NRD [19]. The study showed that compared to other term infants with NRD, infants with PCD had a characteristic clinical picture that should point toward the diagnosis [19].

The neonatal period offers an ideal window for early diagnosis of PCD before long-term damage to the lungs has occurred. However, timely diagnosis has not yet been investigated in an international setting. We used a multicenter dataset from the international PCD (iPCD) cohort to determine the proportion of patients presenting with NRD and the age when PCD was finally diagnosed. We grouped infants into those with and without NRD, and stratified additionally by presence of laterality defects.

2. Methods

2.1. Participants

The iPCD cohort, described in detail elsewhere [21], included 3824 patients as of June 2019 when reviewed for this study [21]. The core dataset of the iPCD cohort is compulsory for all contributors, while specific modules including the one on neonatal history are voluntary. For this analysis, we included only patients from data providers who had also contributed data on the neonatal period for their patients (Figure 1 and Supplementary Materials Table S1). We further excluded patients diagnosed before the year 2000 because PCD diagnosis has evolved considerably during the past 20 years and because we were mainly interested in recent data that are representative of contemporary neonatal care [22].

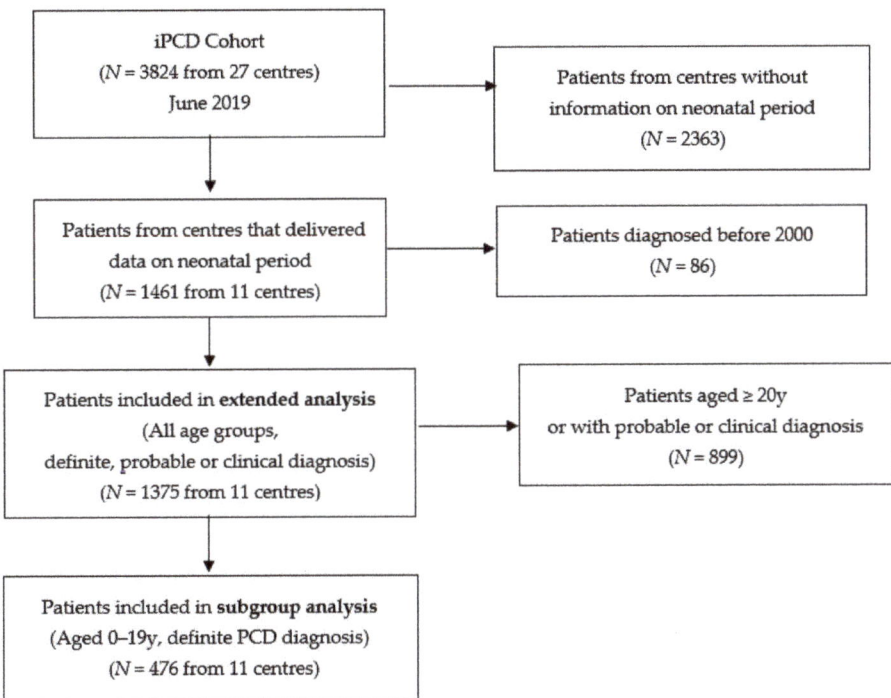

Figure 1. Flow chart showing the patients included for the different analyses performed. PCD: primary ciliary dyskinesia.

2.2. Definition of NRD and PCD Diagnosis

Information on NRD was delivered by data providers and was retrieved from patient charts. NRD was described as a history of hospitalization for respiratory distress during the neonatal period either retrieved from neonatal hospital records or reported to the PCD clinic at diagnosis by patients or their parents. In one of the centers, NRD was defined as the presence of respiratory distress or physician-recorded chest symptoms during the neonatal period, since the data did not distinguish between the two. We also retrieved information on laterality status and defined the presence of situs inversus or heterotaxia as a laterality defect. All patients included in the study had a clinical phenotype consistent with PCD and were under PCD management at the contributing centers.

All patients included in the iPCD cohort had a strong clinical suspicion of PCD and were followed up as PCD cases in the contributing centers after alternative diagnoses such as CF or immunodeficiency had been excluded. However, because the diagnosis of PCD is complex and can sometimes remain inconclusive even after multiple tests, we grouped patients into groups of diagnostic certainty based on the diagnostic guidelines of the European Respiratory Society Task Force [23].

"Definite PCD" diagnosis was defined as a pathogenic biallelic PCD genetic mutation or hallmark structural abnormality in transmission electron microscopy (TEM) [23]. The remaining patients had either abnormal high-speed video microscopy findings or low nasal nitric oxide (probable PCD diagnosis), or were patients with strong clinical suspicion (e.g., Kartagener syndrome) in whom the diagnostic algorithm was not complete (clinical PCD diagnosis). For the diagnostic classification, we reviewed all diagnostic data provided by the centers and contacted the centers where clarifications were required. Age at diagnosis was defined based on information provided by the centers or, when not available, based on the date of positive diagnostic tests. In case several positive tests were available, age of diagnosis corresponded to the date of the first positive test. For patients with only clinical diagnosis, age of diagnosis was defined as the age when the patient started to be managed as PCD at the participating center. We divided the ages at diagnosis into periods, to investigate whether the diagnosis was made in the first three months of life, within infancy (age 3–11 months), during the preschool period (age 1–4 years), or during school years (age 5–9, 10–14, or over 14 years).

2.3. Analysis

We first analyzed data from all patients regardless of age or diagnostic certainty (Figure 1), and assessed the proportions of patients who reported NRD and laterality defects overall and by country. We then stratified the population into four groups and described their ages at diagnosis: patients without NRD and with situs solitus, patients with NRD and situs solitus, patients without NRD and with laterality defects, and patients with both NRD and laterality defects. We assessed the proportion of children diagnosed with PCD within the first three and the first 12 months of life, and the proportion diagnosed later at ages 1–4, 5–9, 10–14, or 15–19 years. We also compared age at diagnosis using a Kruskal–Wallis test [24], followed by pairwise comparisons between groups using a Wilcoxon rank sum test [25].

Second, we repeated all analyses in patients who had "definite PCD" based on recent diagnostic guidelines and were younger than 20 years at the time of investigation, because recall of neonatal problems declines with age (subgroupanalysis, Figure 1) [23,26]. We used STATA 15.1 (StataCorp, College Station, TX, USA) for all analyses. While the first dataset is representative of the majority of patients with PCD currently in treatment, the second includes those for whom quality of information on PCD diagnosis and the neonatal period is best.

2.4. Ethics

In most participating countries, researchers are not required to obtain patient informed consent for retrospectively collected anonymized observational data. In countries where informed consent was needed, primary investigators obtained local ethics approval and informed consent for the contribution of their anonymized data to the iPCD cohort for research purposes [21]. In Switzerland, contribution of anonymized data were approved by the Cantonal Ethics Committee of Bern (KEK-BE: 060/2015).

3. Results

Out of the 3824 patients included in the iPCD cohort at the time of the study, 1461 originated from centers that completed also the module on the neonatal period (Figure 1). After excluding patients diagnosed earlier than 2000, 1375 patients were included in the study (extended analysis). The subgroup analysis included 476 patients who were 0–19 years old and had a definite PCD diagnosis (Figure 1). Data came from 11 centers in nine countries: Argentina, Australia, Colombia, Cyprus, Czech Republic, Italy, Norway, Turkey, and the United Kingdom (UK). Seven countries were represented by one center, while Turkey and UK each had two contributing centers.

Of the entire study population (n = 1375), 45% (95% Confidence Interval (CI): 43–48%) had a history of NRD and 42% (95% CI: 40–45%) a laterality defect (Supplementary Materials Table S2). PCD was diagnosed at a median age of 9.8 years. Only 13% of the 1375 were diagnosed during the first 12 months of life, varying from 4% in those with situs solitus and no NRD to 32% in those with NRD and a laterality defect (Table S2). Median age at diagnosis was 12.4 years for patients without NRD and situs solitus, 10.4 years for those with NRD and situs solitus, 8.8 years for those without NRD but with a laterality defect, and 4.5 years for the group combining a history of NRD and laterality defects. In 14% of patients with NRD and a laterality defect, PCD was diagnosed in the first three months of life (Supplementary Materials Table S3). Among patients with NRD but without a laterality defect, PCD was only diagnosed in the first three months of life only in 2.9%. We found a difference in median age at diagnosis between male and female patients (2.6 compared to 4.4 years) but it disappeared after accounting for NRD and laterality defects.

Results were comparable in the subgroup analyses that included only patients 0–19 years with definite PCD diagnosis. Fifty-five percent (95% CI: 50–59%) reported a history of NRD and 50% (95% CI: 46–55%) had a laterality defect (Table 1). Prevalence of NRD and laterality defects varied between centers (Supplementary Materials Table S4). Age at diagnosis overall was lower than in the whole study population and the differences between the four groups more pronounced. Patients were diagnosed at a median age of 3.4 years, varying from less than one year in Norway and Cyprus to 10 years in Turkey (Table 1). Overall, 30% of children with PCD were diagnosed during the first 12 months of life, varying from 13% in those with no NRD and situs solitus, to 21% in those with NRD and situs solitus, 33% in those with a laterality defect but no NRD, and 52% in those with both NRD and a laterality defect.

Table 1. Characteristics of PCD patients aged 0–19 years with a definite PCD diagnosis (n = 476).

Characteristic	N (%)	Age at Diagnosis (in Years) Median (IQR)	N (%) of Patients Diagnosed at 0–12 m
Total	476 (100)	3.36 (0.69–7.76)	144 (30.3)
Sex			
Male	262 (55.0)	2.62 (0.61–7.06)	87 (33.2)
Female	214 (45.0)	4.38 (0.97–8.34)	57 (26.6)
Country of residence			
Argentina	30 (6.3)	1.5 (0.50–5.00)	10 (33.3)
Australia	19 (4.0)	1.26 (0.40–3.78)	9 (47.4)
Colombia	11 (2.3)	6.61 (4.04–8.34)	1 (9.1)
Cyprus	5 (1.0)	0.61 (0.21–0.67)	4 (80.0)
Czech Republic	21 (4.4)	4.75 (1.49–9.28)	4 (19.0)
Italy	89 (18.7)	1.62 (0.38–5.67)	36 (40.4)
Norway	25 (5.3)	0.63 (0.10–7.17)	14 (56.0)
Turkey	31 (6.5)	10.11 (7.37–12.53)	0 (0.0)
United Kingdom	245 (51.5)	3.53 (0.89–8.08)	66 (26.9)
NRD			
No	193 (40.6)	4.96 (1.10–8.44)	43 (22.3)
Yes	261 (54.8)	1.96 (0.50–6.40)	98 (37.5)
No information	22 (4.6)	2.47 (1.42–9.40)	3 (13.6)
Organ laterality			
Situs solitus	218 (45.8)	5.93 (2.00–9.08)	37 (17.0)
Laterality defect	240 (50.4)	1.44 (0.42–5.07)	103 (42.9)
No information	18 (3.8)	6.35 (1.09–9.54)	4 (22.2)
Clinical characteristics groups			
No NRD, situs solitus	114 (24.0)	6.47 (2.73–9.08)	15 (13.2)
NRD, situs solitus	132 (27.7)	5.44 (1.50–9.41)	27 (20.5)
No NRD, laterality defect	91 (19.1)	2.51 (0.67–6.97)	30 (33.0)
NRD, laterality defect	139 (29.2)	0.91 (0.31–3.17)	72 (52.0)

PCD: primary ciliary dyskinesia, NRD: neonatal respiratory distress, IQR: interquartile range.

Table 2 and Figure 2 show a detailed breakdown of age at diagnosis for the four patient groups. For infants with NRD and a laterality defect, median age at diagnosis was 0.9 years (11 months): 21% were diagnosed within three months of birth, a further 31% before the age of 12 months, and most (80%) before they reached five years. Children with laterality defects not presenting with neonatal respiratory symptoms were also diagnosed relatively early (median age 2.5 years): one-third were diagnosed during infancy and 57% before the age of five years. These results stand in contrast with those for infants with situs solitus. Among infants who presented with NRD and situs solitus, only 6% were diagnosed with PCD within three months, 20% within the first year of life, and only 39% by age five. Of the children who had situs solitus, PCD was diagnosed at a median age of 5.4 years if they had NRD, but of 6.5 years if they had no neonatal symptoms (p = 0.15, Figure 2), suggesting that neonatal symptoms alone, in the absence of situs anomalies, do not lead to diagnostic testing for PCD.

Table 2. Age at diagnosis of PCD patients aged 0–19 years with definite PCD diagnosis, per clinical characteristics group, based on reported NRD and organ laterality (n = 476).

Clinical Characteristics Groups	Age at Diagnosis n (%)						Total
	0–2 m	3–11 m	1–4 yrs	5–9 yrs	10–14 yrs	> 14 yrs	
No NRD, situs solitus	2 (1.7)	13 (11.4)	24 (21.1)	46 (40.4)	26 (22.8)	3 (2.6)	114 (100)
NRD, situs solitus	8 (6.1)	19 (14.4)	25 (18.9)	45 (34.1)	34 (25.7)	1 (0.8)	132 (100)
No NRD, laterality defect	6 (6.6)	24 (26.3)	22 (24.2)	27 (29.7)	11 (12.1)	1 (1.1)	91 (100)
NRD, laterality defect	29 (20.9)	43 (30.9)	39 (28.1)	20 (14.4)	7 (5.0)	1 (0.7)	139 (100)
TOTAL	45 (9.4)	99 (20.8)	110 (23.1)	138 (29.0)	78 (16.4)	6 (1.3)	476 (100)

PCD: primary ciliary dyskinesia, NRD: neonatal respiratory distress, m: months, yrs: years. Age 0–2 months corresponds to 0–2.999 months, similar for all age groups.

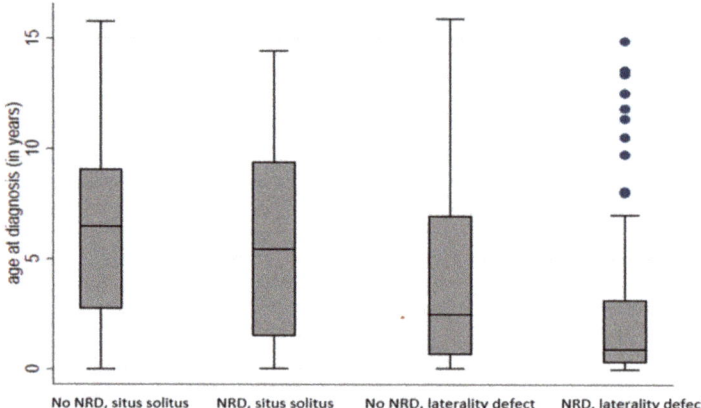

Figure 2. Age at diagnosis of PCD patients (n = 476) aged 0–19 years with definite PCD diagnosis, per clinical characteristics group. PCD: primary ciliary dyskinesia, NRD: neonatal respiratory distress.

Each box represents the median and interquartile range (IQR) of age at diagnosis for the respective group (in years). The whiskers represent the range of age at diagnosis and the dots represent outliers; pairwise comparisons between the four groups using a Wilcoxon rank sum test corrected for multiple testing (Benjamini–Hochberg) resulted in $p \leq 0.003$, with the exemption of the comparison between infants with situs solitus and no NRD and infants with situs solitus and NRD ($p = 0.150$).

4. Discussion

This is the first large multinational study that describes the proportion of infants with PCD who presented with respiratory distress after birth and the age they were diagnosed. Among the 55% of children with PCD in the iPCD cohort who reported NRD, those who also had situs inversus were diagnosed with PCD relatively early, at a median age of 0.9 years. Children who had no laterality defect were diagnosed at a median age of 6 years, independently of whether or not they had presented with NRD. This suggests that although NRD in infants with PCD has typical features, the diagnosis is usually missed by neonatologists and pediatricians unless patients also present with situs anomalies.

The iPCD cohort is the largest dataset on patients with PCD worldwide, and is representative of and follows currently diagnosed PCD patients in developed countries [21]. We analyzed the whole dataset, which was large and representative of the majority of PCD patients in medical follow-up; then, to reduce uncertainties in diagnosis of PCD and of recall bias regarding the neonatal presentation, we repeated all analyses for patients with a definite diagnosis of PCD based on current diagnostic criteria, including those who were younger than 20 when neonatal history was taken. Still, our study has limitations. In particular, since information on NRD was collected retrospectively, there was a lack of standardization for the definition of NRD between centers, and for some participants this information was patient- or parent-reported. This could possibly explain the lower prevalence of NRD compared to previous studies [17–19]. We also lacked detailed information on the characteristics of the neonatal disease presentation, such as onset and duration of respiratory distress, exact diagnoses and treatments given at the hospital, and results of x-rays and other investigations. Thus, we cannot state whether the clinical picture of NRD was as typical as that previously described [19]. There are few other studies to compare our findings with. Prevalence of NRD in our study was lower than in a single-center study from Canada (91%), which was based on a chart review of neonatal records [19]. Similarly, a multicenter study including 205 children with PCD from North American centers reported a higher (81%) prevalence of NRD [18]. In our study, neonatal history was usually obtained from the patients or the parents at the time of PCD diagnosis. NRD prevalence varied between countries and was low in some centers. In several centers the prevalence of NRD was higher (e.g., 68–100%), suggesting that the recorded average might be an underestimation due to a less detailed history in some centers. In another study of consecutively referred and diagnosed patients with PCD from the UK, 56 of 75 patients (75%) reported neonatal chest symptoms [17]. As in our study, these data were also collected from patients or their parents at the first diagnostic visit. The prevalence found was higher than ours (45%). A possible explanation for this difference might be that the definition used for NRD in the UK study was wider, as it included also other neonatal chest symptoms, while in our study it included only history of NRD (with the exception of one center).

What implication does this have for clinical management? Given that up to 5% of term-born infants present with some type of respiratory distress and assuming that 50% of infants with PCD present with NRD while estimating prevalence of PCD as 1 in 10000, it follows that around 1 in 500 term neonates with NRD has PCD [27]. Performing the complex and expensive set of diagnostic tests to diagnose one infant with PCD in 500 is unrealistic, if not impossible. However, the data from the Canadian case-control study suggests (though this needs to be confirmed in other populations) that the clinical picture of NRD is quite typical in PCD, and it differs substantially from much more common diagnoses such as transient tachypnea of the newborn or peripartum pneumothorax, given that infants with PCD often required supplemental oxygen for several days to weeks and had lobar collapse. In that study, the combination of oxygen therapy for more than two days and lobar collapse in the chest x-ray had a sensitivity of 83% for detecting PCD [19]. Thus, term-born infants with late onset but long-duration respiratory distress not needing intubation, and with a radiological picture typical for PCD, could be picked up as suspected PCD candidates and referred for diagnosis from the first days of life. In our study, the average age at diagnosis for children in some centers (e.g., in Norway and Cyprus was 7–8 months) suggests that, although the number of patients was low, earlier diagnosis is possible.

5. Conclusions

We found that only a minority of infants with PCD who present typical symptoms in the neonatal period are diagnosed early, but examples from some countries suggest early diagnosis is possible. In term neonates with NRD, better recognition of the typical clinical picture associated with PCD during the neonatal period could increase the proportion of neonates referred for detailed PCD diagnostic testing. We believe that if the typical clinical picture of PCD in neonates can be better characterized and its recognition improved during the neonatal period, more infants suffering from PCD could receive appropriate care sooner.

Supplementary Materials: The following are available online at http://www.mdpi.com/2077-0383/9/9/2871/s1, Table S1: Inclusion criteria for the total study population and for the subgroup of younger patients with definite PCD, Table S2. Characteristics of PCD patients diagnosed after 2000 ($n = 1375$), Table S3. Age at diagnosis of PCD patients of all ages, per clinical characteristics group, based on reported NRD and organ laterality ($n = 1375$), Table S4. Prevalence of NRD and laterality defects in PCD patients aged 0–19 years with definite PCD diagnosis by country ($n = 476$).

Author Contributions: Conceptualization, M.G. and C.E.K.; data curation, M.G. and F.S.H., methodology, M.G. and F.S.H.; writing—original draft preparation, M.G. and C.E.K.; writing—review and editing, M.G., F.S.H., A.B., S.C., A.H., R.A.H., B.K., V.M., L.M., C.O., U.O., S.S., S.U., P.Y., S.M.S., and C.E.K.; project administration, M.G.; funding acquisition, C.E.K. All authors have read and agreed to the published version of the manuscript.

Funding: This research was funded by the Swiss National Foundation (SNF 320030B_192804). The setting up of the iPCD Cohort (salaries, consumables, and equipment) was funded by the EU FP7 project BESTCILIA (http://bestcilia.eu) and several Swiss funding bodies including the Lung Leagues of Bern, St Gallen, Vaud, Ticino, and Valais, and the Milena Carvajal Pro-Kartagener Foundation. Dr. Goutaki is funded by an Ambizione fellowship by the Swiss National Foundation (PZ00P3_185923). Data collection and management at each site was funded according to local arrangements. The Czech cohort data collection has been supported by the grant No. NV19-07-00210 by the Ministry of Health, Czech Republic. PCD research at the University of Leicester is supported by the NIHR GOSH BRC. The views expressed are those of the author(s) and not necessarily those of the NHS, the NIHR, or the Department of Health. Most participating researchers and data contributors participate in the ERS clinical research collaboration BEAT-PCD and the ERN-LUNG (PCD core).

Acknowledgments: We thank all the patients with PCD in the cohort and their families, and especially the PCD patient organizations for their close collaboration. We also thank all the researchers in the participating centers who were involved in data collection and data entry, and worked closely with us through the whole process of participating to the iPCD Cohort. We thank Christopher Ritter (Institute of Social and Preventive Medicine, University of Bern, Switzerland) for his editorial suggestions to this manuscript.

Conflicts of Interest: The authors declare no conflict of interest.

References

1. Kuehni, C.E.; Frischer, T.; Strippoli, M.P.; Maurer, E.; Bush, A.; Nielsen, K.G.; Escribano, A.; Lucas, J.S.; Yiallouros, P.; Omran, H.; et al. Factors influencing age at diagnosis of primary ciliary dyskinesia in European children. *Eur. Respir. J.* **2010**, *36*, 1248–1258. [CrossRef] [PubMed]
2. Lucas, J.S.; Walker, W.T.; Kuehni, C.E.; Lazor, R. Primary Ciliary Dyskinesia. *Orphan Lung Dis. Eur. Respir. Monogr.* **2011**, *54*, 201–217.
3. O'Callaghan, C.; Chetcuti, P.; Moya, E. High prevalence of primary ciliary dyskinesia in a British Asian population. *Arch. Dis. Child.* **2010**, *95*, 51–52. [CrossRef] [PubMed]
4. Onoufriadis, A.; Paff, T.; Antony, D.; Shoemark, A.; Micha, D.; Kuyt, B.; Schmidts, M.; Petridi, S.; Dankert-Roelse, J.E.; Haarman, E.G.; et al. Splice-site mutations in the axonemal outer dynein arm docking complex gene CCDC114 cause primary ciliary dyskinesia. *Am. J. Hum. Genet.* **2013**, *92*, 88–98. [CrossRef] [PubMed]
5. Bequignon, E.; Dupuy, L.; Zerah-Lancner, F.; Bassinet, L.; Honore, I.; Legendre, M.; Devars du Mayne, M.; Escabasse, V.; Crestani, B.; Maitre, B.; et al. Critical Evaluation of Sinonasal Disease in 64 Adults with Primary Ciliary Dyskinesia. *J. Clin. Med.* **2019**, *8*, 619. [CrossRef]
6. Raidt, J.; Werner, C. Chronic rhinosinusitis in non-cystic fibrosis bronchiectasis and primary ciliary dyskinesia. In *The Nose and Sinuses in Respiratory Disorders (ERS Monograph)*; Bachert, C., Bourdin, A., Chanez, P., Eds.; European Respiratory Society: Sheffield, UK, 2017; pp. 148–161.
7. Shapiro, A.J.; Davis, S.D.; Ferkol, T.; Dell, S.D.; Rosenfeld, M.; Olivier, K.N.; Sagel, S.D.; Milla, C.; Zariwala, M.A.; Wolf, W.; et al. Laterality defects other than situs inversus totalis in primary ciliary dyskinesia: Insights into situs ambiguus and heterotaxy. *Chest* **2014**, *146*, 1176–1186. [CrossRef]
8. Kennedy, M.P.; Omran, H.; Leigh, M.W.; Dell, S.; Morgan, L.; Molina, P.L.; Robinson, B.V.; Minnix, S.L.; Olbrich, H.; Severin, T.; et al. Congenital heart disease and other heterotaxic defects in a large cohort of patients with primary ciliary dyskinesia. *Circulation* **2007**, *115*, 2814–2821. [CrossRef]
9. Halbeisen, F.S.; Goutaki, M.; Spycher, B.D.; Amirav, I.; Behan, L.; Boon, M.; Hogg, C.; Casaulta, C.; Crowley, S.; Haarman, E.G.; et al. Lung function in patients with primary ciliary dyskinesia: An iPCD Cohort study. *Eur. Respir. J.* **2018**, *52*, 1801040. [CrossRef]
10. Kennedy, M.P.; Noone, P.G.; Leigh, M.W.; Zariwala, M.A.; Minnix, S.L.; Knowles, M.R.; Molina, P.L. High-resolution CT of patients with primary ciliary dyskinesia. *AJR Am. J. Roentgenol.* **2007**, *188*, 1232–1238. [CrossRef]
11. Shah, A.; Shoemark, A.; MacNeill, S.J.; Bhaludin, B.; Rogers, A.; Bilton, D.; Hansell, D.M.; Wilson, R.; Loebinger, M.R. A longitudinal study characterising a large adult primary ciliary dyskinesia population. *Eur. Respir. J.* **2016**, *48*, 441–450. [CrossRef]

12. Cohen-Cymberknoh, M.; Weigert, N.; Gileles-Hillel, A.; Breuer, O.; Simanovsky, N.; Boon, M.; De Boeck, K.; Barbato, A.; Snijders, D.; Collura, M.; et al. Clinical impact of Pseudomonas aeruginosa colonization in patients with Primary Ciliary Dyskinesia. *Respir. Med.* **2017**, *131*, 241–246. [CrossRef] [PubMed]
13. Frija-Masson, J.; Bassinet, L.; Honore, I.; Dufeu, N.; Housset, B.; Coste, A.; Papon, J.F.; Escudier, E.; Burgel, P.R.; Maitre, B. Clinical characteristics, functional respiratory decline and follow-up in adult patients with primary ciliary dyskinesia. *Thorax* **2017**, *72*, 154–160. [CrossRef] [PubMed]
14. Kouis, P.; Goutaki, M.; Halbeisen, F.S.; Gioti, I.; Middleton, N.; Amirav, I.; Israeli, P.C.D.C.; Barbato, A.; Italian, P.C.D.C.; Behan, L.; et al. Prevalence and course of disease after lung resection in primary ciliary dyskinesia: A cohort & nested case-control study. *Respir. Res.* **2019**, *20*, 212. [CrossRef]
15. Noone, P.G.; Leigh, M.W.; Sannuti, A.; Minnix, S.L.; Carson, J.L.; Hazucha, M.; Zariwala, M.A.; Knowles, M.R. Primary ciliary dyskinesia: Diagnostic and phenotypic features. *Am. J. Respir. Crit. Care Med.* **2004**, *169*, 459–467. [CrossRef]
16. Kuehni, C.E.; Goutaki, M.; Rubbo, B.; Lucas, J.S. Management of primary ciliary dyskinesia: Current practice and future perspectives. In *Bronchiectasis (ERS Monograph)*; Chalmers, J.D., Polverino, E., Aliberti, S., Eds.; European Respiratory Society: Sheffield, UK, 2018; pp. 282–299.
17. Behan, L.; Dimitrov, B.D.; Kuehni, C.E.; Hogg, C.; Carroll, M.; Evans, H.J.; Goutaki, M.; Harris, A.; Packham, S.; Walker, W.T.; et al. PICADAR: A diagnostic predictive tool for primary ciliary dyskinesia. *Eur. Respir. J.* **2016**, *47*, 1103–1112. [CrossRef]
18. Leigh, M.W.; Ferkol, T.W.; Davis, S.D.; Lee, H.S.; Rosenfeld, M.; Dell, S.D.; Sagel, S.D.; Milla, C.; Olivier, K.N.; Sullivan, K.M.; et al. Clinical Features and Associated Likelihood of Primary Ciliary Dyskinesia in Children and Adolescents. *Ann. Am. Thorac. Soc.* **2016**, *13*, 1305–1313. [CrossRef] [PubMed]
19. Mullowney, T.; Manson, D.; Kim, R.; Stephens, D.; Shah, V.; Dell, S. Primary ciliary dyskinesia and neonatal respiratory distress. *Pediatrics* **2014**, *134*, 1160–1166. [CrossRef]
20. Goutaki, M.; Meier, A.B.; Halbeisen, F.S.; Lucas, J.S.; Dell, S.D.; Maurer, E.; Casaulta, C.; Jurca, M.; Spycher, B.D.; Kuehni, C.E. Clinical manifestations in primary ciliary dyskinesia: Systematic review and meta-analysis. *Eur. Respir. J.* **2016**, *48*, 1081–1095. [CrossRef]
21. Goutaki, M.; Maurer, E.; Halbeisen, F.S.; Amirav, I.; Barbato, A.; Behan, L.; Boon, M.; Casaulta, C.; Clement, A.; Crowley, S.; et al. The international primary ciliary dyskinesia cohort (iPCD Cohort): Methods and first results. *Eur. Respir. J.* **2017**, *49*, 1601181. [CrossRef]
22. Halbeisen, F.S.; Shoemark, A.; Barbato, A.; Boon, M.; Carr, S.; Crowley, S.; Hirst, R.; Karadag, B.; Koerner-Rettberg, C.; Loebinger, M.R.; et al. Time trends in diagnostic testing for PCD in Europe. *Eur. Respir. J.* **2019**, *54*, 1900528. [CrossRef]
23. Lucas, J.S.; Barbato, A.; Collins, S.A.; Goutaki, M.; Behan, L.; Caudri, D.; Dell, S.; Eber, E.; Escudier, E.; Hirst, R.A.; et al. European Respiratory Society guidelines for the diagnosis of primary ciliary dyskinesia. *Eur. Respir. J.* **2017**, *49*, 1601090. [CrossRef] [PubMed]
24. Kruskal, W.H.; Wallis, W.A. Use of Ranks in One-Criterion Variance Analysis. *J. Am. Stat. Assoc.* **1952**, *47*, 583–621. [CrossRef]
25. Wilcoxon, F. Individual Comparisons by Ranking Methods. *Biom. Bull.* **1945**, *1*, 80–83. [CrossRef]
26. Kuehni, C.E.; Lucas, J.S. Diagnosis of primary ciliary dyskinesia: Summary of the ERS Task Force report. *Breathe (Sheffield)* **2017**, *13*, 166–178. [CrossRef] [PubMed]
27. Hermansen, C.L.; Lorah, K.N. Respiratory distress in the newborn. *Am. Fam. Physician* **2007**, *76*, 987–994.

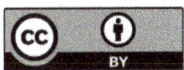

© 2020 by the authors. Licensee MDPI, Basel, Switzerland. This article is an open access article distributed under the terms and conditions of the Creative Commons Attribution (CC BY) license (http://creativecommons.org/licenses/by/4.0/).

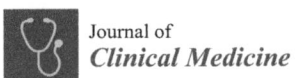 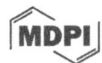

Article

Immunofluorescence Analysis as a Diagnostic Tool in a Spanish Cohort of Patients with Suspected Primary Ciliary Dyskinesia

Noelia Baz-Redón [1,2,†], Sandra Rovira-Amigo [1,2,3,4,†], Mónica Fernández-Cancio [1,4], Silvia Castillo-Corullón [5], Maria Cols [6], M. Araceli Caballero-Rabasco [7], Óscar Asensio [8], Carlos Martín de Vicente [9], Maria del Mar Martínez-Colls [10], Alba Torrent-Vernetta [1,2,3,4], Inés de Mir-Messa [1,3], Silvia Gartner [1,3], Ignacio Iglesias-Serrano [1,3], Ana Díez-Izquierdo [1,3], Eva Polverino [1,11], Esther Amengual-Pieras [12], Rosanel Amaro-Rodríguez [13], Montserrat Vendrell [14,15,16], Marta Mumany [17], María Teresa Pascual-Sánchez [18], Belén Pérez-Dueñas [1,3], Ana Reula [19,20], Amparo Escribano [5,20,21], Francisco Dasí [20,21], Miguel Armengot-Carceller [16,19,20,22], Marta Garrido-Pontnou [23], Núria Camats-Tarruella [1,4,‡] and Antonio Moreno-Galdó [1,2,3,4,*,‡]

1. Vall d'Hebron Institut de Recerca (VHIR), Vall d'Hebron Hospital Universitari, Vall d'Hebron Barcelona Hospital Campus, 08035 Barcelona, Spain; noelia.baz@vhir.org (N.B.-R.); srovi@yahoo.es (S.R.-A.); mfcancio75@gmail.com (M.F.-C.); atorrentvernetta@gmail.com (A.T.-V.); idemir@vhebron.net (I.d.M.-M.); silviagartner@gmail.com (S.G.); nachotela@gmail.com (I.I.-S.); anadiezizquierdo@gmail.com (A.D.-I.); evapo74@gmail.com (E.P.); belen.perez@vhir.org (B.P.-D.); nuria.camats@vhir.org (N.C.-T.)
2. Department of Pediatrics, Obstetrics, Gynecology, Preventative Medicine and Public Health. Universitat Autònoma de Barcelona, 08193 Barcelona, Spain
3. Department of Pediatrics, Vall d'Hebron Hospital Universitari, Vall d'Hebron Barcelona Hospital Campus, 08035 Barcelona, Spain
4. CIBER of Rare Diseases (CIBERER), Instituto de Salud Carlos III (ISCIII), 28029 Madrid, Spain
5. Pediatric Pulmonology Unit, Hospital Clínico Universitario de Valencia, 46010 Valencia, Spain; castillo_sil@gva.es (S.C.-C.); aescribano@separ.es (A.E.)
6. Pediatric Pulmonology Department and Cystic Fibrosis Unit, Hospital Sant Joan de Déu, 08950 Barcelona, Spain; MCols@sjdhospitalbarcelona.org
7. Pediatric Pulmonology Unit, Department of Pediatrics, Hospital del Mar, 08003 Barcelona, Spain; MACaballeroRabasco@parcdesalutmar.cat
8. Pediatric Pulmonology Unit, Hospital Parc Taulí de Sabadell, 08208 Sabadell, Spain; oasensio58@gmail.com
9. Pediatric Pulmonology Unit, Hospital Miguel Servet, 50009 Zaragoza, Spain; carl_zaragoza@yahoo.es
10. Pediatric Pulmonology Unit, Hospital Germans Trias i Pujol, 08916 Badalona, Spain; mimarmartinez@gmail.com
11. Pneumology Department, Vall d'Hebron Hospital Universitari, Vall d'Hebron Barcelona Hospital Campus, 08035 Barcelona, Spain
12. Department of Pediatrics, Hospital Universitario Son Llàtzer, 07198 Palma de Mallorca, Spain; eamengua@hsll.es
13. Pneumology Department, Hospital Clínic, 08036 Barcelona, Spain; ramaro@clinic.cat
14. Pneumology Department, Hospital Josep Trueta, 17007 Girona, Spain; mvendrell.girona.ics@gencat.cat
15. Girona Biomedical Research Institute (IDIBGI), Universitat de Girona, 17190 Girona, Spain
16. CIBER of Respiratory Diseases (CIBERES), Instituto de Salud Carlos III (ISCIII), 28029 Madrid, Spain; miguel.armengot@gmail.com
17. Pediatric Pulmonology Unit, Consorci Sanitari de Terrassa, 08191 Terrassa, Spain; 39769mme@comb.cat
18. Pediatric Pulmonology Unit, Hospital Universitari Sant Joan de Reus, 43204 Tarragona, Spain; maitepasc@gmail.com
19. Grupo de Biomedicina Molecular, Celular y Genómica, IIS La Fe, 46026 Valencia, Spain; areumar91@gmail.com
20. Department of Paediatrics, Obstetrics and Gynecology, Universitat de Valencia, 46010 Valencia, Spain; Dasi@uv.es
21. UCIM, Rare Respiratory Diseases Research Group, Instituto de Investigación Sanitaria INCLIVA, 46010 Valencia, Spain

22 Otorhinolaryngology Department, Hospital Universitario y Politécnico La Fe, 46026 Valencia, Spain
23 Department of Pathology, Vall d'Hebron Hospital Universitari, Vall d'Hebron Barcelona Hospital Campus, 08035 Barcelona, Spain; magarrido@vhebron.net
* Correspondence: amoreno@vhebron.net
† These authors contributed equally to this work.
‡ Co-last authors.

Received: 20 October 2020; Accepted: 6 November 2020; Published: 9 November 2020

Abstract: Primary ciliary dyskinesia (PCD) is an autosomal recessive rare disease caused by an alteration of ciliary structure. Immunofluorescence, consisting in the detection of the presence and distribution of cilia proteins in human respiratory cells by fluorescence, has been recently proposed as a technique to improve understanding of disease-causing genes and diagnosis rate in PCD. The objective of this study is to determine the accuracy of a panel of four fluorescently labeled antibodies (DNAH5, DNALI1, GAS8 and RSPH4A or RSPH9) as a PCD diagnostic tool in the absence of transmission electron microscopy analysis. The panel was tested in nasal brushing samples of 74 patients with clinical suspicion of PCD. Sixty-eight (91.9%) patients were evaluable for all tested antibodies. Thirty-three cases (44.6%) presented an absence or mislocation of protein in the ciliary axoneme (15 absent and 3 proximal distribution of DNAH5 in the ciliary axoneme, 3 absent DNAH5 and DNALI1, 7 absent DNALI1 and cytoplasmatic localization of GAS8, 1 absent GAS8, 3 absent RSPH9 and 1 absent RSPH4A). Fifteen patients had confirmed or highly likely PCD but normal immunofluorescence results (68.8% sensitivity and 100% specificity). In conclusion, immunofluorescence analysis is a quick, available, low-cost and reliable diagnostic test for PCD, although it cannot be used as a standalone test.

Keywords: cilia; primary ciliary dyskinesia; PCD; immunofluorescence; antibody

1. Introduction

Primary ciliary dyskinesia (PCD) is an autosomal recessive rare disease (1/15,000) caused by an alteration of ciliary structure, which impairs mucociliary clearance [1,2]. Symptoms of PCD may include persistent wet cough from early infancy, recurrent respiratory infections, bronchiectasis, chronic rhinosinusitis, persistent otitis media with effusion and associated conductive hearing loss, male infertility, female subfertility, situs inversus in half of PCD patients [1–3] and heterotaxic defects in 6–12% of cases [4].

Diagnosis is often delayed, with the possibility of an impairment of lung function [1], because of non-specificity of PCD symptoms and limitations of the available techniques [5]. According to the European Respiratory Society (ERS), PCD diagnosis is commonly based on studying the ciliary function by high-speed video-microscopy (HSVM) and ciliary ultrastructure by transmission electron microscopy (TEM) [6]. As there is not a unique gold standard diagnostic test, the ERS [6] and the American Thoracic Society (ATS) [7] have recently proposed the use of different diagnostic techniques to improve the accuracy and diagnosis rate of PCD.

Immunofluorescence (IF) is a technique consisting in the use of fluorescently labeled antibodies for the detection of the presence and distribution of different ciliary proteins in human respiratory cells by fluorescence or confocal microscopy, and it has been recently proposed as a tool to improve the diagnosis rate in PCD and facilitate a better understanding of disease-causing genes [6,7]. Motile respiratory cilia (9 + 2 cilia) are composed of nine peripheral microtubular doublets (composed of A and B tubules) and a central pair (C1 and C2) surrounded by a protein central sheath. An important number of protein complexes are distributed among these microtubule structures: the outer (ODA) and inner dynein arms (IDA), the nexin links, the central sheath and the radial spokes [8,9] (Figure 1). The methodology for IF staining of ciliated respiratory epithelial cells was first described by Omran and Loges [10]. Nowadays, an important number of antibodies against different cilia proteins are available, including antibodies against proteins in ODA, IDA, radial spoke head and dynein regulatory complex [6]. IF is cheaper and easier than other techniques and the use of IF as a diagnostic test in PCD is likely to increase as more antibodies become available [6]. However, studies on the use of IF in diagnostic settings and IF validation studies are necessary to consider IF as a diagnostic tool for PCD in diagnostic cohort studies [6]. The ATS considers the IF as one of the emerging PCD diagnosis techniques, although it has emphasized the lack of consensus on a gold standard for diagnosis and the insufficient sensitivity and specificity when applied to the general population [7].

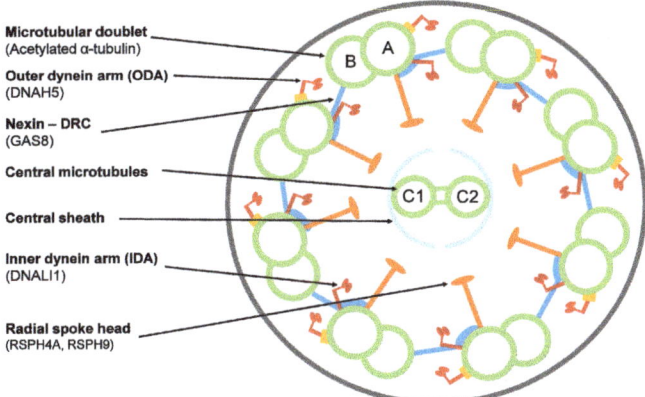

Figure 1. Ciliary axoneme in transverse section indicating the ultrastructural parts and the target proteins by immunofluorescence. Proteins are indicated in parentheses. DRC = dynein regulatory complex. A and B: outer microtubule doublets; C1 and C2: central pair.

A study by Shoemark et al. demonstrated that IF is a useful diagnostic technique and presents the same accuracy as well-performed TEM analysis, which is why the authors support IF as a routine diagnostic test for PCD, especially when TEM expertise or equipment is not available [5]. To our knowledge, this is the only study evaluating the accuracy of conventional IF for the diagnosis of PCD. In a recent study, Liu et al. presented a quantitative super-resolution imaging workflow for the detection of cilia defects thanks to the validation of 21 commercially available IF antibodies. Molecular defects using this super-resolution imaging toolbox were described in 31 clinical PCD cases, including patients with negative TEM results and/or with genetic variants of uncertain significance (VUS) [11].

We hypothesized that an IF panel would be a useful technique to study the cilia structure and improve PCD diagnosis, especially in settings with low availability of TEM results. Our aim was to establish the utility and accuracy for PCD diagnosis of an IF panel in a Spanish cohort of patients with suspected PCD in relation to clinical characteristics, genetics and/or HSVM.

2. Experimental Section

2.1. Patients

This study belongs to a prospective multicentric study including all 74 consecutive patients with a clinical history suggestive of PCD during the period from 2016 to 2020.

This project was approved by the Clinical Research Ethics Committee (CEIC) of Hospital Universitari Vall d'Hebron (PR(AMI)148/2016). Written informed consent was obtained from ≥18-year-old patients, from ≥12-year-old patients and their parents or guardians and from <12-year-old patients' parents or guardians.

The majority of patients attended the Hospital Universitari Vall d'Hebron (HUVH), and patients and samples from other hospitals from Spain were also analyzed: Hospital Sant Joan de Déu (Esplugues de Llobregat, Barcelona), Hospital del Mar (Barcelona), Hospital Parc Taulí (Sabadell, Barcelona), Hospital Germans Trias i Pujol (Badalona, Barcelona), Hospital Clínic (Barcelona), Hospital Miguel Servet (Zaragoza), Hospital Josep Trueta (Girona), Hospital Universitari Sant Joan de Reus (Reus, Tarragona), Consorci Sanitari de Terrassa (Terrasa, Barcelona) and PCD group Valencia (Hospital Universitario y Politécnico la Fe, Hospital Clínico Universitario de Valencia and INCLIVA).

2.2. PCD Diagnostic Evaluation

Patients were evaluated for PCD with a clinical symptoms questionnaire and PICADAR (PrImary CiliARy DyskinesiA Rule) score [12], nasal nitric oxide (nNO), high-speed video-microscopy analysis (HSVM) and genetic testing. In our setting, TEM analysis was available only in a few cases because of logistic difficulties.

ERS guidelines [6] were followed to classify patients as: confirmed PCD (suggestive clinical history with hallmark ciliary ultrastructure defects assessed by TEM and/or presence of pathogenic bi-allelic variants in PCD-associated genes); highly likely PCD (suggestive history with very low nNO and HSVM findings consistently suggestive of PCD after repeated analysis or cell culture); or highly unlikely PCD (weak clinical history, normal nNO and normal HSVM).

Nasal nitric oxide (nNO) measurements were performed using CLD 88sp NO-analyzer (ECO MEDICS, AG, Duerten, Switzerland) according to ERS guidelines [13].

Genetic testing was performed with a high-throughput 44 PCD gene panel using the SeqCap EZ Technology (Roche Nimblegen, Pleasanton, CA, USA) as previously described [14]. Genetic results for most of the patients included in this study have been previously published [14].

HSVM was performed to study ciliary beat frequency (CBF) and ciliary beat pattern (CBP) (local normal values: CBF 8.7–18.8 Hz; CBP ≤20% dyskinetic ciliated cells). Nasal respiratory epithelia were sampled at the inferior nasal meatus with a 2 mm diameter brush submerged in HEPES-supplemented Medium199. A minimum of ten lateral strips with 10 cells each and two overhead axes were captured at 37 °C with an optical microscope coupled to a high-speed video camera (MotionPro® X4, IDT, CA, USA) using MotionPro® X4 software [15].

2.3. Immunofluorescence Technique and Analysis

Nasal-brush respiratory epithelial samples were spread or dropped, air dried and stored at −80 °C until use. Cells were fixed with 4% PFA for 15 min at room temperature (RT), washed 4 times with 1xPBS, permeabilized with 0.2% TritonX100 for 10 min at RT and blocked with 1% fat-free skim milk in PBS overnight at +4 °C to avoid nonspecific binding. Samples were incubated with primary antibodies (all Sigma Aldrich, St. Louis, MO, USA) for 4 h at RT using the following dilutions in 1% skim milk: anti-DNAH5 antibody 1:200, anti-DNALI1 1:100, anti-GAS8 1:200, anti-RSPH4A 1:200 and anti-RSPH9 1:70.

We washed 5 times with 1xPBS at RT (2 washes of 10 min), and all slides were incubated for 45 min at RT with 1:2500 anti-acetylated tubulin antibody (Sigma Aldrich) for cilia localization. After 5 more washes with 1xPBS at RT (2 washes of 10 min), cells were incubated for 30 min at RT with secondary monoclonal anti-rabbit Alexa Fluor 594 and anti-mouse Alexa Fluor 488 antibodies (Thermo Fisher, Waltham, MA, USA). Nuclei DNA was stained with Prolong antifade DAPI (Thermo Fisher).

Slides were analyzed using a fluorescence microscope at X100 magnification. A minimum of ten cells were analyzed for each target protein. The results were considered: (1) normal or present when the protein was present in 8 or more cells, (2) absent or aberrant when the protein was completely absent in the ciliary axoneme or had an abnormal distribution in 8 or more cells, (3) inconclusive when results differed from previously described ones, and (4) insufficient when less than ten cells were observed. In inconclusive or insufficient cases, IF was repeated when possible, following recommendations by Shoemark et al. [5].

Patients were analyzed using antibodies against component proteins for the different structures of the ciliary axoneme: DNAH5 (an ODA component), DNALI1 (an IDA component), GAS8 (a nexin-dynein regulatory complex component) and radial spoke head components RSPH4A (42 patients), RSPH9 (31 patients) or both (1 patient). When this analysis was designed, we specifically chose and optimized these commercial antibodies to detect most cilia defects, following Shoemark et al. [5] and expert recommendations. Anti-acetylated tubulin antibody was used to localize the microtubular doublet (protein location shown in Figure 1).

2.4. Data Analysis

Confirmed and highly likely PCD cases were considered as positive for calculation of sensitivity and specificity. Data were analyzed by using MedCalc Statistical Software version 19.5.3 (MedCalc Software bvba, Ostend, Belgium).

3. Results

Immunofluorescence analysis was performed in a cohort of 74 PCD-suspected patients. Sixty-six percent of patients included in this study were <18 years old (49/74) and the mean age at study was 17.9 years (range 1–63).

After PCD diagnostic evaluation, 25 patients were considered as confirmed PCD, 25 as highly likely and 24 as highly unlikely PCD (Table 1).

Table 1. Immunofluorescence results from 74 primary ciliary dyskinesia (PCD) suspected patients related to the results of the PCD diagnostic evaluation.

		PCD Diagnostic Evaluation		
Immunofluorescence Test Outcome (n = 74)		Confirmed (n = 25)	Highly Likely (n = 25)	Highly Unlikely (n = 24)
Evaluable/Closed	68 (91.9%)	24	24	20
Normal results (all markers presents)	35 (47.3%)	3	12	20
Absent/aberrant results	33 (44.6%)	21	12	0
DNAH5 (-) (ODA)	15			
Proximal DNAH5 (ODA)	3			
DNAH5 (-), DNALI1 (-) (ODA+IDA)	3			
DNALI1 (-), GAS8 (-) (IDA+Nexin-DRC)	7			
GAS8 (-) (Nexin-DRC)	1			
RSPH9 (-) (Radial spoke)	3			
RSPH4A (-) (Radial spoke)	1			
Inconclusive/insufficient results	6 (8.1%)	1	1	4

(-): absent in ciliary axoneme; ODA: outer dynein arm; IDA: inner dynein arm; DRC: dynein regulatory complex.

IF was technically evaluable for all tested antibodies in 68 patients (91.9%), whereas in six, the results were inconclusive/insufficient (8.1%) (Table 1). IF analysis demonstrated an absence or aberrant localization of one or more proteins in the ciliary axoneme in 33 cases: 15 patients presented absent DNAH5; 3 a proximal localization of DNAH5 in ciliary axoneme; 3 patients exhibited absent DNAH5 and DNALI1; 7 showed absent DNALI1 and a cytoplasmatic localization of GAS8; 1 patient presented absent GAS8; 3 showed absent RSPH9; and 1 had absent RSPH4A (Table 1). Figure 2 shows examples of absence/aberrant localization of IF markers in four patients with confirmed PCD.

To evaluate the usefulness of IF analysis as a tool for PCD diagnosis, IF results were compared with those obtained from our PCD gene panel and HSVM analyses (Table 2). The 33 patients with aberrant/absent ciliary axoneme proteins had been diagnosed with confirmed or highly likely PCD. All of them presented a concordant abnormal HSVM and 21 of them presented likely pathogenic variants in PCD-related genes (Table 2). The relation of these abnormal IF results with clinical characteristics and other PCD diagnostic tests for each patient is shown in Table S1.

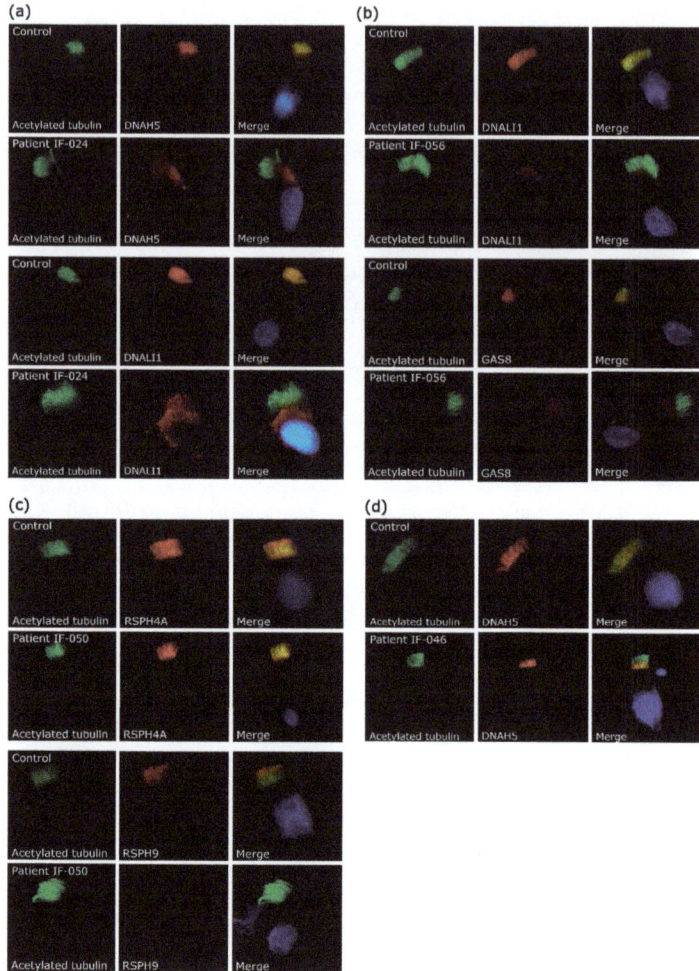

Figure 2. Example results of immunofluorescence technique in control subjects and patients with primary ciliary dyskinesia. The first column shows cilia by acetylated α-tubulin (green); the second column shows the protein of interest (red); and the third column shows the final merged image with the nuclei stained with DAPI (blue). (**a**) Patient IF-024 exhibited absent DNAH5 and DNALI1. (**b**) Patient IF-056 had absent DNALI1 and cytoplasmatic localization of GAS8. (**c**) Patient IF-050 showed a normal axonemal localization of RSPH4A and absent RSPH9. (**d**) Patient IF-046 presented a proximal localization of DNAH5.

Table 2. Correlation among immunofluorescence analysis, high-speed video-microscopy, genetics and clinical characteristics in our PCD patients.

IF Affected Markers (Ultrastructural Part)	#	HSVM	Genetics (#)	PCD Symptoms					
				Neonatal Distress	Upper Respiratory Tract	Lower Respiratory Tract	Bronchiectasis	Chronic Otitis or Hearing loss	Situs Abnormality
DNAH5 (ODA)	15	Completely immotile cilia or residual motility	*CCDC151* (1), *DNAH5* (5), *DNAI2* (4), *TTC25* (1), NA (4)	+/−	+	+	+/−	+/−	+/−
Proximal DNAH5 (ODA)	3	Subtle defects (stiff and disorganized ciliary beat)	*DNAH9* (1), Neg. (2)	−	+	+/−	+/−	+/−	+/−
DNAH5+DNALI1 (ODA+IDA)	3	Completely immotile cilia	Neg. (2), NA (1)	+	+	+	+	+	+/−
DNALI1+GAS8 (IDA+Nexin-DRC)	7	Mainly stiff cilia and immotile cilia	*CCDC39* (3), *CCDC40* (3), NA (1)	+/−	+	+/−	+/−	+/−	+/−
GAS8 (Nexin-DRC)	1	Hyperkinetic stiff cilia	NA (1)	+	+	+	+	+	−
RSPH4A or RSPH9 (Radial spoke)	4	Stiff and circular motion	*RSPH1* (1), *RSPH4A* (1), *RSPH9* (1), NA (1)	+/−	+	+/−	+/−	+/−	−
All markers present (normal result)	3	Hyperkinetic stiff cilia	*DNAH11* (3)	+/−	+	+/−	+/−	+/−	+/−

IF: immunofluorescence; #: number of patients; HSVM: high-speed video-microscopy; ODA: outer dynein arm; IDA: inner dynein arm; DRC: dynein regulatory complex; NA: not available data; Neg.: negative results; +: symptoms present in all patients; −: symptoms absent in all patients; +/−: symptoms present in some patients.

Thirty-five patients had normal distribution or presence of all IF antibodies. The clinical characteristics and results of PCD diagnostic tests for each patient with normal IF are presented in Table S2. We confirmed PCD in three of these patients because they presented likely pathogenic variants in *DNAH11* and hyperkinetic stiff cilia by HSVM (Tables 2 and S2). Another patient presented two variants in *SPAG1*, but there was no concordance with HSVM and IF results (Table S2). Another 11 patients presented normal IF, but abnormal HSVM results together with typical PCD symptoms, so they were considered highly likely PCD (Table S2). Thus far, we have not detected any likely pathogenic genetic variants in these patients. Finally, 20 out of the 33 patients with normal IF were considered highly unlikely to have PCD because of weak clinical history, normal or mild HSVM results and/or negative genetics (Table S2).

It should be mentioned that six (8.1%) samples were not technically evaluable by our IF panel: two cases lacked enough cells to analyze and were considered insufficient; two cases remained inconclusive for one or more antibodies; and two cases resulted in being insufficient for some markers and inconclusive for others (Table S3). Only one patient with insufficient and inconclusive IF sample was diagnosed with PCD because of presenting stiff cilia by HSVM and likely pathogenic variants in *CCDC39*. Among the other cases, four were finally regarded as having no PCD or unlikely to have PCD because of normal or mild HSVM results (Table S3).

Considering all the previous results, IF analysis as a diagnostic test for PCD had a sensitivity of 68.8% (CI 95% 53.7–81.3%) and a specificity of 100% (CI 95% 83.2–100%). In our laboratory, the PCD prevalence (confirmed or highly likely cases) of patients referred for clinical suspicion in the last 4 years was 27.4% (non-published data). Assuming this prevalence, IF positive predictive value would be 100% and the negative predictive value 89.4% (CI 95% 84.8–92.8%).

4. Discussion

In this study, we have explored the diagnostic utility of an immunofluorescence panel of commercial antibodies in 74 patients with clinical suspicion of PCD. A technical evaluable result was possible in 91.9% of cases (Table 1). IF evidenced a protein defect in 44.6% of analyzed patients, all with confirmed or highly likely PCD (Table 1). A normal IF result (47.3% of cases) was seen not only in all non-PCD patients, but also in some patients with confirmed or highly likely PCD. This means that IF detected ciliary structural defects in 68.8% of confirmed or highly likely PCD patients. In our population, IF has shown the highest positive predictive value (a positive value is consistent with a PCD diagnosis) of 100% and a negative predictive value (a normal result may be seen not only in non-PCD patients but also in PCD patients) of 89.4%. Considering our low availability of TEM results, IF was a useful PCD diagnostic test, because it showed a sensitivity (68.8%) close to TEM studies, where 30% of all affected individuals had normal ciliary ultrastructure [16].

To our knowledge, only one previous study by Shoemark et al. [5] evaluated the accuracy of IF in PCD, concluding that IF and TEM have a similar diagnostic rate. Therefore, they proposed IF as a useful diagnostic tool when TEM equipment or expertise is not available, as IF is cheaper, easier to perform, requires more basic equipment and improves the turnaround time [5]. As TEM analysis was not available in most of our cases, we have confirmed that, under these circumstances, IF is a reliable test to study cilia structure. Furthermore, IF may be useful to confirm the results of other diagnostic tests like HSVM and genetics and guide new tests in those cases with absent or aberrant protein/s localization. In Shoemark's study, IF failed to identify 12% of PCD cases [5], which is lower than the 31.3% of normal IF results that we found in our confirmed or highly likely PCD cases. This difference could be related to genetic differences between both series.

DNAH5 absence in ciliary axoneme correlated with immotile cilia by HSVM and variants in genes related to ODA defects concurring with other studies: *DNAH5* [17,18], *DNAI2* [19], *TTC25* [20] and *CCDC151* [21] (Table 2 and Table S1). Moreover, we found proximal axonemal DNAH5 IF staining in three unrelated patients (Figure 2d) with mild clinical symptoms and subtle HSVM defects (mainly stiff and disorganized ciliary beat). One of them presented likely pathogenic variants in *DNAH9*, in concordance with recently published data [22,23] (Tables 2 and S1).

Some of the patients showed absence of both DNAH5 and DNALI1 (Figure 2a) also with completely immotile cilia. We could not find any candidate variant in these patients (Tables 2 and S1). These IF and HSVM results could be explained by genetic alterations in proteins involved in the assembly of both ODA and IDA [24–35] and further studies are warranted.

The patients with absent DNALI1 and abnormal localization (cytoplasmatic) of GAS8 (Figure 2b) had mainly stiff (reduced amplitude) and immotile cilia and likely pathogenic variants in *CCDC39* and *CCDC40* (Tables 2 and S1). These results are consistent with previous description of CCDC39 [36] and CCDC40 [37] as assembling factors of the IDA and the nexin–dynein regulatory complex structures [36–38].

Only one patient presented an absence of GAS8 in ciliary axoneme. This patient had hyperkinetic stiff cilia and respiratory symptoms beginning at neonatal age. These results could be explained by defects in the nexin–dynein regulatory complex (DRC) subunits, as previously described [39–41].

In our IF approach, radial spoke defects were first studied with the RSPH4A antibody and later with RSPH9. We decided to switch to RSPH9 because it is more informative for detecting all radial spoke head defects, and it has been recommended due to its reported absence from ciliary axonemes in radial spoke mutant cells [5,42]. In fact, one of our patients had normal RSPH4A, but absent RSPH9 (Figure 2c). Radial spoke defects in our patients were related to situs solitus and two different HSVM patterns: circular motion and stiff cilia, consistent with previously reported data (Tables 2 and S1) [42–44].

Our IF panel could not detect defects caused by *DNAH11* genetic variants in our patients, consistent with previously reported data [45]. For this reason, it would be interesting to include an anti-DNAH11 antibody in the IF panel, considering that it is commercially available, but it has not been optimized. As it happens with DNAH11, other ciliary proteins have been described to cause none or subtle ultrastructural defects: HYDIN [46], STK36 [47] and, most recently, SPEF2 [48]. STK36 has been described as a protein involved in the interaction between the central pair and the radial spoke [47]. HYDIN and SPEF2 have been functionally described to cause central pair defects in humans, and mutants of both proteins can be detected using antibodies against SPEF2 [48]. These ultrastructural defects could explain some of our normal IF results in highly likely PCD patients.

Some patients could not be resolved by IF as analysis was inconclusive and/or insufficient for some of the target proteins, requiring reevaluation of new brushing samples. Blood and mucus in the IF samples were found to be confounding factors in the analysis in a previous publication [5]. From our experience, we considered the slides with nasal brush sample prepared by dropping a better option than those by spreading. Slides with a dropped sample allowed a faster analysis due to having more cells in a smaller area. In addition, when the sample contained mucus, analysis was more complicated in spread samples, and usually there were not enough viable cells to complete the analysis.

The major limitation of the IF analysis is that, because of the use of primary antibodies directed to specific proteins, defects in unrelated proteins may be missed [5]. Moreover, patients with partial defects or missense mutations have been reported to have normal IF results [5], although we did not have any case with this particular observation in our cohort. As new genes and proteins related to PCD are discovered, the IF antibody panels may need to be revised and expanded in the future for an accurate diagnosis [49]. In fact, antibodies against a high number of ciliary proteins are already commercially available, although most of them have not yet been tested and/or validated for immunofluorescence or in human respiratory tissue [11]. For this reason, the optimization of antibodies in nasal brushing samples is difficult and time-consuming. Furthermore, from our experience, we have not even been able to properly optimize some commercially available antibodies, i.e., DNAH11. Further antibody optimization is necessary, and, as a matter of fact, Liu et al.'s extensive IF technical protocols may help with this [11]. Another pitfall is the lack of consensus regarding the performance of the IF technique and, more importantly, the agreement in the IF considerations when the analysis is performed. Currently, a consensus statement on IF, initiated during the European BEAT-PCD 2019, is on the way.

One important limitation of measuring the accuracy of IF for PCD diagnosis is the lack of a gold standard reference against which to measure it. In our study, we use the ERS task force criteria [6] assuming as a standard for comparison confirmed and highly likely PCD cases, with the added limitation of low availability of TEM analysis.

Moreover, the positive rate of our series was quite high (25 confirmed and 25 highly likely of 74 cases). This is related to a previous pre-screening for IF study of cases with more suggestive clinical symptoms.

Taking all into account, we propose a two-step IF analysis: a first panel with DNAH5, DNALI1, GAS8 and RSPH9 and, in cases with normal IF and consistent PCD suspicion (clinical symptoms and other techniques), a second IF round with antibodies against ciliary components associated with none or subtle ultrastructural defects: DNAH11 [45], STK36 [47] and SPEF2 [48]. Shoemark et al. [5] also recommended a first antibody panel with DNAH5, GAS8 and RSPH9 and omitted DNALI1 because its absence always coexists with an absence of DNAH5 or GAS8 [5]. This recommendation is supported by our cohort results, but as TEM is mostly unavailable and we are using IF results to clarify the genetics, we considered to maintain anti-DNALI1 antibody in our IF studies. Therefore, our proposed two-step IF analysis may be used in cases with non-available TEM. Alternatively, centers with available TEM analysis might use a first step IF panel with DNAH11, SPEF2, GAS8 and RSPH9 antibodies, omitting DNAH5 and DNALI1. For the translation to clinical diagnosis, Liu et al. also proposed a restricted 10-antibody panel (instead of 21) based on proteins which are non-detectable by TEM or those indirectly detecting mislocalization of other proteins (DNAH5, DNAH11, DNALI1, GAS8, CCDC65, RSPH4A, RSPH9, RPGR, OFD1 and SPEF2) [11]. Although a quantitative super-resolution imaging tool, such as the one proposed by Liu et al. [11], gives much more information and may solve so-called difficult or unsolved cases, it would be hard to implement in our clinical setting due to its high costs in time and personnel.

To conclude, the presented results confirm that IF is a reliable diagnosis technique for PCD (with a sensitivity of 68.8% and a specificity of 100%), even when TEM analysis is unavailable, although it cannot be used as a standalone test. Considering our results, we propose IF as a cheap, easy and widely available test to include in PCD diagnosis.

Supplementary Materials: The following are available online at http://www.mdpi.com/2077-0383/9/11/3603/s1, Table S1: Patients with absence or aberrant distribution of target proteins by immunofluorescence and correlation with other PCD analysis techniques, Table S2: Patients with normal localization of target proteins by immunofluorescence and correlation with other PCD analysis techniques, Table S3: Patients with inconclusive and/or insufficient immunofluorescence results and correlation with other PCD analysis techniques.

Author Contributions: A.M.-G. and N.C.-T. were responsible for the conception and design of this study. N.B.-R., N.C.-T., M.F.-C., M.G.-P., S.R.-A., M.A.C.-R, F.D. and A.R. performed immunofluorescence studies and/or diagnostic PCD studies. S.R.-A., S.C.-C., M.C., M.A.C.-R., O.A., C.M.d.V., M.d.M.M.-C., A.T.-V., I.M.-M., S.G., I.I.-S., A.D.-I., E.P., E.A.-P., R.A.-R., M.V., M.M., M.T.P.-S., B.P.-D., A.R., A.E., F.D. and M.A.-C. recruited the patients and undertook the data collection. N.B.-R., N.C.-T. and A.M.-G. performed statistical analysis. N.B.-R., N.C.-T., S.R.-A. and A.M.-G. drafted the manuscript. All remaining authors revised and approved the manuscript before submission. All authors have read and agreed to the published version of the manuscript.

Funding: This research was funded by a grant from the Health Research and Development Strategy (AES) of Instituto de Salud Carlos III (ISCIII) (PI16/01233), co-financed by the European Regional Development Fund, Smart Growth Operational Programme 2014–2020, and with grants from the Spanish Society of Pediatric Pulmonology (SENP, 2016) and the Catalan Pneumology Foundation (FUCAP, 2016). N.C.-T. received a grant for a Short Term Scientific Mission from COST Action BM1407. It was also supported by the CIBER of Rare Diseases (CIBERER, ISCIII) U-712 to N.C.-T. and M.F.-C.

Acknowledgments: The authors have participated in COST Action BM1407 Translational research in primary ciliary dyskinesia: bench, bedside, and population perspectives (BEAT PCD). A.M.-G. and S.R.-A. participate at ERN-LUNG. This work has been carried out within the framework of the Doctorate Program of Pediatrics, Obstetrics and Gynecology of Universitat Autònoma de Barcelona.

Conflicts of Interest: The authors declare no conflict of interest.

References

1. Lucas, J.S.; Burgess, A.; Mitchison, H.M.; Moya, E.; Williamson, M.; Hogg, C. Diagnosis and Management of Primary Ciliary Dyskinesia. *Arch. Dis. Child.* **2014**, *99*, 850–856. [CrossRef] [PubMed]
2. Reula, A.; Lucas, J.S.; Moreno-Galdó, A.; Romero, T.; Milara, X.; Carda, C.; Mata-Roig, M.; Escribano, A.; Dasi, F.; Armengot-Carceller, M. New Insights in Primary Ciliary Dyskinesia. *Expert Opin. Orphan Drugs* **2017**, *5*, 537–548. [CrossRef]
3. Wallmeier, J.; Nielsen, K.G.; Kuehni, C.E.; Lucas, J.S.; Leigh, M.W.; Zariwala, M.A.; Omran, H. Motile Ciliopathies. *Nat. Rev. Dis. Prim.* **2020**, *6*, 1–29. [CrossRef] [PubMed]
4. Shapiro, A.J.; Davis, S.D.; Ferkol, T.; Dell, S.D.; Rosenfeld, M.; Olivier, K.N.; Sagel, S.D.; Milla, C.; Zariwala, M.A.; Wolf, W.; et al. Laterality Defects Other Than Situs Inversus Totalis in Primary Ciliary Dyskinesia. *Chest* **2014**, *146*, 1176–1186. [CrossRef] [PubMed]
5. Shoemark, A.; Frost, E.; Dixon, M.; Ollosson, S.; Kilpin, K.; Patel, M.; Scully, J.; Rogers, A.V.; Mitchison, H.M.; Bush, A.; et al. Accuracy of Immunofluorescence in the Diagnosis of Primary Ciliary Dyskinesia. *Am. J. Respir. Crit. Care Med.* **2017**, *196*, 94–101. [CrossRef] [PubMed]
6. Lucas, J.S.; Barbato, A.; Collins, S.A.; Goutaki, M.; Behan, L.; Caudri, D.; Dell, S.; Eber, E.; Escudier, E.; Hirst, R.A.; et al. European Respiratory Society Guidelines for the Diagnosis of Primary Ciliary Dyskinesia. *Eur. Respir. J.* **2017**, *49*, 1601090. [CrossRef]
7. Shapiro, A.J.; Davis, S.D.; Polineni, D.; Manion, M.; Rosenfeld, M.; Dell, S.D.; Chilvers, M.; Ferkol, T.W.; Zariwala, M.A.; Sagel, S.D.; et al. Diagnosis of Primary Ciliary Dyskinesia. An Official American Thoracic Society Clinical Practice Guideline. *Am. J. Respir. Crit. Care Med.* **2018**, *197*, e24–e39. [CrossRef]
8. Ibañez-Tallon, I.; Heintz, N.; Omran, H. To Beat or Not to Beat: Roles of Cilia in Development and Disease. *Hum. Mol. Genet.* **2003**, *12*, R27–R35. [CrossRef]
9. Olm, M.A.K.; Caldini, E.G.; Mauad, T. Diagnosis of Primary Ciliary Dyskinesia. *J. Bras. Pneumol.* **2015**, *41*, 251–263. [CrossRef]
10. Omran, H.; Loges, N.T. Immunofluorescence Staining of Ciliated Respiratory Epithelial Cells. *Methods Cell Biol.* **2009**, *91*, 123–133. [CrossRef]
11. Liu, Z.; Nguyen, Q.P.H.; Guan, Q.; Albulescu, A.; Erdman, L.; Mahdaviyeh, Y.; Kang, J.; Ouyang, H.; Hegele, R.G.; Moraes, T.J.; et al. A Quantitative Super-Resolution Imaging Toolbox for Diagnosis of Motile Ciliopathies. *Sci. Transl. Med.* **2020**, *12*, eaay0071. [CrossRef]
12. Behan, L.; Dimitrov, B.D.; Kuehni, C.E.; Hogg, C.; Carroll, M.; Evans, H.J.; Goutaki, M.; Harris, A.; Packham, S.; Walker, W.T.; et al. PICADAR: A Diagnostic Predictive Tool for Primary Ciliary Dyskinesia. *Eur. Respir. J.* **2016**, *47*, 1103–1112. [CrossRef]
13. Horváth, I.; Barnes, P.J.; Loukides, S.; Sterk, P.J.; Högman, M.; Olin, A.-C.; Amann, A.; Antus, B.; Baraldi, E.; Bikov, A.; et al. A European Respiratory Society Technical Standard: Exhaled Biomarkers in Lung Disease. *Eur. Respir. J.* **2017**, *49*, 1600965. [CrossRef] [PubMed]
14. Baz-Redón, N.; Rovira-Amigo, S.; Paramonov, I.; Castillo-Corullón, S.; Roig, M.C.; Antolín, M.; Arumí, E.G.; Torrent-Vernetta, A.; Messa, I.D.M.; Gartner, S.; et al. Implementation of a Gene Panel for Genetic Diagnosis of Primary Ciliary Dyskinesia. *Arch. Bronconeumol.* **2020**, *20*, 30073–30079. [CrossRef]
15. Kempeneers, C.; Seaton, C.; Espinosa, B.G.; Chilvers, M.A. Ciliary Functional Analysis: Beating a Path towards Standardization. *Pediatric Pulmonol.* **2019**, *54*, 1627–1638. [CrossRef] [PubMed]
16. Kouis, P.; Yiallouros, P.; Middleton, N.; Evans, J.S.; Kyriacou, K.; Papatheodorou, S.I. Prevalence of Primary Ciliary Dyskinesia in Consecutive Referrals of Suspect Cases and the Transmission Electron Microscopy Detection Rate: A Systematic Review and Meta-Analysis. *Pediatric Res.* **2016**, *81*, 398–405. [CrossRef]
17. Fliegauf, M.; Olbrich, H.; Horvath, J.; Wildhaber, J.H.; Zariwala, M.A.; Kennedy, M.; Knowles, M.R.; Omran, H. Mislocalization of DNAH5 and DNAH9 in Respiratory Cells from Patients with Primary Ciliary Dyskinesia. *Am. J. Respir. Crit. Care Med.* **2005**, *171*, 1343–1349. [CrossRef]

18. Baz-Redón, N.; Rovira-Amigo, S.; Camats-Tarruella, N.; Fernández-Cancio, M.; Garrido-Pontnou, M.; Antolín, M.; Reula, A.; Armengot-Carceller, M.; Carrascosa, A.; Moreno-Galdó, A. Role of Immunofluorescence and Molecular Diagnosis in the Characterization of Primary Ciliary Dyskinesia. *Arch. Bronconeumol.* **2019**, *55*, 439–441. [CrossRef]
19. Loges, N.T.; Olbrich, H.; Fenske, L.; Mussaffi, H.; Horvath, J.; Fliegauf, M.; Kuhl, H.; Baktai, G.; Peterffy, E.; Chodhari, R.; et al. DNAI2 Mutations Cause Primary Ciliary Dyskinesia with Defects in the Outer Dynein Arm. *Am. J. Hum. Genet.* **2008**, *83*, 547–558. [CrossRef] [PubMed]
20. Wallmeier, J.; Shiratori, H.; Dougherty, G.W.; Edelbusch, C.; Hjeij, R.; Loges, N.T.; Menchen, T.; Olbrich, H.; Pennekamp, P.; Raidt, J.; et al. TTC25 Deficiency Results in Defects of the Outer Dynein Arm Docking Machinery and Primary Ciliary Dyskinesia with Left-Right Body Asymmetry Randomization. *Am. J. Hum. Genet.* **2016**, *99*, 460–469. [CrossRef]
21. Hjeij, R.; Onoufriadis, A.; Watson, C.M.; Slagle, C.E.; Klena, N.T.; Dougherty, G.W.; Kurkowiak, M.; Loges, N.T.; Diggle, C.P.; Morante, N.F.; et al. CCDC151 Mutations Cause Primary Ciliary Dyskinesia by Disruption of the Outer Dynein Arm Docking Complex Formation. *Am. J. Hum. Genet.* **2014**, *95*, 257–274. [CrossRef]
22. Loges, N.T.; Antony, D.; Maver, A.; Deardorff, M.A.; Güleç, E.Y.; Gezdirici, A.; Nöthe-Menchen, T.; Höben, I.M.; Jelten, L.; Frank, D.; et al. Recessive DNAH9 Loss-of-Function Mutations Cause Laterality Defects and Subtle Respiratory Ciliary-Beating Defects. *Am. J. Hum. Genet.* **2018**, *103*, 995–1008. [CrossRef]
23. Fassad, M.R.; Shoemark, A.; Legendre, M.; Hirst, R.A.; Koll, F.; Le Borgne, P.; Louis, B.; Daudvohra, F.; Patel, M.P.; Thomas, L.; et al. Mutations in Outer Dynein Arm Heavy Chain DNAH9 Cause Motile Cilia Defects and Situs Inversus. *Am. J. Hum. Genet.* **2018**, *103*, 984–994. [CrossRef]
24. Tarkar, A.; Loges, N.T.; Slagle, C.E.; Francis, R.; Dougherty, G.W.; Tamayo, J.V.; Shook, B.; Cantino, M.; Schwartz, D.; Jahnke, C.; et al. DYX1C1 is Required for Axonemal Dynein Assembly and Ciliary Motility. *Nat. Genet.* **2013**, *45*, 995–1003. [CrossRef]
25. Knowles, M.R.; Ostrowski, L.E.; Loges, N.T.; Hurd, T.; Leigh, M.W.; Huang, L.; Wolf, W.E.; Carson, J.L.; Hazucha, M.J.; Yin, W.; et al. Mutations in SPAG1 Cause Primary Ciliary Dyskinesia Associated with Defective Outer and Inner Dynein Arms. *Am. J. Hum. Genet.* **2013**, *93*, 711–720. [CrossRef]
26. Olcese, C.; UK10K Rare Group; Patel, M.P.; Shoemark, A.; Kiviluoto, S.; Legendre, M.; Williams, H.J.; Vaughan, C.K.; Hayward, J.; Goldenberg, A.; et al. X- Linked Primary Ciliary Dyskinesia Due to Mutations in the Cytoplasmic Axonemal Dynein Assembly Factor PIH1D3. *Nat. Commun.* **2017**, *8*, 14279. [CrossRef]
27. Paff, T.; Loges, N.T.; Aprea, I.; Wu, K.; Bakey, Z.; Haarman, E.G.; Daniels, J.M.; Sistermans, E.A.; Bogunovic, N.; Dougherty, G.W.; et al. Mutations in PIH1D3 Cause X-Linked Primary Ciliary Dyskinesia with Outer and Inner Dynein Arm Defects. *Am. J. Hum. Genet.* **2017**, *100*, 160–168. [CrossRef]
28. Loges, N.T.; Olbrich, H.; Becker-Heck, A.; Häffner, K.; Heer, A.; Reinhard, C.; Schmidts, M.; Kispert, A.; Zariwala, M.A.; Leigh, M.W.; et al. Deletions and Point Mutations of LRRC50 Cause Primary Ciliary Dyskinesia Due to Dynein Arm Defects. *Am. J. Hum. Genet.* **2009**, *85*, 883–889. [CrossRef]
29. Austin-Tse, C.; Halbritter, J.; Zariwala, M.A.; Gilberti, R.M.; Gee, H.Y.; Hellman, N.; Pathak, N.; Liu, Y.; Panizzi, J.R.; Patel-King, R.S.; et al. Zebrafish Ciliopathy Screen Plus Human Mutational Analysis Identifies C21orf59 and CCDC65 Defects as Causing Primary Ciliary Dyskinesia. *Am. J. Hum. Genet.* **2013**, *93*, 672–686. [CrossRef] [PubMed]
30. Mitchison, H.; Schmidts, M.; Loges, N.T.; Freshour, J.; Dritsoula, A.; Hirst, R.A.; O'Callaghan, C.; Blau, H.; Al Dabbagh, M.; Olbrich, H.; et al. Mutations in Axonemal Dynein Assembly Factor DNAAF3 Cause Primary Ciliary Dyskinesia. *Nat. Genet.* **2012**, *44*, 381–389. [CrossRef] [PubMed]
31. Zariwala, M.A.; Gee, H.Y.; Kurkowiak, M.; Al-Mutairi, D.A.; Leigh, M.W.; Hurd, T.W.; Hjeij, R.; Dell, S.D.; Chaki, M.; Dougherty, G.W.; et al. ZMYND10 Is Mutated in Primary Ciliary Dyskinesia and Interacts with LRRC6. *Am. J. Hum. Genet.* **2013**, *93*, 336–345. [CrossRef] [PubMed]
32. Diggle, C.P.; Toddie-Moore, D.; Mali, G.; Lage, P.Z.; Ait-Lounis, A.; Schmidts, M.; Shoemark, A.; Munoz, A.G.; Halachev, M.R.; Gautier, P.; et al. HEATR2 Plays a Conserved Role in Assembly of the Ciliary Motile Apparatus. *PLoS Genet.* **2014**, *10*, e1004577. [CrossRef]

33. Horani, A.; Druley, T.E.; Zariwala, M.A.; Patel, A.C.; Levinson, B.T.; Van Arendonk, L.G.; Thornton, K.C.; Giacalone, J.C.; Albee, A.J.; Wilson, K.S.; et al. Whole-Exome Capture and Sequencing Identifies HEATR2 Mutation as a Cause of Primary Ciliary Dyskinesia. *Am. J. Hum. Genet.* **2012**, *91*, 685–693. [CrossRef] [PubMed]
34. Fassad, M.R.; Shoemark, A.; Le Borgne, P.; Koll, F.; Patel, M.; Dixon, M.; Hayward, J.; Richardson, C.; Frost, E.; Jenkins, L.; et al. C11orf70 Mutations Disrupting the Intraflagellar Transport-Dependent Assembly of Multiple Axonemal Dyneins Cause Primary Ciliary Dyskinesia. *Am. J. Hum. Genet.* **2018**, *102*, 956–972. [CrossRef]
35. Höben, I.M.; Hjeij, R.; Olbrich, H.; Dougherty, G.W.; Nöthe-Menchen, T.; Aprea, I.; Frank, D.; Pennekamp, P.; Dworniczak, B.; Wallmeier, J.; et al. Mutations in C11orf70 Cause Primary Ciliary Dyskinesia with Randomization of Left/Right Body Asymmetry Due to Defects of Outer and Inner Dynein Arms. *Am. J. Hum. Genet.* **2018**, *102*, 973–984. [CrossRef]
36. Merveille, A.-C.; Davis, E.E.; Becker-Heck, A.; Legendre, M.; Amirav, I.; Bataille, G.; Belmont, J.W.; Beydon, N.; Billen, F.; Clément, A.; et al. CCDC39 is Required for Assembly of Inner Dynein Arms and the Dynein Regulatory Complex and for Normal Ciliary Motility in Humans and Dogs. *Nat. Genet.* **2011**, *43*, 72–78. [CrossRef]
37. Becker-Heck, A.; Zohn, I.E.; Okabe, N.; Pollock, A.; Lenhart, K.B.; Sullivan-Brown, J.; McSheene, J.; Loges, N.T.; Olbrich, H.; Haeffner, K.; et al. The Coiled-Coil Domain Containing Protein CCDC40 Is Essential for Motile Cilia Function and Left-Right Axis Formation. *Nat. Genet.* **2011**, *43*, 79–84. [CrossRef]
38. Antony, D.; Becker-Heck, A.; Zariwala, M.A.; Schmidts, M.; Onoufriadis, A.; Forouhan, M.; Wilson, R.; Taylor-Cox, T.; Dewar, A.; Jackson, C.; et al. Mutations in CCDC39 and CCDC40 are the Major Cause of Primary Ciliary Dyskinesia with Axonemal Disorganization and Absent Inner Dynein Arms. *Hum. Mutat.* **2013**, *34*, 462–472. [CrossRef]
39. Olbrich, H.; Cremers, C.; Loges, N.T.; Werner, C.; Nielsen, K.G.; Marthin, J.K.; Philipsen, M.; Wallmeier, J.; Pennekamp, P.; Menchen, T.; et al. Loss-of-Function GAS8 Mutations Cause Primary Ciliary Dyskinesia and Disrupt the Nexin-Dynein Regulatory Complex. *Am. J. Hum. Genet.* **2015**, *97*, 546–554. [CrossRef] [PubMed]
40. Wirschell, M.; Olbrich, H.; Werner, C.; Tritschler, D.; Bower, R.; Sale, W.S.; Loges, N.T.; Pennekamp, P.; Lindberg, S.; Stenram, U.; et al. The Nexin-Dynein Regulatory Complex Subunit DRC1 Is Essential for Motile Cilia Function in Algae and Humans. *Nat. Genet.* **2013**, *45*, 262–268. [CrossRef] [PubMed]
41. Horani, A.; Brody, S.L.; Ferkol, T.W.; Shoseyov, D.; Wasserman, M.G.; Ta-Shma, A.; Wilson, K.S.; Bayly, P.V.; Amirav, I.; Cohen-Cymberknoh, M.; et al. CCDC65 Mutation Causes Primary Ciliary Dyskinesia with Normal Ultrastructure and Hyperkinetic Cilia. *PLoS ONE* **2013**, *8*, e72299. [CrossRef] [PubMed]
42. Frommer, A.; Hjeij, R.; Loges, N.T.; Edelbusch, C.; Jahnke, C.; Raidt, J.; Werner, C.; Wallmeier, J.; Große-Onnebrink, J.; Olbrich, H.; et al. Immunofluorescence Analysis and Diagnosis of Primary Ciliary Dyskinesia with Radial Spoke Defects. *Am. J. Respir. Cell Mol. Biol.* **2015**, *53*, 563–573. [CrossRef]
43. Kott, E.; Legendre, M.; Copin, B.; Papon, J.-F.; Moal, F.D.-L.; Montantin, G.; Duquesnoy, P.; Piterboth, W.; Amram, D.; Bassinet, L.; et al. Loss-of-Function Mutations in RSPH1 Cause Primary Ciliary Dyskinesia with Central-Complex and Radial-Spoke Defects. *Am. J. Hum. Genet.* **2013**, *93*, 561–570. [CrossRef]
44. Castleman, V.H.; Romio, L.; Chodhari, R.; Hirst, R.A.; De Castro, S.C.; Parker, K.A.; Ybot-Gonzalez, P.; Emes, R.D.; Wilson, S.W.; Wallis, C.; et al. Mutations in Radial Spoke Head Protein Genes RSPH9 and RSPH4A Cause Primary Ciliary Dyskinesia with Central-Microtubular-Pair Abnormalities. *Am. J. Hum. Genet.* **2009**, *84*, 197–209. [CrossRef]
45. Dougherty, G.W.; Loges, N.T.; Klinkenbusch, J.A.; Olbrich, H.; Pennekamp, P.; Menchen, T.; Raidt, J.; Wallmeier, J.; Werner, C.; Westermann, C.; et al. DNAH11 Localization in the Proximal Region of Respiratory Cilia Defines Distinct Outer Dynein Arm Complexes. *Am. J. Respir. Cell Mol. Biol.* **2016**, *55*, 213–224. [CrossRef]
46. Olbrich, H.; Schmidts, M.; Werner, C.; Onoufriadis, A.; Loges, N.T.; Raidt, J.; Banki, N.F.; Shoemark, A.; Burgoyne, T.; Al Turki, S.; et al. Recessive HYDIN Mutations Cause Primary Ciliary Dyskinesia without Randomization of Left-Right Body Asymmetry. *Am. J. Hum. Genet.* **2012**, *91*, 672–684. [CrossRef]
47. Edelbusch, C.; Cindrić, S.; Dougherty, G.W.; Loges, N.T.; Olbrich, H.; Rivlin, J.; Wallmeier, J.; Pennekamp, P.; Amirav, I.; Omran, H. Mutation of Serine/Threonine Protein Kinase 36 (STK36) Causes Primary Ciliary Dyskinesia with a Central Pair Defect. *Hum. Mutat.* **2017**, *38*, 964–969. [CrossRef]

48. Cindrić, S.; Dougherty, G.W.; Olbrich, H.; Hjeij, R.; Loges, N.T.; Amirav, I.; Philipsen, M.C.; Marthin, J.K.; Nielsen, K.G.; Sutharsan, S.; et al. SPEF2-and HYDIN-Mutant Cilia Lack the Central Pair–associated Protein SPEF2, Aiding Primary Ciliary Dyskinesia Diagnostics. *Am. J. Respir. Cell Mol. Biol.* **2020**, *62*, 382–396. [CrossRef]
49. Knowles, M.R.; Leigh, M.W. Primary Ciliary Dyskinesia Diagnosis. Is Color Better Than Black and White? *Am. J. Respir. Crit. Care Med.* **2017**, *196*, 9–10. [CrossRef]

Publisher's Note: MDPI stays neutral with regard to jurisdictional claims in published maps and institutional affiliations.

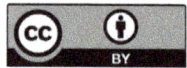

© 2020 by the authors. Licensee MDPI, Basel, Switzerland. This article is an open access article distributed under the terms and conditions of the Creative Commons Attribution (CC BY) license (http://creativecommons.org/licenses/by/4.0/).

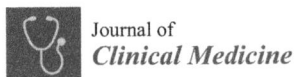

Article

A Revised Protocol for Culture of Airway Epithelial Cells as a Diagnostic Tool for Primary Ciliary Dyskinesia

Janice L. Coles [1,2], James Thompson [1,2], Katie L. Horton [2], Robert A. Hirst [3], Paul Griffin [4], Gwyneth M. Williams [3], Patricia Goggin [5], Regan Doherty [5], Peter M. Lackie [2,5], Amanda Harris [1,2], Woolf T. Walker [1], Christopher O'Callaghan [3,6], Claire Hogg [4], Jane S. Lucas [1,2,*], Cornelia Blume [2,*] and Claire L. Jackson [1,2,*]

[1] Primary Ciliary Dyskinesia Centre, NIHR Biomedical Research Centre, University Hospital Southampton NHS Foundation Trust, Southampton SO16 6YD, UK; j.l.coles@soton.ac.uk (J.L.C.); jt3v12@soton.ac.uk (J.T.); amanda-lea.harris@uhs.nhs.uk (A.H.); woolf.walker@uhs.nhs.uk (W.T.W.)

[2] School of Clinical and Experimental Sciences, University of Southampton Faculty of Medicine, Southampton SO16 6YD, UK; K.Horton@soton.ac.uk (K.L.H.); P.M.Lackie@soton.ac.uk (P.M.L.)

[3] Centre for PCD Diagnosis and Research, Department of Respiratory Sciences, University of Leicester, Robert Kilpatrick Clinical Sciences Building, Leicester LE2 7LX, UK; rah9@leicester.ac.uk (R.A.H.); gmw6@leicester.ac.uk (G.M.W.); c.ocallaghan@ucl.ac.uk (C.O.)

[4] Paediatric Respiratory Department, Royal Brompton and Harefield NHS Foundation Trust, Sydney Street, London SW3 6NP, UK; P.Griffin@rbht.nhs.uk (P.G.); c.hogg@rbht.nhs.uk (C.H.)

[5] Biomedical Imaging Unit, University Hospital Southampton NHS Foundation Trust, Southampton SO16 6YD, UK; p.goggin@soton.ac.uk (P.G.); Regan.Doherty@uhs.nhs.uk (R.D.)

[6] Respiratory, Critical Care and Anaesthesia, UCL Great Ormond Street Institute of Child Health, 30 Guilford Street, London WC1N 1EH, UK

* Correspondence: jlucas1@soton.ac.uk (J.S.L.); C.Blume@soton.ac.uk (C.B.); clj@soton.ac.uk (C.L.J.)

Received: 19 October 2020; Accepted: 19 November 2020; Published: 21 November 2020

Abstract: Air–liquid interface (ALI) culture of nasal epithelial cells is a valuable tool in the diagnosis and research of primary ciliary dyskinesia (PCD). Ex vivo samples often display secondary dyskinesia from cell damage during sampling, infection or inflammation confounding PCD diagnostic results. ALI culture enables regeneration of healthy cilia facilitating differentiation of primary from secondary ciliary dyskinesia. We describe a revised ALI culture method adopted from April 2018 across three collaborating PCD diagnostic sites, including current University Hospital Southampton COVID-19 risk mitigation measures, and present results. Two hundred and forty nasal epithelial cell samples were seeded for ALI culture and 199 (82.9%) were ciliated. Fifty-four of 83 (63.9%) ex vivo samples which were originally equivocal or insufficient provided diagnostic information following in vitro culture. Surplus basal epithelial cells from 181 nasal brushing samples were frozen in liquid nitrogen; 39 samples were ALI-cultured after cryostorage and all ciliated. The ciliary beat patterns of ex vivo samples (by high-speed video microscopy) were recapitulated, scanning electron microscopy demonstrated excellent ciliation, and cilia could be immuno-fluorescently labelled (anti-alpha-tubulin and anti-RSPH4a) in representative cases that were ALI-cultured after cryostorage. In summary, our ALI culture protocol provides high ciliation rates across three centres, minimising patient recall for repeat brushing biopsies and improving diagnostic certainty. Cryostorage of surplus diagnostic samples was successful, facilitating PCD research.

Keywords: PCD; ALI culture; bio-resource; primary nasal epithelium; diagnostics

1. Introduction

Primary ciliary dyskinesia (PCD) is a rare disease usually inherited as an autosomal recessive condition although autosomal dominant and X-linked cases exist [1]. The incidence of PCD is approximately 1:10,000, higher in consanguineous populations [2], and it is associated with impaired function of motile cilia in the airways, embryonic node, and reproductive system [3]. This causes a spectrum of symptoms including unexplained neonatal respiratory distress, persistent wet cough from infancy, repeated respiratory infections, rhino-sinus disease, organ laterality abnormality and subfertility [4]. Early diagnosis is essential to initiate treatment, with the aim of slowing disease progression and improving quality of life [5].

There is no "gold standard" diagnostic test for PCD [6]. European Respiratory Society and American Thoracic Society guidelines both recommend a multidisciplinary approach using a combination of tests to make a diagnosis [7–9]. Ex vivo nasal or bronchial samples obtained by brushing or curette biopsy are imaged by high-speed video microscopy analysis (HSVA) [10,11] and ciliary motility analysed as a frontline functional test [12]. Transmission electron microscopy (TEM) is used to assess and quantify ultrastructural abnormalities of motile cilia [13,14]. Immunofluorescence labelling (IF) can demonstrate the absence or mis-localisation of ciliary proteins [15,16], particularly helpful in cases where no TEM abnormalities are detected such as with DNAH11 [17], DNAH9 [18] and *HYDIN* gene mutations [19]. Genotyping can detect pathogenic bi-allelic or X-linked hemizygous mutations in 50 PCD-related genes to confirm the diagnosis in approximately 70% of well characterized cases [1,3,20]. However, there are still many individuals without a genetic diagnosis. Some genetic defects result in subtle ciliary beat pattern abnormalities, which are difficult to differentiate from secondary defects (e.g., *GAS8* [21], *DNAH9* [18], *CCDC103* [22,23] mutations) by HSVA and appear normal by TEM. *MCIDAS* [24], *CCNO* [25] and *FOXJ1* [26] mutations cause a lack of cilia rather than dyskinesia, and this could be mistaken for severe secondary epithelial damage.

1.1. How Can Cell Culture Be Used in PCD Diagnostics and Research?

Secondary damage of cilia caused by infection, inflammation or sampling trauma is a common feature in ex vivo airway samples [27–29]. In addition, sample yield may not be sufficient to support the growing array of tests required to diagnose difficult cases. Therefore, to address poor quality, low yield or expanded diagnostic testing, cell culture can be used.

Airway epithelial cell monolayer mini-culture methods have been used to reduce secondary ciliary dyskinesia in the nasal brushings (from chronic sinusitis patients) to enable better ciliary function measurements by HSVA following 3 days in culture with 83% culture success and improved ciliary beat pattern visualization [30]. However, following recent infections, the airway cilia may be shed and this culture method does not allow for cilia re-growth.

Likewise, monolayer-suspension methods, initially developed for whole resected tissue [31], have been adapted for nasal brush biopsy [32] and are useful for reducing secondary abnormalities in culture for PCD diagnostics. Briefly, nasal brushing cell suspensions are seeded onto a 1% collagen gel substrate and non-adherent cell aggregates are harvested at 24 h for suspension culture with continuous movement. After 24–48 h, cell spheroids form, which are cultured for at least 21 days before analysis of newly formed cilia on the apical surface of the spheroid. This method confirmed a PCD diagnosis or resolved secondary defects in 46 of 59 cultures (78%) [32]. Pifferi et al., also described a later study in which of 151 subjects, a PCD diagnosis could be confirmed in 36 patients using the suspension model optimally following a 5-day culture process [33].

Marthin et al., (2017) reported a more rapid nasal epithelial cell culture method, where spheroids spontaneously formed from terminally differentiated nasal epithelium, retaining their original cilia [34]. Spheroids formed in 82% of 18 samples, with the median number of days to harvest being 4 (1–5) in 7 healthy volunteers and 2 (1–5) in 8 PCD patients' samples. Whilst retaining their original ciliary beat pattern and frequency, spheroids survived up to 16 days (albeit $n = 1$) and provided ciliated spheroids for HSVA and IF testing of cilia [34]. However, using this method, spheroid numbers are not expanded and are limited by the original sampling yield, which may not support a multitude of tests. Additionally, unhealthy or unciliated samples cannot be re-grown to resolve secondary damage since new cilia are not formed.

Alternatively, basal epithelial cells can be expanded in submerged culture before cells are differentiated on porous membrane inserts within a culture well at an air–liquid interface (ALI) to stimulate cell polarisation and widespread ciliogenesis, which takes 4–6 weeks in vitro. Re-analysis of cilia function after ALI culture gives a further opportunity to carry out HSVA, TEM and IF without secondary health issues [27,35].

Cilia regeneration by spheroid suspension or ALI culture can negate the need for patients, with insufficient or inconclusive test results, to undergo repeat nasal brushing biopsy, reduce the time to a diagnosis of PCD and increase the accuracy of HSVA [7,12]. We have also previously shown how ALI cultures may be used as an airway model to investigate nasal epithelial cell interactions with drugs [36–38], bacterial [37–41] and viral infections [40–43].

1.2. A Revised Protocol with High Diagnostic Efficiency Is Being Used within the UK PCD Service

Here, we present our ALI culture protocol using commercially available expansion and differentiation media, PneumaCult Ex Plus and PneumaCult ALI (STEMCELL Technologies, Vancouver, BC, Canada). We report its efficacy at three UK diagnostic centres. We also report on creating a bio-resource for PCD research and the performance of cell cultures after cryostorage at University Hospital Southampton (UHS). Due to the current COVID-19 pandemic we have additionally described the protocol modifications at UHS used to mitigate risk of SARS CoV2 infection during patient interaction and sample handling since July 2020.

2. Methods

We collected culture data from 70 consecutive patient samples attending the PCD Centre at University Hospital Southampton (UHS) between 1st April 2018 and 1st April 2019 (Table 1). Local and national R&D and ethical approvals were complied with Southampton and South West Hampshire Research Ethics Committee A (approval reference: CHI395, 07/Q1702/109). We further report data from 128 samples processed at Leicester and 45 samples processed at the Royal Brompton Hospital using the same culture protocol (with some minor variations depending on equipment and consumables).

Patients were diagnosed as "PCD highly-unlikely" if they had a non-suggestive clinical history and/or PICADAR score (a diagnostic clinical prediction rule for PCD) [4], normal nNO, and "PCD unlikely" HSVA on ex vivo nasal brushing. Patients with a suggestive clinical history and/or PICADAR score with inconclusive/insufficient or "PCD likely" HSVA on ex vivo nasal brushings underwent further testing. This included TEM of cilia ultrastructure and IF labelling of ciliary proteins, and could include repeat HSVA following ALI culture and/or genetic testing. See HSVA outcome definitions below. Hallmark TEM or genetics diagnosed PCD and "PCD highly-likely" cases were diagnosed according to the ERS guidelines [3,7,44]. All available diagnostic data were discussed at a multidisciplinary team (MDT) meeting to decide the patients' outcome and follow up.

2.1. Nasal Epithelial Cell Culture Protocol (with Additional UHS COVID-19 Modifications)

Nasal brushing biopsies were taken from patients' inferior turbinates, using a 3 mm bronchoscopy cytology brush (Conmed, Utica, NY, USA, #149R). Individually sterile wrapped brushes were opened in clinic and the wire handles were cut to approximately 15 cm to hold (with wire cutters). To maximise chances of a good yield of healthy ciliated tissue, brushings were performed when patients had been free from respiratory exacerbations for at least 6 weeks. Patients were seated (children on parent's laps) and asked to remove spectacles, and to clear mucus secretions from their nose with a tissue. Clinicians placed one brush sequentially into each nostril (without anaesthetic), ensuring that the patients' nostrils were clear. Whilst applying gentle pressure to the inferior turbinate the brush was passed back and forth for approximately 5 s, whilst turning, to ensure coverage. The sample was then placed into a capped 5 mL round bottomed cytology tube (Fisher Scientific, Hampton, NH, USA, #10186400) containing 1.5 mL Medium 199 (Fisher Scientific, Hampton, NH, USA, #22350029) supplemented with 1% penicillin (5000 U/mL)/streptomycin (5000 µg/mL) (Fisher Scientific, Hampton, NH, USA, #15070063).

Table 1. The characteristics of subjects referred for diagnostic testing to University Hospital Southampton primary ciliary dyskinesia (PCD) centre 1st April 2018 to 1st April 2019, grouped by final multidisciplinary team (MDT) diagnostic outcomes.

	PCD Positive/PCD Highly-Likely ($n = 7$)	PCD Highly-Unlikely ($n = 55$)	Equivocal/Ongoing ($n = 8$)
Median age (min, max)	11.15 (0.1, 32.2)	4.5 (0.1, 70.4)	13.5 (4.0, 63.7)
Female n (%)	$n = 5$ (71.4%)	$n = 26$ (47.3%)	$n = 5$ (62.5%)
Chronic wet cough %	100	63.6	87.5
Rhinosinusitis %	85.7	80	75
Situs abnormality %	71.4	12.7	0
Median nNO nl/min	24.4 (Q_1 18.8, Q_3 47.5, min 18, max 67, $n = 6$) $n = 3$ normal	380 (Q_1 240, Q_3 596, min 1.2, max 1280, $n = 49$)	280 (Q_1 93, Q_3 548.5, min 5, max 762, $n = 8$)
TEM	$n = 2$ outer arm defects $n = 2$ outer arm defects with possible inner arm defect	$n = 49$ normal $n = 6$ no data	$n = 7$ normal $n = 1$ no data
Mean ex vivo sample CBF or CBP	$n = 5$ static, 0 Hz $n = 2$ variable dyskinesia	14.8 Hz, SD ± 1.8 ($n = 52$) $n = 2$ variable dyskinesia $n = 1$ insufficient	13.9 Hz, SD ± 1.2 ($n = 6$) $n = 2$ variable dyskinesia
Mean in vitro ALI-culture CBF or CBP	$n = 5$ static, 0 Hz $n = 2$ no data (1 failed due to bacteria, 1 sample frozen)	13.9 Hz, SD ± 2.1 ($n = 52$) $n = 3$ not done	14.4 Hz, SD ± 2.4 ($n = 4$) $n = 2$ became static, 0 Hz $n = 2$ no data (failed due to bacteria)
Causative genes	*RSPH4* homozygous *CCDC151* homozygous *DNAAF3* homozygous *DNAAF5* heterozygous *DNAH11* homozygous $n = 2$ no data	$n = 13$ no mutation found $n = 42$ no data	$n = 4$ no mutation found $n = 1$ *CCDC164* single heterozygous mutation $n = 3$ no data

nasal nitric oxide (nNO); transmission electron microscopy (TEM), ciliary beat frequency (CBF); ciliary beat pattern (CBP).

Since the COVID-19 pandemic, we have adopted several clinical and laboratory modifications to mitigate the risk of acquiring SARS CoV2 infection at UHS, which were approved by UHS and University of Southampton Health, Safety and Risk directorates. We recommend that all those wanting to undertake nasal epithelial cell culture during the COVID-19 pandemic consult their local institute and government policy to ensure health and safety measures are in place. Patients are seen within 48 h of a negative SARS CoV2 polymerase chain reaction (PCR) test. Patients are contacted directly before attending clinic to ensure that they had none of the main COVID-19 symptoms (as cited by http://www.nhs.uk/conditions/coronavirus-covid-19/symptoms/#symptoms including "a high temperature, a new continuous cough and a loss or change to sense of smell or taste"). The clinicians wear full personal protective equipment (PPE) including clinical scrubs with disposable aprons, gloves, FFP3 'filtering face piece' respirator mask (personally fitted) and plastic face shields. The clinical area is ventilated and the number of personnel and patients are restricted to ensure 2 m distancing before and after brushing sampling. To reduce risk of aerosol generation, patients wear disposable surgical face masks whilst in the hospital. Patients enter UHS via a patient-only entrance and are temperature tested on arrival, and escorted to the clinical area directly before their appointment (to minimize interactions with other staff and patients whilst on site). Patient samples are contained and transported at room temperature (within an hour of sampling) to the onsite laboratory within a plastic sample bag within an anti-crush container. Couriered samples from other hospitals are not refrigerated and can take up to 3 h to arrive. Samples received at our containment level 2 laboratory are handled within a class 2 microbiological safety cabinet (MSC). Specific to COVID-19-modified processing: 100 µL of the sample is sent for a SARS CoV2 PCR test via the Public Health England laboratory at UHS and 900 µL of the sample is kept at 4 °C until the test result is returned (24–48 h). Only those samples proven negative are cultured. We have so far not received a nasal brushing sample that has tested positive for SARS CoV2 by PCR. To remove mucus, the remaining 500 µL of sample is washed in 2 mL HBSS without calcium and magnesium, (Gibco, Thermo Fisher Scientific, Waltham, MA, USA, #10532003) and epithelial cells pelleted by centrifugation at 400× g for 7 min. Cell pellets are resuspended in 500 µL Medium 199 (including 1% pen/strep) for HSVA (100 µL), IF diagnostic testing (20 µL/slide, $n = 10$) and the remaining 200 µL is fixed in 4% glutaraldehyde for TEM processing.

To remove mucus, cell suspensions (directly from the brush) intended for culture were washed in 2 mL HBSS without calcium and magnesium, (Gibco, Thermo Fisher Scientific, Waltham, MA, USA, #10532003) and epithelial cells pelleted by centrifugation at 400× g for 7 min. Cell pellets were resuspended in 1 mL PneumaCult Ex plus medium (STEMCELL Technologies, Vancouver, BC, Canada, Ex plus kit #05040) supplemented with hydrocortisone (0.1%) (STEMCELL Technologies, Vancouver, BC, Canada, #07925) to directly seed cell clusters in 1–2 collagen (0.3 mg/mL, PureCol 5005.B CellSystems, Troisdorf, Germany)-coated wells of a 12-well culture plate (Corning Life Sciences, Corning, NY, USA, #3548). We did not digest or quantify cell numbers directly from the brush biopsies, and in our experience cell health is more important than yield. Under-seeding is to be avoided particularly if cell health is considered compromised after microscopic assessment. Cells were cultured in 37 °C incubators with 5% CO_2 and ~100% relative humidity and all culture medium contains additional 1% penicillin (5000 U/mL)/streptomycin (5000 µg/mL) (Fisher Scientific, Hampton, NH, USA, #15070063) and 0.002% nystatin suspension (10,000 U/mL) (Fisher Scientific, Hampton, NH, USA, #15340029). Medium was replaced 3 times weekly and cells were passaged with 0.25% trypsin EDTA (Gibco, Thermo Fisher Scientific, Waltham, MA, USA, #11560626) when at 50–70% confluence for both initial seeding passage 0 and at passage 1 in collagen-coated T25 cm^2 flasks, to give a final basal epithelial cell yield of 1–2 million. All centrifugations were at 400× g for 5 min and cells washed twice in 7 mL HBSS to remove residual trypsin (without use of a trypsin inhibitor). At passage 2,100,000 cells were seeded per collagen-coated 12 mm Transwell® with 0.4 µm pore polyester membrane insert (Corning Life Sciences, Corning, NY, USA, #3460) in a 12-well culture plate. Cells on Transwell® inserts were initially cultured submerged in 250 µL PneumaCult Ex plus medium on the apical side and 650 µL of the same medium on the basolateral side. When a confluent monolayer of basal cells was observed (usually between 1 and 2 days) cells were taken to air–liquid interface (ALI) by apical medium removal and replacement of the basolateral medium with 650 µL PneumaCult ALI medium (STEMCELL Technologies, Vancouver, BC, Canada, ALI kit #05001) supplemented with hydrocortisone (0.5%) and heparin (0.2%) (STEMCELL Technologies, Vancouver, BC, Canada, #07925 and #07980, respectively), replaced 3 times weekly and with apical cell washing (briefly with 100 µL HBSS) aspirated to prevent a build-up of mucus. Cultures were harvested between 3 and 6 weeks to allow for optimal ciliation.

2.2. Bio-Resource

Between March 2018 and August 2020 UHS has cryopreserved surplus diagnostic cells from 181 PCD clinic patient samples and 30 healthy donor samples. Surplus cells from passage 1 were frozen 1 million per cryovial in 1 mL CryoStor® cell cryopreservation medium (Sigma, St. Louis, MO, USA, #C2874). Cells were initially frozen at −80 °C (graduated freezing −1 °C/minute in a Mr. Frosty™ container Thermo Fisher Scientific, Waltham, MA, USA, #5100–0001), then transferred to liquid nitrogen for longer-term storage. After thawing, washed cells were seeded for research in a smaller Transwell® insert format in 24-well plates. Briefly, 50,000 cells per collagen-coated 6.5 mm Transwell® with 0.4 µm pore polyester membrane insert (Corning Life Sciences, Corning, NY, USA, #3470) in 100 µL PneumaCult Ex plus medium supplemented (apical side) and 350 µL of the same medium on the basolateral side. Cultures were taken to ALI after 1–2 days replacing only the basolateral medium with 350 µL PneumaCult ALI medium supplemented and maintained as detailed above.

2.3. Post-ALI Culture High-Speed Video Microscopy Analysis

Motile cilia were usually first observed by day 7 post-ALI by low power light microscopy with normal ciliary function and widespread coverage confirmed by HSVA [12] from day 20. Cultures were analysed between 3 and 6 weeks post-ALI when considered optimally ciliated. Cultures with no discernible cilia were analysed 6 weeks post-ALI, to examine for static cilia or ciliary aplasia. For HSVA, cells were scraped gently from the membrane with a pipette tip, washed and centrifuged to reduce mucus, transferred in 100 µL PneumaCult ALI medium into a 0.5 mm-depth Coverwell imaging chamber (Sigma, St. Louis, MO, USA, #635051) and mounted on a glass slide.

Ciliary beat pattern (CBP) and ciliary beat frequency (CBF) were analysed during HSVA using a ×100 objective lens, with samples equilibrated to 37 °C. Videos were recorded at 500 frames per second and analysed at 30–60 frames per second from a minimum of 6 strips of ciliated epithelium as previously described [27]. Observers with extensive experience [45] in ciliary function analysis then denoted the sample as either "PCD likely", where a widespread "hallmark" beat pattern was observed that was unlikely to be caused by secondary factors alone; "PCD unlikely" where normal ciliary function was observed in at least six areas and any minor abnormalities present could be attributed to obvious secondary factors; "inconclusive" where abnormal ciliary beating was observed which was likely to be due to secondary factors but PCD could not be excluded; or "insufficient" where the quality or quantity of ciliated epithelium was not sufficient for an accurate decision to be made.

2.4. Fast Fourier Transform Analysis of Cilia Coverage

We pseudo-quantified the percentage area of cilia coverage on ALI cultures in-situ on a representative subset of 10 consecutive UHS ciliated samples where cilia were motile (cilia coverage on static cultures requires alternative imaging approaches, e.g., by immunofluorescence labelling or SEM not discussed here). HSVA was carried out at 37 °C with a ×20 objective lens (to acquire larger area mean CBF measurements), imaging every 3rd field of view across the midline of each 12 mm Transwell® insert to collect non-overlapping representative data across the whole membrane. Fields of view with significant moving particulates or mucus debris were avoided. Fast Fourier transform analysis of HSVA.cih Photron video files was performed using an in-house written plugin for https://imagej.net/(by Dr Peter Lackie) to determine the proportion of movement to non-movement (CBF in Hz) detected in the video, using a minimum box size of 4 × 4 pixels (Figure 1). The percentage area of movement detected within 16 fields of view was averaged to give a surrogate for cilia coverage. Of 10 samples the mean cilia coverage was 38.9%, which was within the expected range of 15–50% reported in the respiratory tract in vivo [46].

2.5. Trans-Epithelial Electrical Resistance Measurements

One hour before trans-epithelial electrical resistance (TEER), measurements were taken, PneumaCult ALI medium was replaced on the test ALI cultures (ciliated at passage 2) (using 100 µL PneumaCult Ex plus medium on the apical side and 350 µL on the basolateral side in the Transwell® insert format in 24-well plates) and incubated at 37 °C. A control well with an empty Transwell® insert containing only medium (no cells) was also prepared. A World Precision Instrument EVOM2 epithelial Volt/Ohm meter with STX2 electrode (chopstick probe) (Fisher Scientific, Hampton, NH, USA, #15169112) was used. The chopstick probe was sterilized in 70% industrial methylated spirit for 5 min and rinse in medium before and after use and between test and control wells. The mean of three measurements was taken and background control measurements were subtracted before calculating mean $\Omega.cm^2$ (±SD).

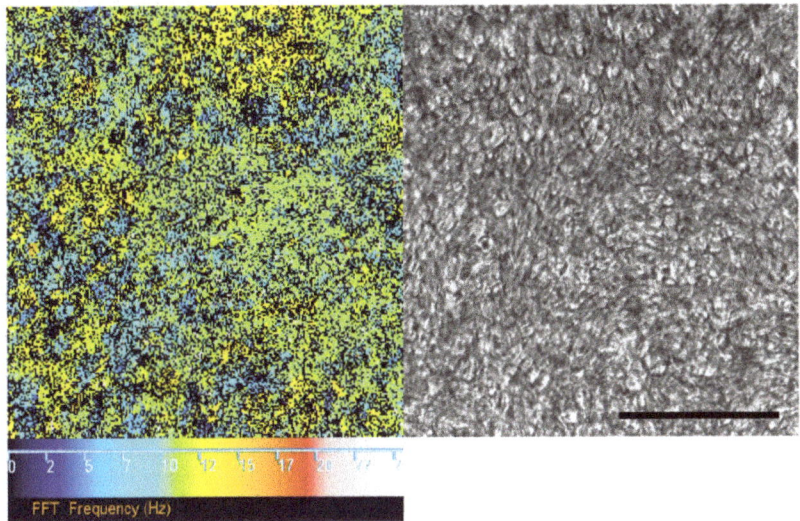

Figure 1. Fast Fourier transform (FFT) analysis of ciliary movement using high-speed video microscopy analysis (HSVA) data. FFT analysis (left) "colour map" corresponding to ciliary movement detected by HSVA (using a 20× objective lens) on the surface of an air–liquid interface (ALI) culture (right). The colour scale (left to right) depicts increasing ciliary beat frequency (CBF) from 0 (black) to 25 Hz (white). Black pixels also represent a CBF measurement outside of the detection threshold (below 2 Hz or above 50 Hz). Normal mean CBF at 37 °C is 11–20 Hz. Scale bar represents 100 μm.

2.6. Immunofluorescence Labelling of Ciliated Ali Cultures

The membranes of ciliated ALI cultures were excised at 4 weeks using a surgical scalpel blade (15) and placed into the well of a 24-well plate submerged in 100 μL PneumaCult Ex plus medium. The ciliated epithelial cells were scraped from the membrane surface using a pipette tip into the medium. Then, 20 μL of cell suspension was dropped onto each coated Shandon™ Cytoslides™ (Fisher Scientific, Hampton, NH, USA, #12026689) and allowed to air dry in the class 2 MSC. Once dry, slides were sealed in slide mailer boxes (Fisher Scientific, Hampton, NH, USA, #11719885) and transferred to a −20 °C freezer for storage for up to 4 months. For immunofluorescence labelling, slides were thawed and fixed with 4% PFA for 15 min, washed in PBS with 0.1% triton X-100 (Fisher Scientific, Hampton, NH, USA, #T/3751/08) then blocked with 5% milk powder in PBS-triton X-100 for 1 h. After washing, primary antibodies (anti-RSPH4a 1:200, Atlas Antibodies, Sigma, St. Louis, MO, USA, #HPA031197; anti-alpha tubulin 1:500, Sigma, St. Louis, MO, USA, #T9026) in PBS-triton X-100 were incubated for 2 h at room temperature, followed by washing and secondary antibody (Alexafluor 488, Life Technologies, Carlsbad, CA, USA, #A21121; Alexafluor 594, Life Technologies, Carlsbad, CA, USA, #A11012) incubation at a dilution of 1:2500 in PBS-triton x-100 for 30 min at room temperature. DAPI (300 nM) (Molecular Probes, Thermo Fisher Scientific, Waltham, MA, USA #D1306) was added to the final wash before mounting onto coverslips with Mowiol aqueous mounting media. The slides were kept in the fridge (at least overnight) until imaging using a Leica SP8 laser scanning confocal microscope with Leica Application Suite X software v3.5.5.19976 (Leica Biosystems, Wetzlar, Germany).

2.7. Statistics

Descriptive statistics are presented in Table 1. Normality was checked using the Shapiro–Wilk test. Two sample comparisons were undertaken using the student t-test when normality test passed or Mann–Whitney test when normality tests failed. Matched samples were analysed using the parametric paired student's *t* test or non-parametric Wilcoxon test. For multiple comparisons One-Way ANOVA was used for parametric samples or Kruskal–Wallis test for non-parametric samples. Statistical analysis was performed in GraphPad Prism 8 (GraphPad, San Diego, CA, USA). A *p*-value less than 0.05 was considered significant.

3. Results

3.1. How Did the Nasal Epithelial Cell Culture Protocol Improve Diagnostic Accuracy at UHS

Sixty-seven of 70 consecutive UHS patients' (Table 1) samples were cultured and 64 of those 67 ALI cultures were successfully ciliated (95.5%). Of three samples that were not cultured, two were not suspected of PCD (due to a weak clinical history, normal nNO and "PCD unlikely" HSVA on the ex vivo nasal brushing) and one was diagnosed as "PCD positive" with hallmark TEM (absent outer dynein arms) with static cilia (by HSVA on the ex vivo sample) as determined at MDT meetings and surplus epithelial cells were cryopreserved.

Of 67 in vitro ALI cultures, only 3 (4.5%) failed (1 insufficient sample, 2 due to infection) and HSVA was performed on the 64 ciliated cultures. The original ex vivo CBP was confirmed in seven normal and six abnormal (PCD likely) ALI-cultured samples (19.4%). Fifty-one original ex vivo samples had an equivocal CBP and ALI culture resolved a normal CBP in 30 (44.8%), an abnormal CBP (PCD likely) in 2 (3%) and remained equivocal in 19 samples (28.4%) (Figure 2). As expected, TEM analysis of ALI cultures demonstrated that normal and PCD hallmark defects were replicated in vitro from representative samples (Figure 3). Example HSVA videos showing the quality of ALI culture after equivocal or abnormal "PCD likely" ex vivo samples are shown in Supplementary Video S1a–d.

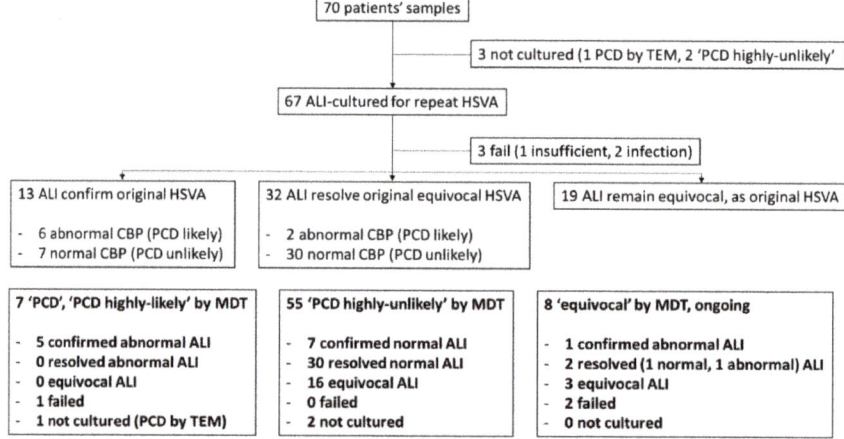

Figure 2. Flow diagram of diagnostic sample processing for ALI culture by repeat HSVA and MDT outcomes. Seventy patients' ex vivo samples evaluated by HSVA (as part of the whole diagnostic process) and their ALI culture outcomes were followed. HSVA on ALI culture either confirmed the original HSVA finding, resolved an originally equivocal HSVA or remained equivocal despite culture. In bold, the ALI culture HSVA outcomes are shown by MDT outcome ("PCD"/"PCD highly-likely"; "PCD highly-unlikely" or "equivocal" pending follow up, repeat tests or further tests (genetics or additional IF for example).

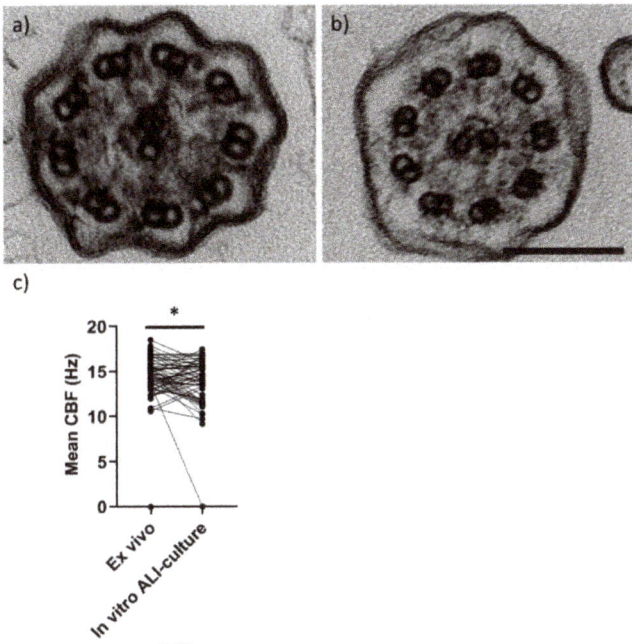

Figure 3. TEM of cilia in transverse section and CBF (by HSVA) in nasal samples and after ALI culture. Representative TEM images (**a**,**b**) of in vitro ALI-cultured cilia in transverse section, showing a "9 + 2" microtubular arrangement. Cilia have normal ciliary ultrastructure in (**a**) a "PCD highly-unlikely" subject (with 3% microtubular defects, 18% inner and 4% outer dynein arm defects quantified from 102 cilia), and (**b**) a "PCD positive" subject (with 11% microtubular defects, 47% inner and 99% outer dynein arm absence quantified from 302 cilia). Scale bar represents 100 nm. Dot plot (**c**) demonstrates the mean CBFs (Hz) of 57 ex vivo nasal brushing samples compared to their matched in vitro ALI cultures (Wilcoxon paired test * p = 0.03). Data from ex vivo samples without a matched ALI sample were excluded (n = 13), which was due to 7 ex vivo samples with a variable ciliary beat pattern (CBP), 3 with failed ALI cultures and 3 that were not cultured. Normal CBF range of ex vivo samples at University Hospital Southampton (UHS) is 11–20 Hz.

The mean CBF was determined in 57 patients' in vitro ALI cultures with unambiguous CBP (completely static cilia were recorded with a mean CBF of 0 Hz). Of the 57, three cases (two "PCD highly-likely" and one "equivocal" at MDT outcome) with mostly static cilia and some residually moving dyskinetic cilia in the original ex vivo sample became completely static in culture, which we have reported before [27]. The Shapiro–Wilk test showed that ex vivo (W = 0.99, p = 0.81) and in vitro (W = 0.96, p = 0.06) sample CBFs were normally distributed only when static samples (three in each group) were excluded. Compared to their matched ex vivo samples (n = 57) the mean CBF of patients samples significantly varied after in vitro ALI culture (median: 14.7 Hz ranging from 0 to 18.5 Hz ex vivo; 13.9 Hz ranging from 0 to 17.5 Hz in vitro) (Wilcoxon matched pairs p = 0.03) (Figure 3). A mean CBF was not considered meaningful in seven patients' ex vivo samples caused by a mixed motile ciliary beat pattern, three samples were not cultured and three failed accounting for the remaining without a CBF.

The in vitro ALI cultures' results were compared by patients' MDT outcome. Of 55 "PCD highly-unlikely" patients, a normal culture CBP was seen in 37 (67.3%) but remained equivocal in 16 (29.1%) and 2 were not cultured. Of seven "PCD"/"PCD highly-likely" patients, an abnormal

"PCD likely" HSVA result was seen in five (71.4%), one was progressing but was deliberately "paused" and frozen due to "hallmark TEM defects" [14] and one patient failed due to infection (Figure 2).

There were eight patients with an equivocal MDT outcome due to inconclusive tests. After all tests, five patients with an unconvincing clinical history were considered to have equivocal diagnostic results at MDT evaluation, with patients advised to seek re-referral if symptoms persisted. Of this group, one patient had a normal CBP, three were equivocal after ALI culture and two failed (insufficiency/infection). Two other patients with normal TEM and "PCD likely" HSVA on in vitro ALI culture are being followed up with genetic testing.

3.2. Was the Nasal Epithelial Cell Culture Protocol Reproducible across the UK PCD Service?

This culture method was simultaneously adopted by the Leicester and Royal Brompton PCD Centres. One hundred and five of 128 (82%) cultures from the Leicester PCD Centre ciliated and of these, 21 of 29 (72.4%) insufficient biopsy samples were successfully differentiated at ALI culture for diagnostic use, providing HSVA results where patients would otherwise have been recalled for repeat biopsy. At the Royal Brompton PCD Centre, 30 of 45 (66.7%) ALI cultures ciliated. Therefore, 199 of 239 consecutive ALI cultures ciliated across 3 UK PCD diagnostic sites, giving a combined ciliation success rate of 83.3%.

Since the COVID-19 pandemic, UHS has cultured 44 patients' samples with protocol modifications to mitigate the risk of acquiring SARS CoV2 infection from nasal brushing samples. This includes storing the nasal cell suspensions in Medium 199 (with 1% pen/strep) at 4 °C for up to 48 h, whilst awaiting the outcome of a SARS CoV2 PCR test. Of the 44 samples cultured during this period, 8 (18%) are still in progress, 28 (64%) ciliated successfully and 8 (18%) failed (3 due to bacteria, 3 due to fungus and 2 as a result of insufficient cell yield).

3.3. Can a Bio-Resource Extend Diagnostic Testing and Research?

Studies have been challenged by the limited number of PCD patients' samples available for research; therefore, since March 2018, UHS has cryopreserved surplus diagnostic cells from PCD clinic patient samples following consent ($n = 181$ to August 2020 including 25 (13.8%) confirmed "PCD positive"/"PCD highly-likely") and 30 healthy donor samples (20 (66.7%) female; median age 37.4, range 21.4–58.3). We have, to date, recovered 6 confirmed "PCD positive"/"PCD highly-likely" samples, 25 confirmed "PCD highly-unlikely" disease control samples and 8 healthy donors from liquid nitrogen storage, with a ciliation success rate of 100% at ALI culture. Here we report representative data from a subset of the thawed samples (Figure 4). The ciliary beat patterns seen on original ex vivo samples (by HSVA) were recapitulated, scanning electron microscopy demonstrated excellent ciliation, and cilia could be immuno-fluorescently labelled in representative cases after cryostorage and ALI culture differentiation (Figure 4).

The physical barrier properties, measured by TEER at 4 weeks post-ALI, of $n = 10$ thawed "PCD highly-unlikely" 383 $\Omega.cm^2$ (SD ± 86.5) and $n = 4$ defrosted "PCD highly-likely" 314 $\Omega.cm^2$ (SD ± 153.9) samples were not significantly different to each other (t test) or to $n = 4$ representative fresh (non-frozen) healthy donor in vitro ALI cultures 299 $\Omega.cm^2$ (SD ± 97.6) (Mann–Whitney test) (Figure 4). HSVA demonstrated that $n = 4$ representative "PCD highly-unlikely" samples with mean nasal brushing CBF of 17.3 Hz, SD ± 2.9 (ex vivo) resolved a normal CBP with mucociliary clearance with a significantly reduced mean CBF of 12.7 Hz, SD ± 2.5 in matched samples that were ALI-cultured (4 weeks) after liquid nitrogen storage (paired t test, $p = 0.01$); while three of these cultures retained a normal CBP, one culture's CBF fell just below the UHS normal range (11–20 Hz) [27] (Figure 4). Six "PCD positive"/"PCD highly-likely" samples that had predominantly static cilia ($n = 4$) or uncoordinated and stiff dyskinetic cilia ($n = 2$) on the ex vivo nasal brushing samples retained their abnormal CBP at week 4 of ALI culture in vitro after freezing (CBF not shown). The quality of ALI cultures prepared for HSVA after samples were defrosted from cryostorage compared to their original ex vivo samples are shown in Supplementary Video S2a–d.

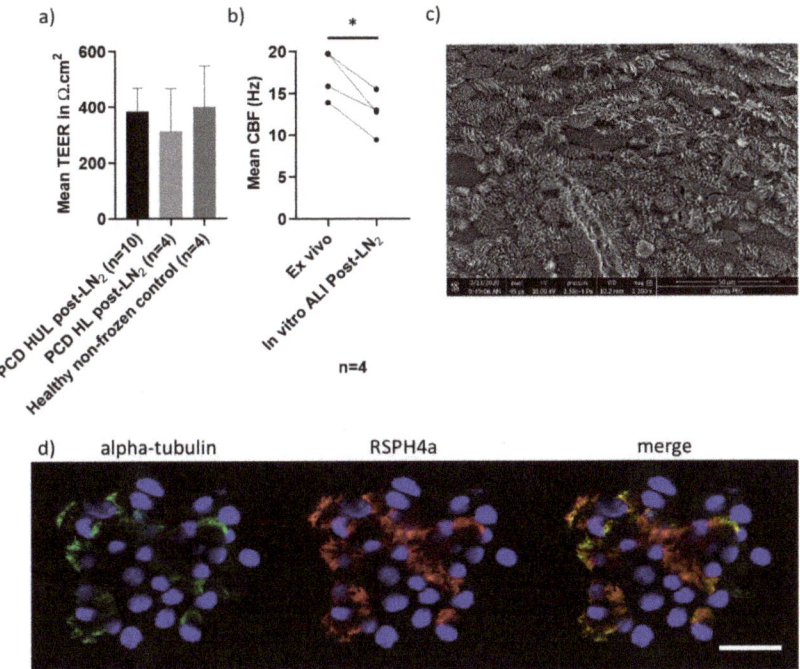

Figure 4. Characteristics of in vitro ALI cultures (ciliated and differentiated at passage 2) derived from frozen liquid nitrogen storage. (**a**) There was no difference in the mean (±SD) trans-epithelial electrical resistance (TEER) ($\Omega.cm^2$) of $n = 10$ "PCD highly-unlikely" and $n = 4$ "PCD highly-likely" ALI cultures recovered from liquid nitrogen cryostorage (post-LN$_2$) (*t* test), or compared to $n = 4$ healthy donor sample (non-frozen) controls (Mann–Whitney test) measured in triplicate per Transwell® insert at 4 weeks ALI culture, when cells were widely ciliated. (**b**) The mean CBF (Hz) of $n = 4$ matched PCD clinic samples differed before (ex vivo) and after liquid nitrogen storage (in vitro ALI culture) * $p = 0.01$ (paired *t* test). (**c**) A representative SEM image from a "PCD highly-unlikely" ALI culture showing typical ciliation at week 4 post-LN$_2$. (**d**) Representative PCD diagnostic immunofluorescence [15] images from an SP8 laser scanning confocal microscope, showing a PCD clinic ALI culture after cryostorage with 4% paraformaldehyde fixation and immunofluorescence labelling with anti-alpha-tubulin (cilia marker-Alexa488 secondary antibody, green), anti-RSPH4a (radial spoke head protein-Alexa549 secondary antibody, red) and DAPI (nuclei DNA stain, blue). Scale 20 µm.

4. Discussion

After revisions to our 2014 [27] culture protocol, employing the commercially available STEMCELL Technologies media system, we demonstrate an excellent 95.5% success rate of ALI cultures differentiating cilia with 38.9% cilia coverage for analysis at the UHS PCD centre. Three UK PCD diagnostic centres share protocols [47,48]. Therefore, this revised protocol was simultaneously adopted, enabling us to confirm a combined success of 83.3% of ALI cultures ciliated across our national service. Differences in success rates between our centres may have been due to several factors such as different patient demographics, sampling variability and physical management of samples due to our logistical setups. For example, the UHS benefits from having laboratories on the same site as the patient clinics and we were able to repeat insufficient samples during clinic, whilst the patient was still onsite as needed. Since we have introduced COVID-19 mitigation measures, to limit our risk of acquiring the illness from our patients and samples, we have cultured 44 nasal brushing samples and 28 (64%) are so far ciliated, 8 (18%) are ongoing and 8 (18%) failed since July 2020. This is encouraging that a high success rate can be maintained during the constraints of the current COVID-19 pandemic. Analyses following ALI culture have negated the need to recall patients for repeat nasal brushing biopsy after inconclusive HSVA results due to secondary factors, and/or insufficient sample for analyses [27,35]. The excellent yield of cilia coupled with the speed at which normally functioning cilia generate allow for repeat HSVA analysis and if needed repeat TEM to be reported within diagnostic time constraints, with sample also available for IF labelling of cilia and RNA extraction for further genetic splice variant screening (as well as genomic DNA genetic screening) if required. Results from ALI cultures gave added confidence for patient discharge as "PCD highly-unlikely" when abnormalities resolved in culture, or a diagnosis of "PCD positive" or "PCD highly-likely" to be given when abnormalities persist after culture.

Cell culture is an important tool in the diagnostic pathway but is a lengthy and technically demanding process. A reliable system for obtaining a good yield of healthy ciliated epithelial cells is vital. In our experience, most failures occur early in the culture process due to either a lack of viable epithelial cells from nasal brush biopsy or viral/bacteria/fungal infections. To minimise failure rates, we recommend nasal brush biopsies are taken only from patients free from symptoms of infection for the previous six weeks. Basal epithelial cell survival, proliferation and differentiation in vitro rely on high cell densities [49]. With the patients still in clinic, typically cell yields from biopsies can quickly be checked by low power light microscopy to ensure enough material is present for all tests needed. In the event of a poor yield of healthy cells the patient may be approached for another brushing if tolerated. However, in light of the current COVID-19 pandemic, we are not practicing this to limit our exposure to nasal brushing samples in the laboratory. Although this could potentially be circumvented if microscope equipment can be housed within a customized class 2 MSC. As with all long-term cell culture, infection risks are high, maintaining the cultures in a designated culture facility with limited numbers of experienced users is important to maximise success rates.

Airway cells stored in a bio-resource and cultured at ALI retain their pre-frozen characteristics and provide a model for PCD diagnostic testing and investigating the pathogenesis and treatments of respiratory disease (particularly for rare samples) without needing to recall patients for repeat brushings [36–39,50]. Exceptionally, 100% of samples recovered from liquid nitrogen successfully ciliated ($n = 6$ "PCD positive"/"PCD highly-likely", $n = 25$ "PCD highly-unlikely" and $n = 8$ healthy donor samples). In $n = 4$ "PCD highly-unlikely" samples with normal CBP and normal CBF (11–20 Hz at UHS) ex vivo, the CBF of ALI cultures significantly ($p = 0.01$) reduced after freezing despite maintaining normal CBP, either due to low sample numbers or the freezing/defrosting process (Figure 4). The CBF reduction was not pronounced after the ALI culture process in 56 patients' samples that were not previously stored in liquid nitrogen (Figure 3). We believe this method provides great scope for studies of both healthy and diseased ciliated epithelia, yet we advise for CBF studies that a baseline CBF of ALI cultures derived from cryostored cells be established in-house. However, limitations of the model are the reliance upon commercially obtained culture media, and the undisclosed nature of the culture media components. In summary, we have presented an updated protocol for culture of airway epithelial cells, which has been stable and reliable, with consistently high success rates over the course of one year, based on the experience at three PCD diagnostic centres within a national service. Long-term, our patients will benefit directly from reduced recall for repeat samples, and advances in our understanding of disease phenotype and new treatment efficacy. Bio-resourcing will enable us to participate in national and international networks (https://bestcilia.eu/ and https://beat-pcd.squarespace.com/) that are collaborating to better characterise and treat PCD.

Supplementary Materials: The following are available online at http://www.mdpi.com/2077-0383/9/11/3753/s1. Video S1: Removing secondary dyskinesia in "PCD highly-unlikely" and confirming "PCD highly-likely" in ex vivo clinic samples before and after in vitro ALI culture. Video S2: Removing secondary dyskinesia in "PCD highly-unlikely" and confirming "PCD highly-likely" in ex vivo clinic samples before and after in vitro ALI culture post LN_2. All UHS videos were recorded at 500 fps and are shown at 30 fps playback.

Author Contributions: Conceptualization, C.L.J., C.B. and J.L.S.; methodology, C.L.J, J.L.C., C.B., R.A.H. and P.G. (Paul Griffin); software, P.M.L.; validation, C.L.J., J.L.C., R.A.H., G.M.W. and P.G. (Paul Griffin); formal analysis, J.L.C., C.B. and C.L.J.; investigation, C.L.J., J.L.C., J.T., K.L.H., P.G. (Patricia Goggin), R.D., A.H., W.T.W., R.A.H., G.M.W. and P.G. (Paul Griffin); data curation, C.L.J., J.L.C., J.T., K.L.H., P.G. (Patricia Goggin), R.D., R.A.H., G.M.W. and P.G. (Paul Griffin); writing—original draft preparation, J.L.C, C.L.J., and J.S.L.: writing—all authors reviewed and edited; supervision, J.S.L., C.L.J. and C.B.; funding acquisition, J.S.L., C.H., C.O., C.L.J. and C.B. All authors have read and agreed to the published version of the manuscript.

Funding: This research was funded by AAIR Charity: "Expansion of an ex vivo primary respiratory epithelial cell model to facilitate primary ciliary dyskinesia airway research" and the NIHR Research for Patient Benefit Programme: 200470. The National PCD Service is commissioned and funded by NHS England.

Acknowledgments: PCD research in Southampton is supported by NIHR Southampton Biomedical Research Centre, NIHR Welcome Trust Clinical Research Facility). PCD research in Leicester is supported by the NIHR GOSH BRC. Authors are members of BEAT-PCD (supported by COST Action BM1407 and ERS Clinical Research Collaboration). UHS and RBH are members of the European Reference Network for Rare Respiratory Diseases (ERN-LUNG)—Project ID No 739546. The views expressed in this publication are those of the authors and not necessarily those of the NHS, the National Institute for Health Research, or other organisations.

Conflicts of Interest: All authors certify that they have no conflicts of interest to declare.

References

1. Wallmeier, J.; Nielsen, K.G.; Kuehni, C.E.; Lucas, J.S.; Leigh, M.W.; Zariwala, M.A.; Omran, H. Motile ciliopathies. *Nat. Rev. Dis. Prim.* **2020**, *6*, 1–29. [CrossRef]
2. O'Callaghan, C.; Chetcuti, P.; Moya, E. High prevalence of primary ciliary dyskinesia in a British Asian population. *Arch. Dis. Child.* **2010**, *95*, 51–52. [CrossRef] [PubMed]
3. Lucas, J.S.; Davis, S.D.; Omran, H.; Shoemark, A. Primary ciliary dyskinesia in the genomics age. *Lancet Respir. Med.* **2020**, *8*, 202–216. [CrossRef]
4. Behan, L.; Dimitrov, B.D.; Kuehni, C.E.; Hogg, C.; Carroll, M.; Evans, H.J.; Goutaki, M.; Harris, A.; Packham, S.; Walker, W.T.; et al. PICADAR: A diagnostic predictive tool for primary ciliary dyskinesia. *Eur. Respir. J.* **2016**, *47*, 1103–1112. [CrossRef] [PubMed]
5. Lucas, J.S.; Alanin, M.C.; Collins, S.; Harris, A.; Johansen, H.K.; Nielsen, K.G.; Papon, J.F.; Robinson, P.; Walker, W.T. Clinical care of children with primary ciliary dyskinesia. *Expert Rev. Respir. Med.* **2017**, *11*, 779–790. [CrossRef] [PubMed]
6. Lucas, J.S.; Leigh, M.W. Diagnosis of primary ciliary dyskinesia: Searching for a gold standard. *Eur. Respir. J.* **2014**, *44*, 1418–1422. [CrossRef] [PubMed]
7. Lucas, J.S.; Barbato, A.; Collins, S.A.; Goutaki, M.; Behan, L.; Caudri, D.; Dell, S.; Eber, E.; Escudier, E.; Hirst, R.A.; et al. European Respiratory Society guidelines for the diagnosis of primary ciliary dyskinesia. *Eur. Respir. J.* **2017**, *49*. [CrossRef]
8. Shapiro, A.J.; Davis, S.D.; Polineni, D.; Manion, M.; Rosenfeld, M.; Dell, S.D.; Chilvers, M.; Ferkol, T.W.; Zariwala, M.A.; Sagel, S.D.; et al. Diagnosis of Primary Ciliary Dyskinesia. An Official American Thoracic Society Clinical Practice Guideline. *Am. J. Respir. Crit. Care Med.* **2018**, *197*, e24–e39. [CrossRef]
9. Shoemark, A.; Dell, S.; Shapiro, A.; Lucas, J. ERS and ATS diagnostic guidelines for primary ciliary dyskinesia: Similarities and differences in approach to diagnosis. *Eur. Respir. J.* **2019**, *54*. [CrossRef]
10. Jackson, C.L.; Behan, L.; Collins, S.A.; Goggin, P.M.; Adam, E.C.; Coles, J.L.; Evans, H.J.; Harris, A.; Lackie, P.M.; Packham, S.; et al. Accuracy of diagnostic testing in primary ciliary dyskinesia. *Eur. Respir. J.* **2016**, *47*, 837–848. [CrossRef]
11. Kempeneers, C.; Seaton, C.; Chilvers, M.A. Variation of Ciliary Beat Pattern in Three Different Beating Planes in Healthy Subjects. *Chest* **2017**, *151*, 993–1001. [CrossRef] [PubMed]
12. Rubbo, B.; Shoemark, A.; Jackson, C.L.; Hirst, R.; Thompson, J.; Hayes, J.; Frost, E.; Copeland, F.; Hogg, C.; O'Callaghan, C.; et al. Accuracy of High-Speed Video Analysis to Diagnose Primary Ciliary Dyskinesia. *Chest* **2019**, *155*, 1008–1017. [CrossRef] [PubMed]
13. Shoemark, A.; Dixon, M.; Corrin, B.; Dewar, A. Twenty-year review of quantitative transmission electron microscopy for the diagnosis of primary ciliary dyskinesia. *J. Clin. Pathol.* **2011**, *65*, 267–271. [CrossRef] [PubMed]

14. Shoemark, A.; Boon, M.; Brochhausen, C.; Bukowy-Bieryllo, Z.; De Santi, M.M.; Goggin, P.; Griffin, P.; Hegele, R.G.; Hirst, R.A.; Leigh, M.W.; et al. International consensus guideline for reporting transmission electron microscopy results in the diagnosis of Primary Ciliary Dyskinesia (BEAT PCD TEM Criteria). *Eur. Respir. J.* **2020**, *55*. [CrossRef]
15. Shoemark, A.; Frost, E.; Dixon, M.; Ollosson, S.; Kilpin, K.; Patel, M.; Scully, J.; Rogers, A.V.; Mitchison, H.M.; Bush, A.; et al. Accuracy of Immunofluorescence in the Diagnosis of Primary Ciliary Dyskinesia. *Am. J. Respir. Crit. Care Med.* **2017**, *196*, 94–101. [CrossRef]
16. Liu, Z.; Nguyen, Q.P.H.; Guan, Q.; Albulescu, A.; Erdman, L.; Mahdaviyeh, Y.; Kang, J.; Ouyang, H.; Hegele, R.G.; Moraes, T.J.; et al. A quantitative super-resolution imaging toolbox for diagnosis of motile ciliopathies. *Sci. Transl. Med.* **2020**, *12*. [CrossRef]
17. Dougherty, G.W.; Loges, N.T.; Klinkenbusch, J.A.; Olbrich, H.; Pennekamp, P.; Menchen, T.; Raidt, J.; Wallmeier, J.; Werner, C.; Westermann, C.; et al. DNAH11 Localization in the Proximal Region of Respiratory Cilia Defines Distinct Outer Dynein Arm Complexes. *Am. J. Respir. Cell Mol. Biol.* **2016**, *55*, 213–224. [CrossRef]
18. Loges, N.T.; Antony, D.; Maver, A.; Deardorff, M.; Güleç, E.Y.; Gezdirici, A.; Nöthe-Menchen, T.; Höben, I.M.; Jelten, L.; Frank, D.; et al. Recessive DNAH9 Loss-of-Function Mutations Cause Laterality Defects and Subtle Respiratory Ciliary-Beating Defects. *Am. J. Hum. Genet.* **2018**, *103*, 995–1008. [CrossRef]
19. Cindrić, S.; Dougherty, G.W.; Olbrich, H.; Hjeij, R.; Loges, N.T.; Amirav, I.; Philipsen, M.C.; Marthin, J.K.; Nielsen, K.G.; Sutharsan, S.; et al. SPEF2- and HYDIN-Mutant Cilia Lack the Central Pair–associated Protein SPEF2, Aiding Primary Ciliary Dyskinesia Diagnostics. *Am. J. Respir. Cell Mol. Biol.* **2020**, *62*, 382–396. [CrossRef]
20. Marshall, C.R.; Scherer, S.W.; Zariwala, M.A.; Lau, L.; Paton, T.A.; Stockley, T.L.; Jobling, R.K.; Ray, P.N.; Knowles, M.R.; Hall, D.A.; et al. Whole-Exome Sequencing and Targeted Copy Number Analysis in Primary Ciliary Dyskinesia. *G3 Genes Genomes Genet.* **2015**, *5*, 1775–1781. [CrossRef]
21. Olbrich, H.; Cremers, C.; Loges, N.T.; Werner, C.; Nielsen, K.G.; Marthin, J.K.; Philipsen, M.; Wallmeier, J.; Pennekamp, P.; Menchen, T.; et al. Loss-of-Function GAS8 Mutations Cause Primary Ciliary Dyskinesia and Disrupt the Nexin-Dynein Regulatory Complex. *Am. J. Hum. Genet.* **2015**, *97*, 546–554. [CrossRef] [PubMed]
22. Panizzi, J.R.; Becker-Heck, A.; Castleman, V.H.; Al-Mutairi, D.A.; Liu, Y.; Loges, N.T.; Pathak, N.; Austin-Tse, C.; Sheridan, E.; Schmidts, M.; et al. CCDC103 mutations cause primary ciliary dyskinesia by disrupting assembly of ciliary dynein arms. *Nat. Genet.* **2012**, *44*, 714–719. [CrossRef] [PubMed]
23. Shoemark, A.; Moya, E.; Hirst, R.A.; Patel, M.P.; Robson, E.A.; Hayward, J.; Scully, J.; Fassad, M.R.; Lamb, W.; Schmidts, M.; et al. High prevalence of CCDC103 p.His154Pro mutation causing primary ciliary dyskinesia disrupts protein oligomerisation and is associated with normal diagnostic investigations. *Thorax* **2018**, *73*, 157–166. [CrossRef] [PubMed]
24. Boon, M.; Wallmeier, J.; Ma, L.; Loges, N.T.; Jaspers, M.; Olbrich, H.; Dougherty, G.W.; Raidt, J.; Werner, C.; Amirav, I.; et al. MCIDAS mutations result in a mucociliary clearance disorder with reduced generation of multiple motile cilia. *Nat. Commun.* **2014**, *5*, 4418. [CrossRef]
25. Wallmeier, J.; Al-Mutairi, D.A.; Chen, C.-T.; Loges, N.T.; Pennekamp, P.; Menchen, T.; Ma, L.; Shamseldin, H.; Olbrich, H.; Dougherty, G.W.; et al. Mutations in CCNO result in congenital mucociliary clearance disorder with reduced generation of multiple motile cilia. *Nat. Genet.* **2014**, *46*, 646–651. [CrossRef]
26. Wallmeier, J.; Frank, D.; Shoemark, A.; Nöthe-Menchen, T.; Cindric, S.; Olbrich, H.; Loges, N.T.; Aprea, I.; Dougherty, G.W.; Pennekamp, P.; et al. De Novo Mutations in FOXJ1 Result in a Motile Ciliopathy with Hydrocephalus and Randomization of Left/Right Body Asymmetry. *Am. J. Hum. Genet.* **2019**, *105*, 1030–1039. [CrossRef]
27. Hirst, R.A.; Jackson, C.L.; Coles, J.L.; Williams, G.; Rutman, A.; Goggin, P.M.; Adam, E.C.; Page, A.; Evans, H.J.; Lackie, P.M.; et al. Culture of Primary Ciliary Dyskinesia Epithelial Cells at Air-Liquid Interface Can Alter Ciliary Phenotype but Remains a Robust and Informative Diagnostic Aid. *PLoS ONE* **2014**, *9*, e89675. [CrossRef]
28. Dixon, M.; Shoemark, A. Secondary defects detected by transmission electron microscopy in primary ciliary dyskinesia diagnostics. *Ultrastruct. Pathol.* **2017**, *41*, 390–398. [CrossRef]
29. O'Callaghan, C.; Rutman, A.; Williams, G.; Kulkarni, N.; Hayes, J.; Hirst, R.A. Ciliated conical epithelial cell protrusions point towards a diagnosis of primary ciliary dyskinesia. *Respir. Res.* **2018**, *19*, 125. [CrossRef]
30. Toskala, E.; Haataja, J.; Shirasaki, H.; Rautiainen, M. Culture of cells harvested with nasal brushing: A method for evaluating ciliary function. *Rhinology* **2005**, *43*, 121–124.

31. Willems, T.; Jorissen, M. Sequential monolayer-suspension culture of human airway epithelial cells. *J. Cyst. Fibros.* **2004**, *3* (Suppl. 2), 53–54. [CrossRef] [PubMed]
32. Pifferi, M.; Montemurro, F.; Cangiotti, A.M.; Ragazzo, V.; Di Cicco, M.; Vinci, B.; Vozzi, G.; Macchia, P.; Boner, A.L. Simplified cell culture method for the diagnosis of atypical primary ciliary dyskinesia. *Thorax* **2009**, *64*, 1077–1081. [CrossRef] [PubMed]
33. Pifferi, M.; Bush, A.; Montemurro, F.; Pioggia, G.; Piras, M.; Tartarisco, G.; Di Cicco, M.E.; Chinellato, I.; Cangiotti, A.M.; Boner, A.L. Rapid diagnosis of primary ciliary dyskinesia: Cell culture and soft computing analysis. *Eur. Respir. J.* **2013**, *41*, 960–965. [CrossRef] [PubMed]
34. Marthin, J.K.; Stevens, E.; Larsen, L.A.; Christensen, S.T.; Nielsen, K.G. Patient-specific three-dimensional explant spheroids derived from human nasal airway epithelium: A simple methodological approach for ex vivo studies of primary ciliary dyskinesia. *Cilia* **2017**, *6*, 3. [CrossRef] [PubMed]
35. Hirst, R.A.; Rutman, A.; Williams, G.; O'Callaghan, C. Ciliated Air-Liquid Cultures as an Aid to Diagnostic Testing of Primary Ciliary Dyskinesia. *Chest* **2010**, *138*, 1441–1447. [CrossRef] [PubMed]
36. Ong, H.X.; Jackson, C.L.; Cole, J.L.; Lackie, P.M.; Traini, D.; Young, P.M.; Lucas, J.; Conway, J. Primary Air–Liquid Interface Culture of Nasal Epithelium for Nasal Drug Delivery. *Mol. Pharm.* **2016**, *13*, 2242–2252. [CrossRef]
37. Collins, S.A.; Kelso, M.J.; Rineh, A.; Yepuri, N.R.; Coles, J.; Jackson, C.L.; Halladay, G.D.; Walker, W.T.; Webb, J.S.; Hall-Stoodley, L.; et al. Cephalosporin-3′-Diazeniumdiolate NO Donor Prodrug PYRRO-C3D Enhances Azithromycin Susceptibility of Nontypeable Haemophilus influenzae Biofilms. *Antimicrob. Agents Chemother.* **2017**, *61*, 02086-16. [CrossRef]
38. Walker, W.T.; Jackson, C.L.; Allan, R.N.; Collins, S.A.; Kelso, M.J.; Rineh, A.; Yepuri, N.R.; Nicholas, B.; Lau, L.; Johnston, D.; et al. Primary ciliary dyskinesia ciliated airway cells show increased susceptibility to Haemophilus influenzae biofilm formation. *Eur. Respir. J.* **2017**, *50*. [CrossRef]
39. Walker, W.T.; Jackson, C.L.; Coles, J.; Lackie, P.M.; Faust, S.N.; Hall-Stoodley, L.; Lucas, J. Ciliated cultures from patients with primary ciliary dyskinesia produce nitric oxide in response to Haemophilus influenzae infection and proinflammatory cytokines. *Chest* **2014**, *145*, 668–669. [CrossRef]
40. Smith, C.M.; Kulkarni, H.; Radhakrishnan, P.; Rutman, A.; Bankart, M.J.; Williams, G.; Hirst, R.A.; Easton, A.J.; Andrew, P.W.; O'Callaghan, C. Ciliary dyskinesia is an early feature of respiratory syncytial virus infection. *Eur. Respir. J.* **2014**, *43*, 485–496. [CrossRef]
41. Smith, C.M.; Sandrini, S.; Datta, S.; Freestone, P.; Shafeeq, S.; Radhakrishnan, P.; Williams, G.; Glenn, S.M.; Kuipers, O.P.; Hirst, R.A.; et al. Respiratory syncytial virus increases the virulence of Streptococcus pneumoniae by binding to penicillin binding protein 1a. A new paradigm in respiratory infection. *Am. J. Respir. Crit. Care Med.* **2014**, *190*, 196–207. [CrossRef] [PubMed]
42. Blume, C.; Swindle, E.J.; Dennison, P.; Jayasekera, N.P.; Dudley, S.; Monk, P.; Behrendt, H.; Schmidt-Weber, C.; Holgate, S.T.; Howarth, P.H.; et al. Barrier responses of human bronchial epithelial cells to grass pollen exposure. *Eur. Respir. J.* **2012**, *42*, 87–97. [CrossRef] [PubMed]
43. Blume, C.; Jackson, C.L.; Spalluto, C.M.; Legebeke, J.; Nazlamova, L.A.; Conforti, F.; Perotin-Collard, J.M.; Frank, M.; Crispin, M.; Coles, J.; et al. A novel isoform of *ACE2* is expressed in human nasal and bronchial respiratory epithelia and is upregulated in response to RNA respiratory virus infection. *BioRxiv* **2020**. [CrossRef]
44. Kuehni, C.E.; Lucas, J.S. Diagnosis of primary ciliary dyskinesia: Summary of the ERS Task Force report. *Breathe* **2017**, *13*, 166–178. [CrossRef] [PubMed]
45. Lucas, J.; Evans, H.J.; Haarman, E.G.; Hirst, R.A.; Hogg, C.; Jackson, C.L.; Nielsen, K.G.; Omran, H.; Papon, J.-F.; Robinson, P.; et al. Exploring the Art of Ciliary Beating. *Chest* **2017**, *152*, 1348–1349. [CrossRef] [PubMed]
46. Serafini, S.M.; Michaelson, E.D. Length and distribution of cilia in human and canine airways. *Bull. Eur. Physiopathol. Respir.* **1977**, *13*, 551–559.
47. Lucas, J.S.; Burgess, A.; Mitchison, H.M.; Moya, E.; Williamson, M.; Hogg, C.; National PCD Service, UK. Diagnosis and management of primary ciliary dyskinesia. *Arch. Dis. Child.* **2014**, *99*, 850–856. [CrossRef]
48. Lucas, J.; Chetcuti, P.; Copeland, F.; Hogg, C.; Kenny, T.; Moya, E.; O'Callaghan, C.; Walker, W.T. Overcoming challenges in the management of primary ciliary dyskinesia: The UK model. *Paediatr. Respir. Rev.* **2014**, *15*, 142–145. [CrossRef]

49. Fulcher, M.L.; Gabriel, S.; Burns, K.A.; Yankaskas, J.R.; Randell, S.H. Well-Differentiated Human Airway Epithelial Cell Cultures. *Methods Mol. Med.* **2005**, *107*, 183–206. [CrossRef]
50. Lai, M.; Pifferi, M.; Bush, A.; Piras, M.; Michelucci, A.; Di Cicco, M.; Del Grosso, A.; Quaranta, P.; Cursi, C.; Tantillo, E.; et al. Gene editing of DNAH11 restores normal cilia motility in primary ciliary dyskinesia. *J. Med. Genet.* **2016**, *53*, 242–249. [CrossRef]

Publisher's Note: MDPI stays neutral with regard to jurisdictional claims in published maps and institutional affiliations.

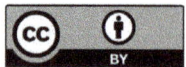

© 2020 by the authors. Licensee MDPI, Basel, Switzerland. This article is an open access article distributed under the terms and conditions of the Creative Commons Attribution (CC BY) license (http://creativecommons.org/licenses/by/4.0/).

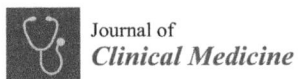

Article

Serum Levels of Glutamate-Pyruvate Transaminase, Glutamate-Oxaloacetate Transaminase and Gamma-Glutamyl Transferase in 1494 Patients with Various Genotypes for the Alpha-1 Antitrypsin Gene

José María Hernández Pérez [1], Ignacio Blanco [2], Agustín Jesús Sánchez Medina [3], Laura Díaz Hernández [4] and José Antonio Pérez Pérez [5,*]

1. Pulmonology Department, University Hospital Nuestra Señora de Candelaria, Santa Cruz de Tenerife, 38010 Canary Islands, Spain; jmherper@hotmail.com
2. Spanish Registry of Alpha-1 Antitrypsin Deficiency (REDAAT), Respira Foundation, Spanish Society of Pulmonology and Thoracic Surgery (SEPAR), 08029 Barcelona, Spain; ignablanco@yahoo.es
3. University Institute of Sciences and Cybernetic Technologies, University of Las Palmas de Gran Canaria, 35018 Las Palmas, Spain; agustin.sanchez@ulpgc.es
4. Digestive System Department, University Hospital Nuestra Señora de Candelaria, Santa Cruz de Tenerife, 38010 Canary Islands, Spain; lauradiazhdez@hotmail.com
5. Institute of Tropical Diseases and Public Health of the Canary Islands, University of La Laguna, Genetic Area, 38206 Canary Islands, Spain
* Correspondence: joanpere@ull.edu.es; Tel.: +34-922-316-502 (ext. 8678/6891); Fax: +34-922-318-311

Received: 6 November 2020; Accepted: 1 December 2020; Published: 3 December 2020

Abstract: Background: Patients with liver disease associated with alpha-1 antitrypsin deficiency (AATD) are homozygous for the Z mutation, leading to chronic liver damage. Objective: To assess the serum levels of glutamate-oxaloacetate transaminase (GOT), glutamate-pyruvate transaminase (GPT), and gamma-glutamyl transpeptidase (GGT) in patients with different genotypes for the alpha-1 antitrypsin (AAT) gene. Methods: Patients (n = 1494) underwent genotyping of the *SERPINA1* gene, together with a determination of AAT and GOT and GPT and GGT transaminase levels. Patients with a deficient allele (n = 476) and with a normal genotype were compared. Results: A statistically significant association was found between deficient genotypes and GOT ($p < 0.0003$), GPT ($p < 0.002$), and GGT ($p < 0.006$). Comparing GOT levels in patients with PI*Z deficient variant versus those with normal genotype, an odds ratio (OR) of 2.72 (CI: 1.5–4.87) ($p < 0.0005$) was obtained. This finding was replicated with the *PI*Z* allele and the GPT values (OR = 2.31; CI: 1.45–3.67; $p < 0.0003$). In addition, a statistically significant association was found between liver enzymes and AAT values. Conclusion: The *PI*Z* allele seemed to be a risk factor for the development of liver damage. AAT deficient genotypes were associated with GOT, GPT, and GGT altered values. Low AAT levels were associated with high GPT and GGT levels.

Keywords: Alpha-1 antitrypsin deficiency; liver disease; glutamate-oxaloacetate transaminase; glutamate-pyruvate transaminase; gamma-glutamyl transpeptidase

1. Introduction

Alpha-1 antitrypsin (AAT) is a glycoprotein synthesized and secreted primarily by hepatocytes, whose main function is to neutralize excess elastase released by activated neutrophils, thereby protecting the extracellular matrix of the lungs from the harmful effects of this protease [1].

The two alleles that an individual possesses for this genetic locus are transmitted by autosomal Mendelian inheritance. The phenotypic relationship between normal and deficient alleles is partial dominance when circulating AAT levels are analyzed, or codominance when different protein variants are detected by isoelectric focusing (becoming complete dominance in the case of null alleles). Normal alleles, found in 85–90% of individuals, are called *PI*M*, while the most common deficient alleles are *PI*S* and *PI*Z*, with a prevalence among Caucasians of 3–10% and 1–3%, respectively [2].

Severe alpha-1 antitrypsin deficiency (AATD) is a hereditary condition, typically associated with *PI*ZZ* genotypes, which promotes the development of various diseases, including: chronic obstructive pulmonary disease (COPD), with onset in early adulthood in up to 50% of deficient subjects (from the age of 40, as opposed to 50–60 years for common COPD); childhood-juvenile cirrhosis in 2.5% of individuals with the *PI*ZZ* genotype; adult cirrhosis in 30% (generally men from the age of 50 years); hepatocarcinoma in 2–3% of elderly individuals with *PI*ZZ* genotype; systemic vasculitis (Wegener's) in 2–3%; and neutrophilic panniculitis (in 1% of *PI*ZZ* individuals in the UK registry and 0.1% in the American registry) [3].

In clinical practice, most patients with AATD-associated liver disease are homozygous for the Z mutation (Glu342Lys). This genetic defect causes an abnormal folding of the PiZ protein, 80–90% of which is retained in the rough endoplasmic reticulum [4] of hepatocytes, forming highly stable polymer accumulations, which lead to a cellular stress response and chronic liver damage in some individuals [5]. The PiS protein polymerizes moderately, but its inhibitory capacity remains unchanged. However, the S and Z proteins of *PI*SZ* heterozygotes can form hepatic heteropolymers that can cause cirrhosis [6].

The transaminases glutamate-oxaloacetate transaminase (GOT), glutamate-pyruvate transaminase (GPT), and gamma-glutamyl transpeptidase (GGT) are enzymes routinely used as general laboratory markers of liver disease. GPT and GGT are expressed in hepatocytes. As well as in the liver, GOT is expressed in the myocardium, skeletal muscle, kidneys, brain, pancreas, lung, leukocytes, and erythrocytes [7].

The objective of this study was to determine whether patients with AAT deficiency have a higher risk of liver involvement according to the different genotypes.

2. Experimental Section

2.1. Study Design

An observational, cross-sectional, and descriptive study was carried out, in which a total of 1494 patients who attended the pulmonology outpatient clinic for any reason were included and analysed. They were divided into two comparable groups, those with a normal genotyping result (*Pi*MM*) and another group of subjects whose genotyping result was different *(Pi* ≠ MM)*. In addition, two comparable age-based groups were created (≤25 years and >25 years). The study was conducted in accordance with the Declaration of Helsinki. This study was approved by the ethics committee of the hospital, and all patients were informed of the study objectives and signed an informed consent. In the case of minors, their parent or guardian signed the consent.

Inclusion criteria: Patients who attended the pulmonology outpatient clinic consecutively, regardless of the reason for doing so, patients who had undergone genotyping of the SERPINA1 gene, patients whose GOT, GPT, and GGT values had been measured via blood clinical chemistry, and patients who expressed their participation in the study by signing the informed consent.

Exclusion criteria: Patients with severe chronic alcoholism or diagnosed with previous alcoholic liver disease, a history of drug-related liver toxicity, autoimmune or viral liver cirrhosis, fatty liver, viral hepatitis, haemochromatosis, or Wilson's disease were excluded. Various analytical studies were carried out (serological determination of hepatitis virus, autoimmunity, iron levels, and copper levels). In addition, imaging studies were performed using liver ultrasound or computed axial tomography in some patients with abnormal laboratory tests to rule out involvement from other causes (neoplasms, malformations, infections, etc.).

2.2. Patients

Each patient underwent genotyping to check for PI*S alleles, PI*Z alleles, and rare variants of the SERPINA1 gene. To make comparisons, the sample of patients was subdivided into two groups: 476 patients with a genetic diagnosis of AATD and 1018 with a normal genotype for the SERPINA1 gene.

2.3. Genetic Analysis

The genotype was determined using so-called hybridization probes or HybProbes [8], which allow both real-time PCR to be performed and, after the initial amplification process, the genetic variants present in a certain region within the amplified DNA fragment to be identified. Specifically, the genotyping protocol described by Hernández-Pérez et al. was followed [9].

Determination of AAT and Transaminase Serum Levels

The AAT serum levels of each patient were quantified by immunonephelometry, while the serum concentrations of the enzymes GOT, GPT, and GGT were determined by standard clinical analysis procedures. Cut-off levels were those determined by the reference laboratories.

2.4. Statistical Analysis

The descriptive analyses of the variables were expressed as median (interquartile range (IQR)) or number (%). Differences in the distributions of patient characteristics by subgroups of outcomes were reported using differences with a 95% CI. Categorical data were compared using the χ^2 test or Fisher's exact test. Continuous variables were expressed as absolute (n) and variables (%). Differences between both groups were evaluated by univariate analysis and multiple logistic regression to calculate odds ratios (ORs). The different ORs are shown with their respective 95% confidence intervals (CIs). Multivariate logistic regression was used to assess independent associations. Linear correlations between clinical variables and biomarkers were evaluated by Pearson's or Spearman's correlation coefficient. A significant difference was considered when $p < 0.05$. Statistical analysis was performed with the IBM® SPSS Statistics version 25 program.

3. Results

3.1. Baseline Characteristics

Of the 1494 patients, elevated GOT levels were observed in 5.7%, elevated GPT in 10.6%, and elevated GGT in 20.3%. Most cases were male, with a mean age of 51.4 years and a range between 1–94, a weight of 76.14 kg ranging between 36 and 152, and a median BMI of 27.67 kg/m^2 with a range between 14.9 and 53.6. The median AAT level of the patients was 82.14 mg/dL with a range between 5 and 308.2. The rest of the baseline characteristics of the patients are shown in Table 1.

Table 1. Baseline characteristics of study patients. N/S: not significant. BMI: body mass index. AAT: Alpha-1 antitrypsin.

	Pi*MM n = 1018	Pi*MS n = 287	Pi*SS n = 23	Pi*MZ n = 112	Pi*SZ n = 26	Pi*ZZ n = 7	Rare Variants n = 21	Degree of Significance PiMM-Pi ≠ MM
Male, n	612 (59.18%)	142 (49.47%)	10 (43.47%)	62 (53.35%)	11 (42.30%)	4 (57.14%)	6 (28.57%)	$p < 0.0001$
Age, years, median (range)	57 (11–94)	52.05 (1–86)	57.13 (16–86)	48.68 (1–89)	46.54 (10–81)	57.86 (45–87)	40.57 (1–75)	$p < 0.004$
Weight, kg median (range)	82.22 (39–152)	79.94 (3.6–135)	74.76 (49–116)	79.67 (4.6–119)	80.52 (54–115)	65.67 (47–97)	70.22 (4.4–92)	N/S
BMI, kg/m^2 median (range)	30.16 (14.9–53.6)	29.06 (15–52.5)	27.43 (19–40.1)	28.67 (17.9–42.2)	29.14 (21.4–44.1)	23.03 (16.3–31.3)	26.20 (19.6–37)	N/S
Serum AAT levels, mg/dL median (range)	135.9 (82.8–308.2)	115.05 (76.2–126.6)	90.31 (74.6–125)	85.15 (62.3–137.6)	60.18 (43.9–82.1)	18.94 (5–36.3)	69.51 (7–111)	$p < 0.05$

3.2. Relationship between Genotypes and Transaminase Levels

A statistically significant association was found between genotypes for the SERPINA1 gene and serum levels of liver enzymes, in the sense that the more deficient the genotype, the higher the enzyme elevation observed (odds ratio (OR): GOT = 25.32, $p < 0.0003$; GPT = 20.19, $p < 0.002$; GGT = 17.78, $p < 0.006$). It was found that serum GPT and GGT values changed more frequently the more deficient the genotypes (Figure 1). Similar results were observed with GOT values, excluding the Pi*ZZ genotype, although this was not so marked.

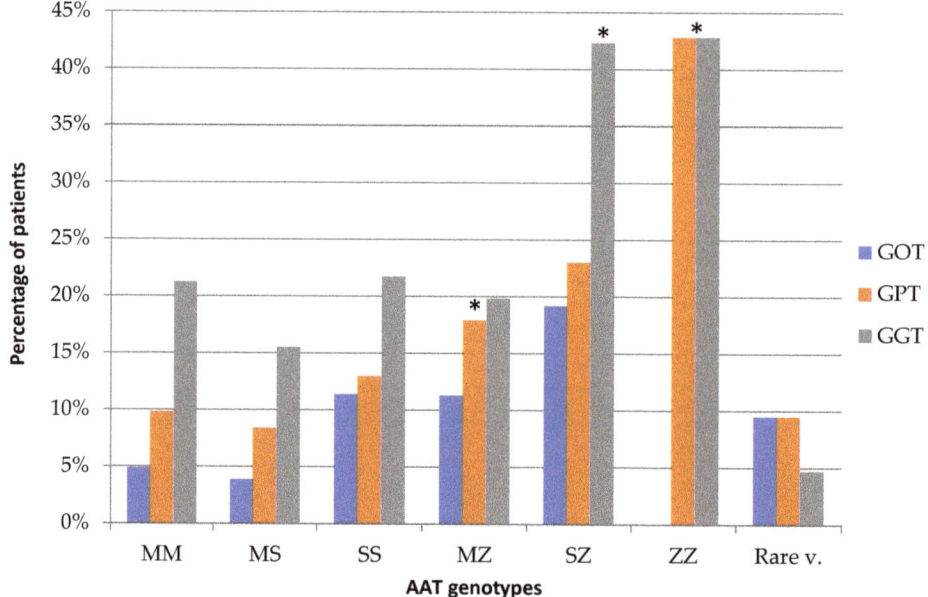

Figure 1. Relationship between genotypes and transaminase levels (IU/L). Transaminases (GOT > 37 U/L), (GPT > 38 U/L), and (GGT > 40 U/L). It can be seen that the most deficient genotypes are those that cause the greatest significant increases in transaminases levels ($p < 0.05$). * In the Pi*ZZ genotype, no changes in GOT levels were observed.

Regarding the GOT and GPT serum levels, when measuring the prevalence of exposure in patients who had a genotype with the Pi*Z allele and comparing them with patients of normal genotype

($Pi*MM$), an OR of 2.72 (CI: 1.5–4.87) was obtained for GOT with a significance level of $p < 0.0005$, and for GPT an OR of 2.31 (CI: 1.45–3.67) with a level of statistical significance of $p < 0.0003$ was obtained. When analyzing the GGT levels, an OR of 1.25 (CI: 0.82–1.88) was obtained, but this time without reaching statistical significance. Table 2 describes the results for genotypes containing the $Pi*Z$ allele in more detail.

Table 2. Odds ratio relationship between the genotypes that include the $PI*Z$ allele and the serum transaminase levels. GOT: glutamate-oxaloacetate transaminase. GPT: glutamate-pyruvate transaminase. GGT: gamma-glutamyl transpeptidase. N/S: not significant.

Genotype	GOT	GPT	GGT
$Pi*MZ$	2.49 (CI: 1.28–4.85) $p < 0.005$	4.65 (CI: 1.68–12.84) $p < 0.001$	0.91 (0.55–1.51) N/S
$Pi*SZ$	2 (CI: 1.17–3.42) $p < 0.01$	2.75 (CI: 1.07–7) $p < 0.02$	6.87 (CI: 1.52–31.15) $p < 0.003$
$Pi*ZZ$	Not applicable N/S	2.72 (1.23–6) $p < 0.01$	2.78 (0.61–12.52) N/S

No statistically significant relationship was found between the $PI*S$ allele and altered transaminase levels, with OR values for GOT, GPT, and GGT levels of 1.003 (CI: 0.55–1.81), 0.88 (CI: 0.56–1.37), and 0.70 (CI: 0.50–1), respectively.

3.3. Relationship between Transaminases and Serum AAT Levels

Finally, a statistically significant association was found between the transaminase values and the different AAT values, with a chi-squared statistical value of 14.06 for GOT ($p < 0.002$) and 17.12 for GPT ($p < 0.0007$). The result was not significant for GGT ($p > 0.05$). Our study found that low levels of AAT were associated with high levels of GPT and GGT transaminases (Figure 2).

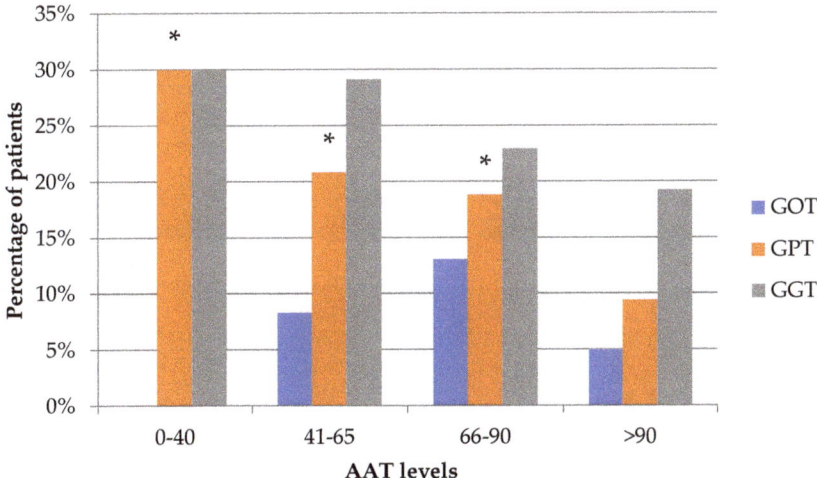

Figure 2. Relationship between transaminase levels (IU/L) and the different ranges of AAT levels (mg/dL). Transaminases (GOT > 37 U/L), (GPT > 38 U/L), and (GGT > 40 U/L). It can be seen that lower AAT levels were associated with statistically significant increases in transaminase levels ($p < 0.05$) *. However, in the group with the lowest AAT values (0–40), no changes were observed in GOT.

Correlation studies showed a statistically significant ($p < 0.001$) negative correlation between AAT levels and GOT, GPT, and GGT levels.

4. Discussion

The liver damage associated with AAT deficiency and caused mainly by the deposition of AAT polymers is well-known, having been confirmed in the literature with various articles that all reach similar conclusions [2,10,11]. Our study shows that having the *Pi*Z* allele is a risk factor for developing liver damage, which is reflected in abnormal transaminase serum levels, especially GOT and GPT. In our results, the association of abnormal transaminase levels and the *PI*ZZ* genotype was only statistically significant with GPT, mainly due to the small number of these patients in the sample.

Although several studies cast doubt on the association of heterozygous *PI*MZ* or *PI*SZ* genotypes and liver impairment [12,13], our results suggest that heterozygous states of the *Pi*Z* allele are a risk factor for the development of abnormal serum levels of some transaminases. As such, these patients require stricter liver enzyme control, albumin levels, and coagulation status throughout their lives, and imaging tests, such as abdominal ultrasound or fibroscan, that allow for early detection of abnormalities suggestive of cirrhosis could even be considered. In addition, healthy lifestyle habits, such as physical exercise, a fat-free diet, and avoiding alcohol are advisable in patients homozygous or heterozygous for the Z allele. These findings are in line with various liver function studies and the development of cirrhosis in patients with deficient genotypes, especially with the *Pi*ZZ* genotype, showing that it is a risk factor for the development of liver cirrhosis 20 times greater than in normal individuals [14–16]. However, our low number of *PI*ZZ* patients is not representative to confirm the results reported in those studies. This association has also been described in *PI*MZ* and *PI*SZ* heterozygous individuals, reporting ORs that can vary between 1.8–3.1, especially in men [17,18].

Similarly, it is generally accepted that the *PI*MS* or *PI*SS* genotypes do not pose a risk of liver disease due to deposits of AAT polymers [19,20], mainly due to the fact that the polymerization of PiS polypeptides occurs in a lower percentage of molecules and more slowly than in PiZs, in which cellular inclusion bodies responsible for liver damage are not formed. The results obtained in our study show that the presence of the *PI*S* allele by itself is not a risk factor for the development of liver disease. Polymerization of mutated Z-AAT is an inhomogeneous phenomenon. In the liver, undamaged hepatocytes can coexist with hepatocytes presenting large accumulations of polymer. The cause of this difference is unknown, although it is postulated that it may be related to the different secretion capacity of AAT by the hepatocytes of the same liver [20]. Some studies have described that heteropolymers are common in heterozygous patients for the Z allele [6,21]. We believe that heterozygous patients have a risk of developing elevated transaminases in response to intrahepatic damage due to varied accumulation of polymers, although it will be necessary to assess whether this damage is evolutionary or self-limiting and does not have pathological implications.

Low levels of AAT are associated with elevated levels of GPT and GGT transaminases. Specifically, AAT values between 0–40 mg/dL were associated with the most altered GPT and GGT levels, which indicates that the most deficient genotypes and, therefore, that have lower AAT levels, are frequently associated with liver involvement, with the exception of the presence of null alleles where no liver damage has been reported.

The study by Mostafavi et al. [22] reports that GOT is the liver enzyme with the highest serum levels in *PI*ZZ* and *PI*SZ* individuals up to the age of 30 years. In the elderly, GGT is affected to a greater extent, concluding that GGT plasma levels are a more useful marker to measure liver involvement. Our study revealed similar data, probably due to the fact that most of our patients were older than 30 years. However, other authors [23] have found that in patients with the *PI*ZZ* genotype, being male and over 50 years of age, having repeated elevation of plasma transaminase levels, and having been diagnosed with diabetes mellitus or COPD were associated with the development of liver disease, so these variables are proposed as risk factors.

Patients were subsequently stratified into two groups (≤25 years and >25 years), and no statistically significant results were found for any of the three transaminases (GOT, GPT, GGT) that indicated that our patients had a higher degree of liver disease in childhood and that it progressively disappeared as adulthood was reached, although our sample was lacking a significant population of patients aged 25 or under (9.86%).

Our analysis has the limitations of a cross-sectional observational study. The temporal sequence of the variables studied could not be established, making it difficult to separate risk factors from prognostic factors. Furthermore, as no imaging study was performed using fibroscan or serial abdominal ultrasound over time, it is impossible to know which patients with altered transaminases developed liver fibrosis or cirrhosis. Despite this major limitation, our data indicate that it must be considered that patients with a *PI*Z* allele may not only have altered lung function (determined by spirometry), but also that, in these patients, liver involvement is more frequent than expected, often going unnoticed, and transaminase alteration may be the first indication of underlying liver disease. For this reason, closer long-term follow-up should be considered with serial analytical controls that include, in addition to transaminase levels, levels of bilirubin and albumin, and a complete blood count with coagulation, to detect abnormalities that guide us towards established liver damage. The influence of potential confounding factors, such as toxic habits affecting the liver, including alcoholism and drug-related liver toxicity, as well as hepatotropic viral infections, was minimized by the application of exclusion criteria.

5. Conclusions

In conclusion, the results of this study indicate that the presence of a *PI*Z* allele seems to be a risk factor for the development of liver involvement, since the different genotypes of AAT deficiency were associated with abnormal GOT, GPT, and GGT values. Furthermore, lower levels of AAT imply a greater involvement of GOT and GPT transaminases.

Author Contributions: Conceptualization, J.M.H.P., I.B. and J.A.P.P.; methodology, J.M.H.P., A.J.S.M. and J.A.P.P.; software, A.J.S.M.; validation, resources, data curation writing—review and editing: J.M.H.P., I.B., A.J.S.M., L.D.H. and J.A.P.P.; formal analysis, J.M.H.P. and A.J.S.M.; investigation, J.M.H.P., A.J.S.M. and J.A.P.P.; writing—original draft preparation, J.M.H.P., I.B. and J.A.P.P.; visualization, J.M.H.P., I.B. and J.A.P.P.; supervision and project administration, J.M.H.P. and J.A.P.P.; funding acquisition, J.M.H.P. All authors have read and agreed to the published version of the manuscript.

Funding: This research was funded by Grifols, manufacturer of plasma alpha-1 antitrypsin.

Acknowledgments: The authors thank Grifols for funding this research project. The authors also thank Jordi Bozzo, and Eugenio Rosado (Grifols) for their help preparing the manuscript.

Conflicts of Interest: This research was funded by Grifols, manufacturer of plasma alpha-1 antitrypsin. There is no other conflict of interest to disclose.

References

1. American Thoracic Society; European Respiratory Society statement. American Thoracic Society/European Respiratory Society statement: Standards for the diagnosis and management of individuals with alpha-1 antitrypsin deficiency. *Am. J. Respir. Crit. Care Med.* **2003**, *168*, 818–900. [CrossRef] [PubMed]
2. Stoller, J.K.; Aboussouan, L.S. Alpha1-antitrypsin deficiency. *Lancet* **2005**, *365*, 2225–2236. [CrossRef]
3. de Serres, F.; Blanco, I. Role of alpha-1 antitrypsin in human health and disease. *J. Intern. Med.* **2014**, *276*, 311–335. [CrossRef] [PubMed]
4. Mela, M.; Smeeton, W.; Davies, S.E.; Miranda, E.; Scarpini, C.; Coleman, N.; Alexander, G.J. The Alpha-1 Antitrypsin Polymer Load Correlates with Hepatocyte Senescence, Fibrosis Stage and Liver-Related Mortality. *Chronic Obstr. Pulm. Dis.* **2020**, *7*, 151–162. [CrossRef]
5. Teckman, J.H.; Blomenkamp, K.S. Pathophysiology of Alpha-1 Antitrypsin Deficiency Liver Disease. *Methods Mol. Biol.* **2017**, *1639*, 1–8. [CrossRef]
6. Mahadeva, R.; Chang, W.S.W.; Dafforn, T.R.; Oakley, D.J.; Foreman, R.C.; Calvin, J.; Wight, D.G.; Lomas, D.A. Heteropolymerization of S, I, and Z α1-antitrypsin and liver cirrhosis. *J. Clin. Investig.* **1999**, *103*, 999–1006. [CrossRef]
7. Nelson, D.L.; Cox, M.M. *Lehninger Principles of Biochemistry*, 3rd ed.; Worth Publishers: New York, NY, USA, 2000; pp. 628–631.

8. Lay, M.J.; Wittwer, C.T. Real-time fluorescence genotyping of factor V Leiden during rapid-cycle PCR. *Clin. Chem.* **1997**, *43*, 2262–2267. [CrossRef]
9. Hernández, P.J.; Ramos, D.R.; Fumero, G.S.; Pérez, P.J. Description of alpha-1-antitrypsin deficiency associated with PI* Q0ourém allele in La Palma Island (Spain) and a genotyping assay for its detection. *Arch. Bronconeumol.* **2015**, *51*. [CrossRef]
10. Tanash, H.A.; Nystedt-Düzakin, M.; Montero, L.C.; Sveger, T.; Piitulainen, E. The Swedish α1-Antitrypsin Screening Study: Health Status and Lung and Liver Function at Age. *Ann. Am. Thorac. Soc.* **2015**, *12*, 807–812. [CrossRef]
11. Alagille, D. α-1-Antitrypsin deficiency. *Hepatology* **1984**, *4* (Suppl. 1), 11–14. [CrossRef]
12. Silverman, E.K.; Sandhaus, R.A. Alpha1-antitrypsin deficiency. *N. Engl. J. Med.* **2009**, *360*, 2749–2757. [CrossRef] [PubMed]
13. Regev, A.; Guaqueta, C.; Molina, E.G.; Conrad, A.; Mishra, V.; Brantly, M.L.; Torres, M.; De Medina, M.; Tzakis, A.G.; Schiff, E.R. Does the heterozygous state of alpha-1 antitrypsin deficiency have a role in chronic liver diseases? Interim results of a large case-control study. *J. Pediatr. Gastroenterol. Nutr.* **2006**, *43* (Suppl. 1), 30–35. [CrossRef] [PubMed]
14. Berg, N.O.; Eriksson, S. Liver disease in adults with alpha-1 -antitrypsin deficiency. *N. Engl. J. Med.* **1972**, *287*, 1264–1267. [CrossRef] [PubMed]
15. Mandorfer, M.; Bucsics, T.; Hutya, V.; Schmid-Scherzer, K.; Schaefer, B.; Zoller, H.; Ferlitsch, A.; Peck-Radosavljevic, M.; Trauner, M.; Ferenci, P.; et al. Liver disease in adults with α1-antitrypsin deficiency. *United Eur. Gastroenterol. J.* **2018**, *6*, 710–718. [CrossRef]
16. Larsson, C. Natural history and life expectancy in severe alpha1-antitrypsin deficiency, Pi Z. *Acta Med. Scand.* **1978**, *204*, 345–351. [CrossRef]
17. Eigenbrodt, M.L.; McCashland, T.M.; Dy, R.M.; Clark, J.; Galati, J. Heterozygous α1-antitrypsin phenotypes in patients with end stage liver disease. *Am. J. Gastroenterol.* **1997**, *92*, 602–607.
18. Strnad, P.; Buch, S.; Hamesch, K.; Fischer, J.; Rosendahl, J.; Schmelz, R.; Brueckner, S.; Brosch, M.; Heimes, C.V.; Woditsch, V.; et al. Heterozygous carriage of the alpha1-antitrypsin Pi*Z variant increases the risk to develop liver cirrhosis. *Gut* **2019**, *68*, 1099–1107. [CrossRef]
19. Sveger, T. The natural history of liver disease in α1-antitrypsin deficient children. *Acta Paediatr. Scand.* **1988**, *77*, 847–851. [CrossRef]
20. Blanco, I.; Lara, B. *Déficit de Alfa-1 Antitripsina: Fisiopatología, Enfermedades Relacionadas y Tratamiento*; Issuu Inc.: Copenhagen, Denmark, 2017.
21. Tan, L.; Dickens, J.A.; DeMeo, D.L.; Miranda, E.; Perez, J.; Rashid, S.T.; Day, J.; Ordoñez, A.; Marciniak, S.J.; Haq, I.; et al. Circulating polymers in α1-antitrypsin deficiency. *Eur. Respir. J.* **2014**, *43*, 1501–1504. [CrossRef]
22. Mostafavi, B.; Diaz, S.; Tanash, H.A.; Piitulainen, E. Liver function in alpha-1-antitrypsin deficient individuals at 37 to 40 years of age. *Medicine* **2017**, *96*. [CrossRef]
23. Tanash, H.A.; Piitulainen, E. Liver disease in adults with severe alpha-1-antitrypsin deficiency. *J. Gastroenterol.* **2019**, *54*, 541–548. [CrossRef] [PubMed]

Publisher's Note: MDPI stays neutral with regard to jurisdictional claims in published maps and institutional affiliations.

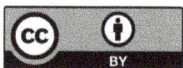

© 2020 by the authors. Licensee MDPI, Basel, Switzerland. This article is an open access article distributed under the terms and conditions of the Creative Commons Attribution (CC BY) license (http://creativecommons.org/licenses/by/4.0/).

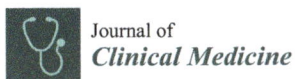 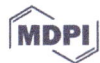

Article

Physical Activity and Mental Health of Patients with Pulmonary Hypertension during the COVID-19 Pandemic

Carolin Leoni Dobler [1], Britta Krüger [2], Jana Strahler [3,4], Christopher Weyh [1], Kristina Gebhardt [1], Khodr Tello [5], Hossein Ardeschir Ghofrani [5], Natascha Sommer [5], Henning Gall [5], Manuel Jonas Richter [5] and Karsten Krüger [1,*]

1. Department of Exercise Physiology and Sports Therapy, Institute of Sports Science, Justus Liebig University Giessen, 35394 Giessen, Germany; Carolin.Dobler@sport.uni-giessen.de (C.L.D.); christopher.weyh@sport.uni-giessen.de (C.W.); kristina.gebhardt@sport.uni-giessen.de (K.G.)
2. Nemolab, Institute of Sports Science, Justus Liebig University Giessen, 35394 Giessen, Germany; g51130@uni-giessen.de
3. Department of Psychotherapy and Systems Neuroscience, University of Giessen, 35394 Giessen, Germany; Jana.Strahler@psychol.uni-giessen.de
4. Bender Institute of Neuroimaging, Justus Liebig University Giessen, 35394 Giessen, Germany
5. Department of Internal Medicine, Universities of Giessen and Marburg Lung Center (UGMLC), Member of the German Center for Lung Research (DZL), Excellence Cluster Cardio-Pulmonary Institute (CPI), Justus-Liebig University, 35394 Giessen, Germany; Khodr.Tello@innere.med.uni-giessen.de (K.T.); ardeschir.ghofrani@innere.med.uni-giessen.de (H.A.G.); Natascha.Sommer@innere.med.uni-giessen.de (N.S.); Henning.gall@innere.med.un-giessen.de (H.G.); Manuel.Richter@innere.med.uni-giessen.de (M.J.R.)
* Correspondence: Karsten.krueger@sport.uni-giessen.de; Tel.: +49-641-992-52210

Received: 24 November 2020; Accepted: 10 December 2020; Published: 12 December 2020

Abstract: The aim of the study was to analyze the effect of personal restrictions on physical activity, mental health, stress experience, resilience, and sleep quality in patients with pulmonary hypertension (PH) during the "lockdown" period of the COVID-19 pandemic. In total, 112 PH patients and 52 age-matched healthy control subjects completed a questionnaire on the topics of physical activity, mental health, resilience, and sleep quality. PH patients had significantly lower physical activity, mental health, and sleep quality compared to age-matched healthy controls. Physical activity positively correlated with mental health and sleep quality in the PH group. Mental wellbeing and life satisfaction could be predicted by total physical activity, sleep, stress level, and resilience. PH patients appeared as an especially vulnerable group, demanding interventions to promote an active lifestyle and protect mental health in these patients. This could be helpful in counseling on how to carry out physical activity while maintaining infection control.

Keywords: resilience; active lifestyle; stress levels; infection control measure; self-quarantine

1. Introduction

Pulmonary hypertension (PH) is a multifactorial chronic pulmonary disease which is defined by an elevated mean pulmonary arterial pressure, which untreated eventually can lead to right heart failure and death [1]. Depending on the clinical classification and risk stratification PH patients have quite a different prognoses, treatment options, and impairment in daily life [2]. Patients with PH experience symptoms such as shortness of breath, exertion, fatigue, chest pain that restrict physical activity, which in turn impairs quality of life and favors mental disorders such as depression [3–6].

Accordingly, PH patients experience a high degree of functional limitations, which was shown to be almost comparable to those reported by cancers patients [7].

In January 2020, the outbreak of COVID-19 was declared as a "Public Health Emergency of International Concern" by the WHO. On January 27th, the first COVID-19 infection in Germany was detected. By end of March 2020, the COVID-19 was classified as a pandemic. Since "socio-physical distancing" is seen as one of the most effective strategies to reduce the number of infections, Robert-Koch Institute (RKI) called on the population in Germany to keep their distance from other people [8]. As elderly and patients with specific risk factors and pre-existing diseases are at a higher risk of severe COVID-19 course of disease and mortality [8], these groups, including PH patients, were prompted to be particularly careful to reduce individual infection risks. One can therefore assume that many persons at risk stayed at home, reduced their physical activity, and performed a social distancing to protect themselves.

Recent studies indicate that common reactions to the COVID-19 pandemic and the protection measures are elevated levels of anxiety [9–11], depression [12,13], and stress [14]. Being a woman and having a (chronic) disease [15] are factors associated with stronger mental burdens during COVID-19 relate to shock and lockdown measures amongst others. Those identifying themselves as a high-risk group when being infected with COVID-19 also showed higher levels of anxiety, depression, and stress symptoms [10]. Furthermore, it seems reasonable that high-risk patients are particularly careful and isolate themselves, which ultimately may result in physical deconditioning [12–14]. Decreased exercise capacity and emotional difficulties such as anxiety, depression, and stress correlate with a negative HRQoL of patients with pulmonary arterial hypertension (PAH) [6]. Research also shows that this relationship works in both directions with PH symptoms reinforcing stress and anxiety [10]. Data suggests that PH patients might be very susceptible to mental impairment due to pandemic restrictions and protection measures. Remaining physically active though has been associated with better mental health scores during this pandemic [13,16]. Whether this also applies to PH patients is currently unknown. Related knowledge would however be of utmost importance to better understand risk factors of lockdown measure-related vulnerabilities and possible therapeutic approaches.

On this background, the present study aimed to investigate the quality of life of PH patients during the first weeks of the lockdown period of the COVID-19 pandemic in Germany. More specifically, associations between mental health, stress experience, physical activity, sleep quality, and sociodemographic factors were analyzed. As the individual's resilience (i.e., adapting, managing, and negotiating adversity) [17] is another important factor supporting mental health and wellbeing as it for example moderates physical activity effects, we also assessed resilience. We analyzed whether and to which degree resilience, physical activity, stress experience, and sleep behavior determined mental health issues. We further explored whether the subjective stress level is related to the perceived mental well- or illbeing of PH patients compared to an age and education-matched control group. We hypothesize that PH patients experience a stronger reduction of physical activity, sleep quality, and resilience as well as an increased subjective stress experience during the pandemic than healthy subjects, which is at the same time associated with a higher psychological burden.

2. Methods

2.1. Subjects Characteristics

In this cross-sectional study, subjects diagnosed with pulmonary hypertension were compared to a healthy control group concerning to their mental health represented by WHO-5, PHQ-4, L-1, physical activity, resilience, stress experience, and sleep quality during the COVID-19 associated lockdown. The control group was matched by age.

Subjects of the PH group had to have their residence inside of Germany and a medical diagnosis of PH. To be eligible for the control group, subjects must not have had a confirmed infection or symptoms of COVID-19, any comorbidities, or a residence outside of Germany. Only subjects declaring consent were included in this study.

PH patients of the University Hospital of Gießen and Marburg (UKGM) were directly contacted. The questionnaire was promoted during online consultation hours of the UKGM and in PH support groups (https://pulmonale-hypertonie-selbsthilfe.de/). If necessary, the questionnaire was sent to patients per mail due to lacking access to the internet and was entered into the online survey by hand.

In total, 251 PH patients followed the invitation to participate in the survey. There were 139 cases that were excluded, 111 of those for not completing the questionnaire, 25 for reporting to have no medical diagnosis of PH, and three because their residence was outside of Germany. This left us with questionnaires of 112 subjects being valid for the PH group. The mean age in the PH group was 54.4 ± 14.0 years with 77.7% being female. The average number of comorbidities was 2.6 ± 2.0. 52 healthy subjects were recruited into the control group in dependence of their eligibility criteria and age matching. The mean age of the control group was 52.3 ± 8.9 years with 67.3% being female. The sociodemographic characteristics of both groups are presented in Table 1.

Table 1. Sociodemographic characteristics of patients with pulmonary hypertension (PH group) and subjects of the control group.

	Subcategory	PH Group		Control Group	
Age		54.4	± 14.0	52.3	± 8.9
Gender	Female	77.7	(69.6; 84.8)	67.3	(53.8; 80.7)
	Male	22.3	(15.2; 30.4)	32.7	(19.3; 46.2)
Relationship status	Single	19.8	(12.6; 27.9)	11.5	(3.8; 19.2)
	Partnership	68.5	(60.4; 76.6)	86.5	(76.9; 94)
	Other	11.7	(6.3; 18.0)	1.9	(0.0; 5.8)
Living situation 1	Rural	54.1	(45.0; 63.1)	44.2	(30.8; 57.7)
	Suburban	23.4	(15.3; 31.5)	21.2	(11.5; 32.7)
	Urban	22.5	(15.3; 30.6)	34.6	(23.1; 48.1)
Living situation 2	None	6.3	(2.7; 11.7)	7.7	(1.9; 15.4)
	Balcony	23.4	(15.3; 31.5)	25.0	(13.5; 36.5)
	Garden	43.2	(33.3; 53.2)	42.3	(28.8; 57.7)
	Balcony and garden	27.0	(18.9; 35.1)	25.0	(13.5; 36.5)
Residents	Residents per household	2.1	± 1.1	3.0	± 1.3
	Children per household	0.3	± 0.6	0.7	± 1.0
Level of education	Certificate of secondary education	10.1	(4.6; 15.6)	3.8	(0.0; 9.6)
	General certificate of secondary education	18.3	(11.9; 25.7)	5.8	(0.0; 13.5)
	Completed apprenticeship	29.4	(21.2; 38.5)	19.2	(9.6; 30.8)
	Advanced vocational certificate of education	19.3	(11.9; 27.5)	9.6	(1.9; 17.3)
	A level	5.5	(1.8; 10.1)	17.3	(7.7; 28.8)
	Bachelor's degree	8.3	(3.7; 13.8)	3.8	(0.0; 9.6)
	Master's degree	9.2	(4.6; 14.7)	30.8	(19.2; 42.3)
	PhD	0		9.6	(1.9; 19.2)
Occupational status	Student/articled	0.9	(0.0; 2.8)	0	
	Full-time equivalent	19.8	(12.3; 27.4)	46.2	(32.7; 59.6)
	Half-time equivalent	7.5	(2.8; 13.2)	7.7	(1.9; 15.4)
	Public official	0.9	(0.0; 2.8)	13.5	(5.8; 23.1)
	Self-employed	2.8	(0.0; 6.6)	9.6	(1.9; 17.3)
	Unemployed	1.9	(0.0; 4.7)	0	
	Retired	45.3	(35.8; 55.6)	15.4	(5.8; 25.0)
	Other	20.8	(13.2; 28.3)	7.7	(1.9; 15.4)
Comorbidities		2.61	± 2.0	0	± 0

Data are presented as an arithmetic mean ± SD or % (n/N) and (95%-CI). The PH group is lacking data >2% in four variables: children per household (6), level of education (3), occupational status (6), comorbidities (3). There were no missing cases in the control group regarding the listed variables.

2.2. Questionnaire and Outcomes

The survey contained several questions and validated questionnaires to evaluate study variables. In the beginning, sociodemographic data such as age, gender, relationship status, living situation, the number of residents per household, educational level, occupational status, worries about health, and satisfaction with sports behavior were gathered. The living situation covered the living area and the availability of a garden or a balcony. The number of residents per household was divided into the total number of residents and those younger than 18 years. The category comorbidity included sub-categories of comorbidities (apart from PH for the PH group). Every sub-category could be answered with "No", "Yes, medical diagnosis", or "Yes, self-assessment", although a self-assessed diagnosis was counted as a "No" in the analysis. The number of "Yes, medical diagnosis" was counted and summed up to create the variable "Comorbidities". Possible SARS-CoV-2 infection or symptoms were also evaluated.

Physical activity data were collected through items three to six of the BSA-F which was shown to be a valid tool for the measurement of physical activity and sports behavior [18]. The outcome scores were *total physical activity, the activity of daily living, sports activity,* and *climbing stairs*. The variable *total physical activity* is a sum of the *activity of daily living* and *sports activity*. The amount of different physical activity, exercise and sports modalities are calculated by multiplying the duration and frequency of the corresponding items and then summating them. The examined period for all scores was four weeks in the PH group. The scores *total physical activity, activity of daily living* and *sports activity* were converted into the unit minutes/week as designated and were thereby made comparable. The item *climbing stairs* was converted into unit floors/week.

Mental health was assessed by using the WHO-5 Well-Being Index (WHO-5), the Patient Health Questionnaire-4 (PHQ-4), the L-1-scale, one question on perceived stress, and four items measuring state resilience [19]. The 5-item WHO-5 scale, which assesses subjective wellbeing but is also a valid tool for the screening of depression [20], was converted into a score ranging from 0 to 100 for comparison with other studies. Zero represents the worst mental health and a score ≤50 was used as sign for depression. Another valid and reliable score for the investigation of depression and anxiety in the general population is the PHQ-4 [3]. The PHQ-4 was added up to create a single score ranging between 0 and 12 with 0 indicating good mental health. The PHQ-4 consists of the Patient Health Questionnaire-2 (PHQ-2) measuring depression and the Generalized Anxiety Disorder 2 (GAD-2) quantifying anxiety. The overall life satisfaction was measured by the valid and reliable eleven-point L-1-scale [21] with 0 indicating no satisfaction and 10 representing a strong overall life satisfaction. Resilience was measured by four eight-point Likert-scales that were then averaged to a total score [19]. The subjective stress-level was assessed by a further eight-point Likert-scale rating the statement "I feel stressed out".

Sleep data were divided into general sleep quality and current sleep quality. Both scores were measured through a ten-point Likert-scale with 1 indicating bad sleep quality and 10 indicating excellent sleep quality.

2.3. Statistical Analysis

First, descriptive statistics were performed for both groups. Prior to this, we z-standardized all variables.

In the next step, we tested all observed variables regarding their distribution features. As none of the variables were normally distributed, the Mann–Whitney-U-Test was used to identify differences between the PH and the control group regarding mental health scores (WHO-5, PHQ-4, L-1), physical activity (*total physical activity, the activity of daily living, sports activity, climbing stairs*) resilience, stress experience, and quality of sleep.

We further used Spearman's rank correlation coefficients to determine the relationship between mental health (as indicated by WHO-5, L-1, and PHQ-4), physical activity (*total physical activity, the activity of daily living, sports activity, climbing stairs*), resilience, feelings of stress, and sleep quality for the PH and the control group separately.

Lastly, we analyzed the impact of resilience, total physical activity, sleep quality and feelings of stress as potential predictors of mental health using multiple regression analyses for the PH group as well as over both groups. We, therefore, further added four product terms to the model to test for an interaction between total physical, resilience, stress, sleep, and group membership. SPSS 22 was used for statistical analysis and partly for graphical illustration. For further illustration of the data, we used Python 3. p values < 0.05 will be considered significant. Bonferroni-correction was used to correct for multiple comparisons.

3. Results

3.1. Mental Health Indicated by WHO-5, PHQ-4, and L-1

For the PH group, the level of mental health was represented through the WHO-5 scoring 11.9 ± 5.6, the PHQ-4 being 3.9 ± 3.0, and the L-1 being 5.6 ± 2.7 on average. In the present cohort, a prevalence of depression ranged from 36.4% and 53.6% derived from the WHO-5 score (score less than or equal to 50 as depressed), the PHQ-2 yellow flag (score greater than or equal to 3), and PHQ-2 red flag. Symptoms of anxiety were found in about one-third of the PH patients. The assessment of mental health revealed significantly lower life satisfaction (L1), well-being (WHO-5) as well as increased levels of depression and anxiety (PHQ-4) in the PH group regarding WHO-5, PHQ-4 and its subscores PHQ-2 and GAD-2 and L-1 (all $p < 0.001$) (Table 2).

Table 2. Characteristics and group differences of subjects of the PH and control group.

Variable	Subcategory	PH Group		Control Group		p-Value
Physical activity	Activity of daily living (ADL) (min/week)	551.4	±816.9	707.0	±686.8	<0.001
	Sports activity (min/week)	129.4	±219.8	407.5	±314.7	<0.001
	Total physical activity (min/week)	684.3	±954.3	1103.8	±851.4	<0.001
	Climbing stairs (floors/week)	14.3	±23.0	38.0	±56.6	<0.001
Mental health	WHO-5	11.9	±5.4	16.0	±4.1	<0.001
	PHQ-4	3.9	±3.0	1.6	±1.7	<0.001
	L-1	5.6	±2.7	7.5	±1.6	<0.001
Resilience (z-standard.)		−0.2	±0.85	0.0	±0.88	n.s.
Stress (z-standard.)		0.0	±1.01	0.0	±1.0	n.s.
Support of surrounding people	Respected	2.8	±1.1	3.3	±0.6	0.002
	Supported	2.9	±1.0	3.2	±0.7	n.s.
	Liked	3.1	±1.0	3.3	±0.7	n.s.
	Sum	8.7	±2.7	9.8	±1.7	n.s.
Sleep	General sleep quality	5.7	±2.4	7.5	±1.8	<0.001
	Acute sleep quality	5.3	±2.5	7.3	±1.9	<0.001
Lifestyle estimation	Satisfaction with nutrition	3.8	±1.7	4.3	±1.3	n.s.
	Worries about health	4.5	±1.6	2.5	±1.7	<0.001
	Satisfaction with sports behavior	2.3	±1.8	3.9	±1.6	<0.001
	Worries about finances	2.4	±2.3	1.8	±1.6	n.s.

Data are presented as the arithmetic mean ± SD. p-values were adjusted to $p < 0.0026$ through the level for multiple comparisons. WHO-5: The World Health Organization-Five Well-Being Index, PHQ-4: Patient Health Questionnaire-4; L-1: Likert-scale rating-1.

3.2. Resilience, Stress Experience, and Sleep Quality

The level of resilience was rated on average 4.1 ± 1.6, subjective stress experience was rated on average 2.9 ± 2.1 in the PH group. The general sleep quality was rated as 5.7 ± 2.4 on average, while the current sleep quality was only 5.3 ± 2.5. The level of resilience as well as the subjective stress experience in the PH group did not differ significantly compared to the control group. The general and current sleep quality were both significantly lower in the PH group compared to the control group (both $p < 0.001$). The estimation of one's living standard showed a statistically significant increased score in the PH group regarding the item "worries about health" and a decreased score in the PH group regarding the item "satisfaction with sports behavior" ($p < 0.001$). Results are depicted in Figure 1 and Table 2.

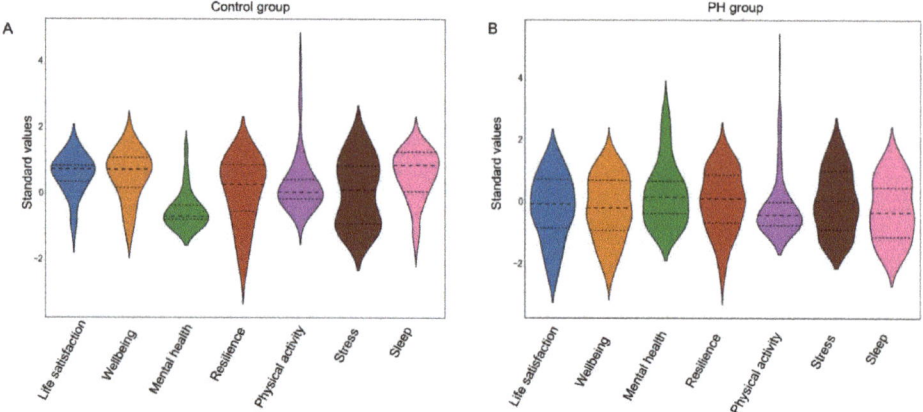

Figure 1. Z-standardized values of mental health variables. (**A**): z-standardized values of life satisfaction, mental wellbeing, mental health, resilience, total physical activity, stress experience, and sleep habits of healthy controls during the lockdown. The dashed inner line of each violin graph reflects the quartiles of each health variable. (**B**): z-standardized values of life satisfaction, mental wellbeing, mental health, resilience, total physical activity, stress experience and sleep habits of PH patients. The dashed inner line of each violin graph reflects the quartiles of each health variable.

3.3. Physical Activity

The average *total physical activity* of the PH group was 684.3 ± 954.3 (min/week), whereby 551.4 ± 816.9 (min/week) were accounted for by the *activity of daily living* and 129.4 ± 219.8 (min/week) for *sports activities*. The mean score of *climbing stairs* was 14.3 ± 23.0 (floors/week). All modalities of physical activity were significantly lower compared to the control group (all $p < 0.001$, Table 2).

3.4. Associations between Subjects' Characteristics, Physical Activity, Mental Health (Reflected by L-1, WHO-5, PHQ-4), Resilience, and Stress Experience in PH Patients

The four activity indices were correlated with the mental health scores, resilience, stress experience, sleep quality, and sociodemographic data in the PH group (Table 3 for a detailed description). *Total physical activity* showed a significant positive correlation with WHO-5 ($r = 0.26$, $p = 0.016$), L-1 ($r = 0.30$, $p = 0.005$), general sleep quality ($r = 0.31$, $p = 0.003$), and current sleep quality ($r = 0.25$, $p = 0.018$). The subcategory *activity of daily living* significantly correlated with WHO-5 ($r = 0.33$, $p = 0.002$), L1 ($r = 0.33$, $p = 0.001$), general ($r = 0.33$, $p = 0.001$), resilience ($r = 0.236$, $p = 0.027$), and acute sleep quality ($r = 0.32$, $p = 0.002$). *Sports activity* though only showed a significant correlation with age ($r = -0.23$, $p = 0.020$) and educational level ($r = 0.27$, $p = 0.007$) but not with any of the self-report measures. Significant correlations regarding *climbing stairs* were found with WHO-5 ($r = 0.33$, $p = 0.002$,), PHQ-4 ($r = 0.23$, $p = 0.031$), L-1 ($r = 0.31$, $p = 0.003$), general sleep quality ($r = 0.39$, $p < 0.001$), resilience ($r = 0.312$; $p = 0.004$), and current sleep quality ($r = 0.32$ $p = 0.002$). These associations were not found in the control group. All correlations for the PH group can be found in Table 3.

Table 3. Spearman's rank correlation coefficients for associations between activity scores, sociodemographic data, mental health, and sleep quality of PH patients. Significant associations are depicted in bold.

	Activity of Daily Living		Sports Activity		Total Physical Activity		Climbing Stairs	
Age	−0.19	(0.080)	−0.23	(0.020)	−0.22	(0.041)	0.22	(0.041)
Level of education	0.06	(0.570)	0.27	(0.007)	0.14	(0.202)	0.06	(0.575)
Residents per household	0.20	(0.052)	0.09	(0.353)	0.20	(0.067)	0.21	(0.049)
Children per household	0.18	(0.101)	−0.00	(0.945)	0.19	(0.093)	0.19	(0.080)
Comorbidities	−0.20	(0.062)	0.03	(0.787)	−0.17	(0.116)	0.13	(0.234)
WHO-5	0.33	(0.002)	0.09	(0.396)	0.26	(0.016)	0.33	(0.002)
PHQ-4	−0.16	(0.130)	0.13	(0.207)	−0.11	(0.300)	0.23	(0.031)
L-1	0.33	(0.001)	0.04	(0.716)	0.30	(0.005)	0.31	(0.003)
General sleep quality	0.33	(0.001)	0.11	(0.263)	0.31	(0.003)	0.39	(<0.001)
Acute sleep quality	0.32	(0.002)	0.09	(0.385)	0.25	(0.018)	0.32	(0.002)
Resilience (z-standard.)	0.24	(0.027)	0.058	(0.572)	0.20	(0.076)	0.31	(0.004)
Stress (z-standard.)	0.06	(0.578)	0.074	(0.461)	0.85	(0.438)	0.05	(0.649)

WHO-5: The World Health Organization-Five Well-Being Index, PHQ-4: Patient Health Questionnaire-4; L-1: Likert-scale rating-1.

3.5. Regression Analysis: Prediction of the Mental Health by Resilience, Stress Experience, and Sleep Quality during the Lockdown

In a first step, we calculated regression models for the PH group only to investigate whether life satisfaction, mental well- and illbeing (represented by L1, WHO-5, and PHQ-4) could be predicted by total physical activity, sleep, stress, and resilience.

The present data revealed that life satisfaction of PH patients is significantly predicted by sleep quality (B = 0.327, beta = 0.321, $p = 0.001$), total physical activity (B = 0.190, beta = 0.178, $p = 0.012$), stress experience (B = −0.215, beta = −0.184, $p = 0.017$), and resilience (B = 0.465, beta = 0.438, $p < 0.001$). The total variance explained by the full model as a whole was $R^2 = 0.632$, $F(4, 82) = 36.260$, $p < 0.001$. For psychological wellbeing, we found significant associations for sleep quality (B = 0.248, beta = 0.264, $p = 0.001$), stress experience (B = −0.195, beta = −0.181, $p = 0.006$), and resilience (B = 0.579, beta = 0.591, $p < 0.001$) in the PH group. The total variance explained by the model as a whole was $R^2 = 0.739$, $F(4, 80) = 57.596$, $p < 0.001$. With regard to mental health, we found significant associations for sleep quality (B = −0.182, beta = −0.175, $p = 0.03$), stress experience (B = 0.348, beta = 0.293, $p < 0.001$), and resilience (B = −0.601, beta = −0.555, $p < 0.001$) in the PH group. The total variance explained by the model as a whole was $R^2 = 0.682$, $F(4, 81) = 44.379$, $p < 0.001$. These data revealed that especially resilience, sleep quality, and stress experience are relevant predictors of mental health outcomes and wellbeing. The patients' total physical activity only seem to impact variables related to life satisfaction (Figure 2A–C).

When considering the total sample and including the group variable in order to reveal differences between the PH group and healthy controls, linear regression analysis revealed that the mental health issues and mental wellbeing could be predicted by the diagnosis of PH, resilience, stress experience, total physical activity, and the current sleep quality. Total physical activity level had an albeit smaller impact on mental wellbeing.

Regarding life satisfaction, results showed that the L1-score was significantly lower for PH patients compared to healthy controls (B = −0.482, beta = −0.226, $p < 0.001$). Moreover, increases in L1-scores correlated significantly with increases in resilience (B = 0.444, beta = 0.449, $p < 0.001$), increases in sleep quality (B = 0.288, beta = 0.291, $p < 0.001$), increases in total physical activity (B = 0.168, beta = 0.165, $p = 0.004$), as well as decreases in stress experience (B = −0.157, beta = −0.149, $p = 0.014$) The total variance explained by the model as a whole was $R^2 = 0.627$, $F(5, 129) = 44.431$, $p < 0.001$. The inclusion of the product terms did not explain significant additional variance in the L1 score, corrected $R^2 = 0.649$, $F(9, 129) = 27.505$, $p < 0.001$, revealing no significant interactions between PH and control group.

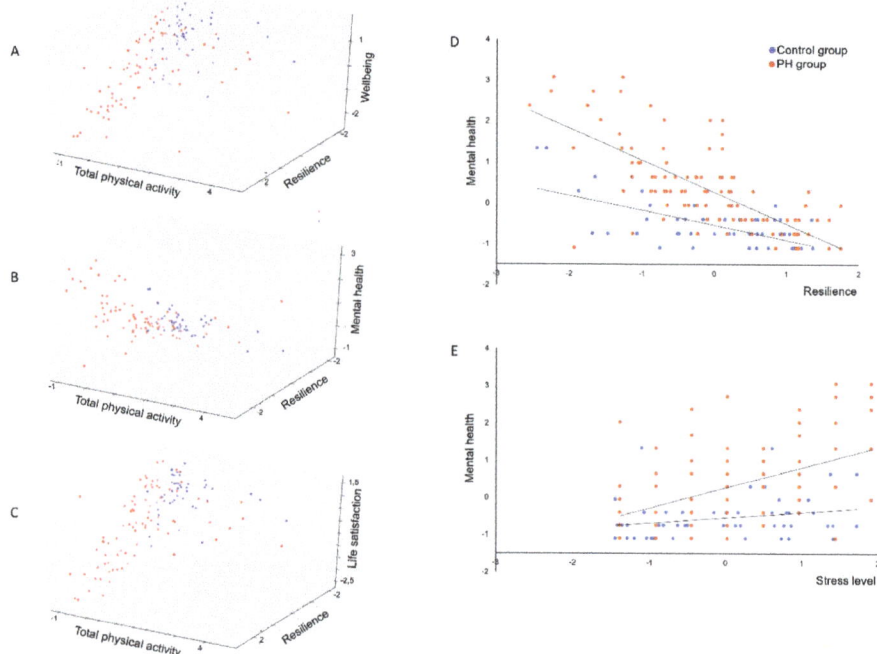

Figure 2. Associations between mental health dimensions, daily activity, and resilience for PH and control group. (**A**): Association between total physical activity, resilience, and wellbeing for PH and control group. (**B**): Association between total physical activity, resilience, and mental health for PH and control group. (**C**): Association between total physical activity, resilience, and life satisfaction for PH and control group. (**D**): Association between resilience and mental health for PH and control group. (**E**): Association between stress and mental health for PH and control group.

Results further showed that the WHO-5 score was significantly lower for the PH group compared to healthy controls (B = −0.511, beta = −0.246, $p = 0.001$). Like for the PH group only, the WHO-5 score was significantly moderated by the individual resilience (B = 0.522, beta = 0.539, $p < 0.001$), subjective stress level (B = −0.179, beta = −0.172, $p = 0.001$), and sleep quality (B = 0.269, beta = 0.278, $p < 0.001$) in the total sample analysis. Total physical activity had also a small significant impact on wellbeing (B = 0.096, beta = 0.097, $p = 0.044$) The total variance explained by the model as a whole was $R^2 = 0.740$, $F(5, 127) = 73.393$, $p < 0.001$. The inclusion of product terms reflecting interaction by group did not explain significant additional variance in the WHO-5 score, $R^2 = 0.738$, $F(9, 127) = 40.809$, $p < 0.001$, revealing no significant interactions between PH and control group.

Regarding mental health, results showed that the PHQ-4 score was significantly higher for PH patients compared to healthy controls (B = 0.638, beta = 0.295, $p < 0.001$). Moreover, increases in PHQ-4 scores correlated significantly with decreases in resilience (B = −0.505, beta = −0.504, $p < 0.001$), decreases in sleep quality (B = −0.196, beta = −0.196, $p = 0.004$) and increases in stress (B = 0.235, beta = 0.219, $p < 0.001$). The total variance explained by the model as a whole was $R^2 = 0.640$, $F(5, 128) = 46.508$, $p < 0.001$. The inclusion of the product terms did explain significant additional variance in the PHQ-4 score, $R^2 = 0.685$, $F(9, 128) = 31.85$, $p < 0.001$, revealing that significant interactions between group and resilience (B = −0.251, beta = −0.201, $p = 0.034$) as well as group and stress experience (B = 0.299, beta = 0.218, $p = 0.014$) reflecting a lower resilience as well as a higher stress experience during lockdown in patients with PH leading to a stronger rate of change of mental disorders in PH patients (Figure 2C,D).

4. Discussion

The present data showed that during the COVID-19 pandemic PH patients had significantly lower physical activity, mental health, and sleep quality compared to age-matched healthy subjects. Being physically active positively correlated with mental health and sleep quality in the PH group. The inclusion of product terms reflecting interaction by group did not explain significant additional variance in the WHO-5 score, revealing no significant interactions between PH and control group. Using multiple regression, data revealed for the PH group that mental health issues could be predicted by total physical activity, sleep, stress level, and resilience indicating that especially resilience, sleep quality and stress experience are relevant predictors of mental health outcomes and wellbeing. The patients' total physical activity levels, however, only seem to impact life satisfaction. When comparing both groups, we found that in PH patients as well as healthy controls lower resilience, higher stress experience, lower sleep quality as well as reduced physical activity leading to a diminishment of life satisfaction and mental wellbeing. Furthermore, the present data demonstrate that lower resilience and higher stress experience were even leading to a stronger increase of mental illbeing in PH patients compared to healthy controls.

Previous studies documented that PH patients are significantly less active compared to healthy subjects in non-pandemic living conditions [22,23]. During the lockdown period of the pandemic, PH patients seemed to further reduce their activity levels to about 50% compared to accelerometry data from Gonzales-Saiz et al. [22]. Here, one has to keep in mind that accelerometer data are difficult to compare with questionnaire data. However, due to social desirability, most people are even more positive about themselves in surveys than they are [24]. Interestingly, these results are in contrast to recent findings in healthy subjects. Here, it has been demonstrated for a large group of participants that lockdown restrictions did not lead to a decrease in sports activity levels in previously low active subjects [16]. From a therapeutic point of view, this seems to be problematic for PH patients, because a daily activity is an important prognostic factor for the symptomatology and progression of the disease [25].

Concerning mental health issues, PH patients show a significantly decreased mental wellbeing compared to healthy controls. The present data further implicate a prevalence of depression ranging from 36.4% and 53.6% during the pandemic. In contrast, during non-pandemic times, depression prevalence of 7.5 to 55% was reported, with an average prevalence of depression of 36% [5,26,27]. Hence, the prevalence of depressive symptoms of PH patients during the pandemic was found in the upper half of the occurrence under normal circumstances. These findings suggest that social distancing and self-isolation only slightly favor the development of depressive symptoms. However, the more significant factor seems to be the functional limitations of PH patients [26]. Mental impairments that promote depression, are represented by anxious symptoms which were found in about one-third of the PH patients. Compared to the given control group, this prevalence is significantly higher. However, previous studies found anxiety disorders in PH patients in a range of 13 to 45.5% in non-pandemic situations [27–29]. Accordingly, the level of anxiety seems to be not significantly higher during the COVID-19 pandemic.

A potential driver of mental disorders seems be the worse sleep quality of PH patients. The self-reported general sleep quality indicates an about 25% lower level compared to subjects of the control group. Similar results were found for the current sleep quality during the COVID-19 pandemic, where the PH group scored 27% lower levels compared to the control group. PH patients seem to suffer also during non-pandemic conditions from a reduced sleep quality compared to healthy subjects [26]. Quality of sleep and the mental health scores WHO-5 and L-1 positively correlated with total physical activity, total activity and climbing stairs. These associations once again underline the close connection between different lifestyle factors. However, it has to be stated that the participation in sports activities is generally low in PH patients, even if there is sufficient evidence available that regular exercise training has an overall positive effect on the physiological and psychological components of PH [25]. The positive relationship between sports activity and mental wellbeing and life satisfaction holds for the PH and the control group as revealed by the missing interaction in the multiple regression analysis which is not surprising given the tremendous evidence for physical activity and sports to promote wellbeing and buffer stress [30]. However, correlations for the control group failed to reach significance. Here, we speculate that this effect is driven by the rather small size of this sub-group.

The present data revealed that especially subjective stress experience as well as individual resilience seem to be strong predictors of mental illbeing of PH patients as well as healthy controls. We assume that subjects of the control group also experience more stress during the pandemic and that their resilience suffers. Therefore, they are approaching the lower level of PH patients. As one major antecedent of mental health issues, like depression, is life stress, both daily hassles [31] and major negative life events [32], it is not surprising that the subjective stress level is strongly associated with mental wellbeing in both groups. Our data revealed that lower resilience and higher stress experience even lead to a stronger increase of mental illbeing in PH patients than in healthy controls reflecting that the present pandemic hit PH patients even harder as their adaptive capacity and resources to react on the situation are lower and mental health might be impaired even more.

The observed impact of resilience on mental health seems plausible and has already been confirmed in healthy subjects [33]. Theory suggests that resilient individuals bounce back from negative experiences quicker and more effectively [34]. As it is demonstrated by a broad body of literature, physical activity is positively associated with a person's resilience [35]. Recent research showed that especially individuals with high trait anxiety, which may be a risk factor for developing clinically significant mental health problems, may preferentially show psychological, as well as physiological, benefit from physical activity [36]. In the present study, however, this could only partly be confirmed as we found only a small relationship between the activity level and life satisfaction and mental wellbeing.

A limitation of our study is that we used the hemodynamic PH definition of the current European Society of Cardiology (ESC)/European Respiratory Society (ERS) guidelines. The impact of the newly proposed hemodynamic PH criteria on mental health, physical activity, and resilience merit further investigation [2].

5. Clinical Implications

Given current research [25] and the present data, we suggest that patients should be encouraged to remain physically active even in pandemic times, although they should certainly do so in consideration of infection control. Vulnerable populations should also receive therapeutic support to improve their sleep quality and stress management as well as psychological resilience factors. All these interventions should also have a positive effect on mental wellbeing accompanied by less anxiety and depressive symptoms [37,38]. Of note, scheduling of appointments of PH patients in specialized outpatient PH expert centers was significantly reduced during the lockdown period [39].

6. Conclusions

Current data showed that PH patients showed significantly lower physical activity, mental health, and sleep quality compared to the healthy subjects during the lockdown period of the COVID-19 pandemic. While levels of depression seem to be only slightly affected during the COVID-19 pandemic, significantly lower resilience and higher stress experience lead to an albeit stronger diminishment of wellbeing in PH patients. Hence, it seems desirable to pay special attention to PH patients. Especially in this situation, patients should receive increased therapeutic support to improve lifestyle factors such as sleep quality, stress management and physical activity levels. This could be helpful, for example, in counseling on how to carry out physical activity while observing infection control.

Author Contributions: Conceptualization, K.K., J.S., M.J.R.; Methodology, C.L.D., K.G., K.K., B.K., J.S., K.T., M.J.R.; Software, C.W., K.G., K.K., M.J.R.; Validation, C.W., K.K., B.K.; Formal Analysis, C.L.D, C.W., K.K., B.K., M.J.R.; Investigation, C.L.D., C.W., K.G., K.K., B.K., J.S., K.T., H.A.G., N.S., H.G., M.J.R.; Resources, K.K., J.S., K.T., H.A.G., N.S., H.G., M.J.R.; Data Curation, C.W., K.K., B.K., J.S., M.J.R.; Writing-Original Draft Preparation, C.L.D., K.K., B.K.; Writing-Review & Editing, K.K., B.K., J.S., K.T., H.A.G., N.S., H.G., M.J.R.; Visualization, B.K.,; Supervision, K.K., M.J.R.; Project Administration, K.K., M.J.R. All authors have read and agreed to the published version of the manuscript.

Funding: We got no funding for the study.

Acknowledgments: We thank Ralf Schmiedel and the study participants for their support of the study.

Conflicts of Interest: There is no conflict of interest.

Data Availability Statement: All data are available upon request.

References

1. Galiè, N.; Humbert, M.; Vachiery, J.-L.; Gibbs, S.; Lang, I.; Torbicki, A.; Simonneau, G.; Peacock, A.; Vonk Noordegraaf, A.; Beghetti, M.; et al. 2015 ESC/ERS Guidelines for the Diagnosis and Treatment of Pulmonary Hypertension: The Joint Task Force for the Diagnosis and Treatment of Pulmonary Hypertension of the European Society of Cardiology (ESC) and the European Respiratory Society (ERS): Endorsed by: Association for European Paediatric and Congenital Cardiology (AEPC), International Society for Heart and Lung Transplantation (ISHLT). *Eur. Heart J.* **2016**, *37*, 67–119. [CrossRef] [PubMed]
2. Simonneau, G.; Montani, D.; Celermajer, D.S.; Denton, C.P.; Gatzoulis, M.A.; Krowka, M.; Williams, P.G.; Souza, R. Haemodynamic Definitions and Updated Clinical Classification of Pulmonary Hypertension. *Eur. Respir. J.* **2019**, *53*. [CrossRef] [PubMed]
3. Löwe, B.; Wahl, I.; Rose, M.; Spitzer, C.; Glaesmer, H.; Wingenfeld, K.; Schneider, A.; Brähler, E. A 4-Item Measure of Depression and Anxiety: Validation and Standardization of the Patient Health Questionnaire-4 (PHQ-4) in the General Population. *J. Affect. Disord.* **2010**, *122*, 86–95. [CrossRef]
4. McDonough, A.; Matura, L.A.; Carroll, D.L. Symptom Experience of Pulmonary Arterial Hypertension Patients. *Clin. Nurs. Res.* **2011**, *20*, 120–134. [CrossRef] [PubMed]
5. Shafazand, S.; Goldstein, M.K.; Doyle, R.L.; Hlatky, M.A.; Gould, M.K. Health-Related Quality of Life in Patients with Pulmonary Arterial Hypertension. *Chest* **2004**, *126*, 1452–1459. [CrossRef] [PubMed]
6. Gu, S.; Hu, H.; Dong, H. Systematic Review of Health-Related Quality of Life in Patients with Pulmonary Arterial Hypertension. *Pharmacoeconomics* **2016**, *34*, 751–770. [CrossRef]
7. Taichman, D.B.; Shin, J.; Hud, L.; Archer-Chicko, C.; Kaplan, S.; Sager, J.S.; Gallop, R.; Christie, J.; Hansen-Flaschen, J.; Palevsky, H. Health-related quality of life in patients with pulmonary arterial hypertension. *Respir. Res.* **2005**, *6*, 92. [CrossRef]
8. Robert-Koch-Institut. *COVID-19: Jetzt Handeln, Vorausschauend Planen—Strategie-Ergänzung zu Empfohlenen Infektionsschutzmaßnahmen und Zielen (2. Update)*; Robert-Koch-Institut: Berlin, Germany, 2020. [CrossRef]
9. Zhang, Y.; Zhang, H.; Ma, X.; Di, Q. Mental Health Problems during the COVID-19 Pandemics and the Mitigation Effects of Exercise: A Longitudinal Study of College Students in China. *Int. J. Environ. Res. Public Health* **2020**, *17*, 3722. [CrossRef]
10. Rodríguez-Rey, R.; Garrido-Hernansaiz, H.; Collado, S. Psychological Impact and Associated Factors During the Initial Stage of the Coronavirus (COVID-19) Pandemic Among the General Population in Spain. *Front. Psychol.* **2020**, *11*, 1540. [CrossRef]
11. Petzold, M.B.; Bendau, A.; Plag, J.; Pyrkosch, L.; Mascarell Maricic, L.; Betzler, F.; Rogoll, J.; Große, J.; Ströhle, A. Risk, Resilience, Psychological Distress, and Anxiety at the Beginning of the COVID-19 Pandemic in Germany. *Brain Behav.* **2020**, *10*. [CrossRef]
12. Jacob, L.; Tully, M.A.; Barnett, Y.; Lopez-Sanchez, G.F.; Butler, L.; Schuch, F.; López-Bueno, R.; McDermott, D.; Firth, J.; Grabovac, I.; et al. The Relationship between Physical Activity and Mental Health in a Sample of the UK Public: A Cross-Sectional Study during the Implementation of COVID-19 Social Distancing Measures. *Ment. Health Phys. Act.* **2020**, *19*, 100345. [CrossRef] [PubMed]
13. Pierce, M.; Hope, H.; Ford, T.; Hatch, S.; Hotopf, M.; John, A.; Kontopantelis, E.; Webb, R.; Wessely, S.; McManus, S.; et al. Mental Health before and during the COVID-19 Pandemic: A Longitudinal Probability Sample Survey of the UK Population. *Lancet Psychiatry* **2020**, *7*, 883–892. [CrossRef]

14. Vindegaard, N.; Benros, M.E. COVID-19 Pandemic and Mental Health Consequences: Systematic Review of the Current Evidence. *Brain Behav. Immun.* **2020**, *89*, 531–542. [CrossRef] [PubMed]
15. Lesser, I.A.; Nienhuis, C.P. The Impact of COVID-19 on Physical Activity Behavior and Well-Being of Canadians. *Int. J. Environ. Res. Public Health* **2020**, *17*, 3899. [CrossRef]
16. Brand, R.; Timme, S.; Nosrat, S. When Pandemic Hits: Exercise Frequency and Subjective Well-Being During COVID-19 Pandemic. *Front. Psychol.* **2020**, *11*, 570567. [CrossRef]
17. Southwick, S.M.; Bonanno, G.A.; Masten, A.S.; Panter-Brick, C.; Yehuda, R. Resilience Definitions, Theory, and Challenges: Interdisciplinary Perspectives. *Eur. J. Psychotraumatol.* **2014**, *5*. [CrossRef]
18. Fuchs, R.; Klaperski, S.; Gerber, M.; Seelig, H. Messung Der Bewegungs-Und Sportaktivität Mit Dem BSA-Fragebogen: Eine Methodische Zwischenbilanz. [Measurement of Physical Activity and Sport Activity with the BSA Questionnaire]. *Z. Gesundh.* **2015**, *23*, 60–76. [CrossRef]
19. Schwerdtfeger, A.R.; Dick, K. Episodes of Momentary Resilience in Daily Life Are Associated with HRV Reductions to Stressful Operations in Firefighters: An Ambulatory Assessment Approach Using Bayesian Multilevel Modeling. *J. Posit. Psychol.* **2019**, *14*, 593–602. [CrossRef]
20. Topp, C.W.; Østergaard, S.D.; Søndergaard, S.; Bech, P. The WHO-5 Well-Being Index: A Systematic Review of the Literature. *Psychother. Psychosom.* **2015**, *84*, 167–176. [CrossRef]
21. Beierlein, C.; Kovaleva, A.; László, Z.; Kemper, C.J.; Rammstedt, B. *Eine Single-Item-Skala Zur Erfassung Der Allgemeinen Lebenszufriedenheit: Die Kurzskala Lebenszufriedenheit-1 (L-1)*; GESIS-Working Papers; GESIS-Leibniz-Institut für Sozialwissenschaften: Mannheim, Germany, 2014; Volume 2014/33.
22. González-Saiz, L.; Santos-Lozano, A.; Fiuza-Luces, C.; Sanz-Ayán, P.; Quezada-Loaiza, C.A.; Ruiz-Casado, A.; Alejo, L.B.; Flox-Camacho, A.; Morán, M.; Lucia, A.; et al. Physical Activity Levels Are Low in Patients with Pulmonary Hypertension. *Ann. Transl. Med.* **2018**, *6*, 205. [CrossRef]
23. Pugh, M.E.; Buchowski, M.S.; Robbins, I.M.; Newman, J.H.; Hemnes, A.R. Physical Activity Limitation as Measured by Accelerometry in Pulmonary Arterial Hypertension. *Chest* **2012**, *142*, 1391–1398. [CrossRef] [PubMed]
24. Skender, S.; Ose, J.; Chang-Claude, J.; Paskow, M.; Brühmann, B.; Siegel, E.M.; Steindorf, K.; Ulrich, C.M. Accelerometry and Physical Activity Questionnaires—A Systematic Review. *BMC Public Health* **2016**, *16*, 515. [CrossRef] [PubMed]
25. Waller, L.; Krüger, K.; Conrad, K.; Weiss, A.; Alack, K. Effects of Different Types of Exercise Training on Pulmonary Arterial Hypertension: A Systematic Review. *J. Clin. Med.* **2020**, *9*, 1689. [CrossRef] [PubMed]
26. Harzheim, D.; Klose, H.; Pinado, F.P.; Ehlken, N.; Nagel, C.; Fischer, C.; Ghofrani, A.; Rosenkranz, S.; Seyfarth, H.-J.; Halank, M.; et al. Anxiety and Depression Disorders in Patients with Pulmonary Arterial Hypertension and Chronic Thromboembolic Pulmonary Hypertension. *Respir. Res.* **2013**, *14*, 104. [CrossRef]
27. Wilkens, H.; Grimminger, F.; Hoeper, M.; Stähler, G.; Ehlken, B.; Plesnila-Frank, C.; Berger, K.; Resch, A.; Ghofrani, A. Burden of Pulmonary Arterial Hypertension in Germany. *Respir. Med.* **2010**, *104*, 902–910. [CrossRef]
28. Zhou, X.; Shi, H.; Yang, Y.; Zhang, Z.; Zhai, Z.; Wang, C. Anxiety and Depression in Patients with Pulmonary Arterial Hypertension and Chronic Thromboembolic Pulmonary Hypertension: Results from a Chinese Survey. *Exp. Ther. Med.* **2020**, *19*, 3124–3132. [CrossRef]
29. McCollister, D.H.; Beutz, M.; McLaughlin, V.; Rumsfeld, J.; Masoudi, F.A.; Tripputi, M.; Yaeger, T.; Weintraub, P.; Badesch, D.B. Depressive Symptoms in Pulmonary Arterial Hypertension: Prevalence and Association with Functional Status. *Psychosomatics* **2010**, *51*, 339–339.e8. [CrossRef]
30. Craike, M.J.; Coleman, D.; MacMahon, C. Direct and Buffering Effects of Physical Activity on Stress-Related Depression in Mothers of Infants. *J. Sport Exerc. Psychol.* **2010**, *32*, 23–38. [CrossRef]
31. Kanner, A.D.; Coyne, J.C.; Schaefer, C.; Lazarus, R.S. Comparison of Two Modes of Stress Measurement: Daily Hassles and Uplifts versus Major Life Events. *J. Behav. Med.* **1981**, *4*, 1–39. [CrossRef]
32. Sarason, I.G.; Johnson, J.H.; Siegel, J.M. Assessing the Impact of Life Changes: Development of the Life Experiences Survey. *J. Consult Clin. Psychol.* **1978**, *46*, 932–946. [CrossRef]
33. Silverman, M.N.; Deuster, P.A. Biological Mechanisms Underlying the Role of Physical Fitness in Health and Resilience. *Interface Focus* **2014**, *4*, 20140040. [CrossRef] [PubMed]
34. Tugade, M.M.; Fredrickson, B.L. Resilient Individuals Use Positive Emotions to Bounce Back from Negative Emotional Experiences. *J. Pers. Soc. Psychol.* **2004**, *86*, 320–333. [CrossRef] [PubMed]

35. Forcier, K.; Stroud, L.R.; Papandonatos, G.D.; Hitsman, B.; Reiches, M.; Krishnamoorthy, J.; Niaura, R. Links between Physical Fitness and Cardiovascular Reactivity and Recovery to Psychological Stressors: A Meta-Analysis. *Health Psychol.* **2006**, *25*, 723–739. [CrossRef] [PubMed]
36. Hegberg, N.J.; Tone, E.B. Physical Activity and Stress Resilience: Considering Those at-Risk for Developing Mental Health Problems. *Ment. Health Phys. Act.* **2015**, *8*, 1–7. [CrossRef]
37. Yoshikawa, E.; Nishi, D.; Matsuoka, Y.J. Association between Regular Physical Exercise and Depressive Symptoms Mediated through Social Support and Resilience in Japanese Company Workers: A Cross-Sectional Study. *BMC Public Health* **2016**, *16*, 553. [CrossRef] [PubMed]
38. Wermelinger, S.; Gampe, A.; Daum, M.M. The Dynamics of the Interrelation of Perception and Action across the Life Span. *Psychol. Res.* **2019**, *83*, 116–131. [CrossRef]
39. Yogeswaran, A.; Gall, H.; Tello, K.; Grünig, E.; Xanthouli, P.; Ewert, R.; Kamp, J.C.; Olsson, K.M.; Wißmüller, M.; Rosenkranz, S.; et al. Impact of SARS-CoV-2 Pandemic on Pulmonary Hypertension out-Patient Clinics in Germany: A Multi-Centre Study. *Pulm. Circ.* **2020**, *10*, 2045894020941682. [CrossRef]

Publisher's Note: MDPI stays neutral with regard to jurisdictional claims in published maps and institutional affiliations.

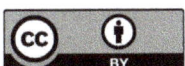

© 2020 by the authors. Licensee MDPI, Basel, Switzerland. This article is an open access article distributed under the terms and conditions of the Creative Commons Attribution (CC BY) license (http://creativecommons.org/licenses/by/4.0/).

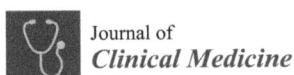

Article

New Laboratory Protocol to Determine the Oxidative Stress Profile of Human Nasal Epithelial Cells Using Flow Cytometry

Ana Reula [1,2], Daniel Pellicer [1,2], Silvia Castillo [2,3], María Magallón [1,2], Miguel Armengot [4,5], Guadalupe Herrera [6], José-Enrique O'Connor [7], Lucía Bañuls [1,2], María Mercedes Navarro-García [2], Amparo Escribano [2,3,8] and Francisco Dasí [1,2,*]

Citation: Reula, A.; Pellicer, D.; Castillo, S.; Magallón, M.; Armengot, M.; Herrera, G.; O'Connor, J.-E.; Bañuls, L.; Navarro-García, M.M.; Escribano, A.; et al. New Laboratory Protocol to Determine the Oxidative Stress Profile of Human Nasal Epithelial Cells Using Flow Cytometry. *J. Clin. Med.* **2021**, *10*, 1172. https://doi.org/10.3390/jcm10061172

Academic Editors: Antonio Spanevello, Luis Garcia-Marcos and Davide Chiumello

Received: 23 January 2021
Accepted: 5 March 2021
Published: 11 March 2021

Publisher's Note: MDPI stays neutral with regard to jurisdictional claims in published maps and institutional affiliations.

Copyright: © 2021 by the authors. Licensee MDPI, Basel, Switzerland. This article is an open access article distributed under the terms and conditions of the Creative Commons Attribution (CC BY) license (https://creativecommons.org/licenses/by/4.0/).

1. Department of Physiology, School of Medicine, University of Valencia, Avda. Blasco Ibáñez, 17, 46010 Valencia, Spain; ana.reula@uv.es (A.R.); dpellicerroig@gmail.com (D.P.); mariamagallon94@gmail.com (M.M.); lucia.banyuls.soto@gmail.com (L.B.)
2. Rare Respiratory Diseases Research Group, IIS INCLIVA, Fundación Investigación Hospital Clínico Valencia, Avda. Menéndez y Pelayo, 4, 46010 Valencia, Spain; sccorullon@gmail.com (S.C.); mer_navarro2002@yahoo.es (M.M.N.-G.); aescribano@separ.es (A.E.)
3. Pediatrics Unit, Hospital Clínico Universitario Valencia, 46004 Valencia, Spain
4. Department of Surgery, School of Medicine, University of Valencia, Avda. Blasco Ibáñez, 17, 46010 Valencia, Spain; miguel.armengot@uv.es
5. ENT Unit, Hospital La Fe, 46026 Valencia, Spain
6. Flow Cytometry Unit, IIS INCLIVA, Fundación Investigación Hospital Clínico Valencia, Avda. Menéndez y Pelayo, 4, 46010 Valencia, Spain; guadalupe.herrera@uv.es
7. Department of Biochemistry, School of Medicine, University of Valencia, Avda. Blasco Ibáñez, 17, 46010 Valencia, Spain; jose.e.oconnor@uv.es
8. Department of Pediatrics, Obstetrics and Gynecology, School of Medicine, University of Valencia, Avda. Blasco Ibáñez, 17, 46010 Valencia, Spain
* Correspondence: Francisco.Dasi@uv.es; Tel.: +34-676-515598

Abstract: Several studies have shown the importance of oxidative stress (OS) in respiratory disease pathogenesis. It has been reported that the nasal epithelium may act as a surrogate for the bronchial epithelium in several respiratory diseases involving OS. However, the sample yields obtained from nasal biopsies are modest, limiting the number of parameters that can be determined. Flow cytometry has been widely used to evaluate cellular OS profiles. It has the advantage that analyses can be performed using a small amount of sample. Therefore, we aimed to set up a new method based on flow cytometry to assess the oxidative profile of human nasal epithelial cells which could be used in research on respiratory diseases. Levels of total nitric oxide, superoxide anion, peroxynitrite, and intracellular peroxides were measured. Reduced thiol levels, such as antioxidant-reduced glutathione and oxidative damaged lipids and proteins, were also analysed. The intracellular calcium levels, plasma membrane potential, apoptosis, and percentage of live cells were also studied. Finally, a strategy to evaluate the mitochondrial function, including mitochondrial hydrogen peroxide, superoxide anion, mitochondrial mass, and membrane potential, was set up. Using small amounts of sample and a non-invasive sampling technique, the described method enables the measurement of a comprehensive set of OS parameters in nasal epithelial cells, which could be useful in research on respiratory diseases.

Keywords: flow cytometry; rare respiratory diseases; nasal epithelium; oxidative stress; reactive oxygen species

1. Introduction

Free radicals are molecules with at least one unpaired electron in their outer layer. The need to acquire an electron to achieve electrochemical stability drives reactions of free radicals with other biomolecules. Free radicals react with DNA, lipids, and proteins, producing oxidation and a loss of activity in these biomolecules [1]. As a by-product of cellular aerobic metabolism, various reactive species are generated, including reactive oxygen species (ROS), such as superoxide (O_2^-) or hydrogen peroxide (H_2O_2), and reactive nitrogen species (RNS), such as nitric oxide (NO) or peroxynitrite ($ONOO^-$) [2,3]. The primary intracellular sources of ROS and RNS are mitochondria, lysosomes, peroxisomes, nuclear and cytoplasmic membranes, and the endoplasmic reticulum [4]. ROS and RNS are also generated by external factors, such as tobacco or environmental pollution [5]. Eukaryotic cells possess defence mechanisms to avoid biomolecular oxidative damage, with vitamin C, vitamin E, and glutathione all relevant examples of simple defence mechanisms [6]. Cells also have complex enzymatic systems, such as superoxide dismutase (SOD), catalase (CAT), glutathione peroxidase (GPx), and glutathione reductase (GR), which evolved to reduce ROS levels [7,8]. Under physiological conditions, basal ROS and RNS levels are necessary for cells' function by acting as regulatory and signalling molecules. Thus, cells need these species to maintain the cellular reduction-oxidation (REDOX) balance [9].

Oxidative stress (OS) is produced when there is an imbalance toward pro-oxidation between pro-oxidant and antioxidant systems. When defensive mechanisms cannot prevent ROS and RNS accumulation, signalling pathways are activated and gene expression and protein synthesis changes occur [9]. In response to DNA oxidative damage, cells react by repairing the damage, activating different cell cycle checkpoints, or inducing apoptosis [10]. These conditions are linked to numerous pathological processes, such as cancer, chronic inflammation, ageing, neurodegenerative and cardiovascular disease, and asthma, among others [11,12].

Nasal epithelial cells represent the first line of defence against various environmental factors. These cells clean, humidify, and warm inhaled air and produce mucus, which attaches to particles transported by cilia present on some cells to the digestive tract, where they are eliminated. Nasal epithelial cells are not only a physical barrier but were also shown to respond by producing inflammatory mediators that can affect the local immune response [13]. These cells are suitable in vitro models for the study of novel defence mechanisms [14]. Thus, the nasal epithelium may act as a surrogate for the bronchial epithelium in asthma studies [15].

On the other hand, numerous studies have shown the importance of OS as a factor involved in the pathogenesis of several diseases of the respiratory system, such as Chronic Obstructive Pulmonary Disease (COPD) [16], asthma [17], alpha-1 antitrypsin deficiency (AATD) [18–21] and primary ciliary dyskinesia (PCD) [22]. Therefore, it is essential to know the underlying mechanisms by which OS directs pathogenesis in these diseases to develop more effective therapies. There are currently no methods based on flow cytometry that allow the analysis of different OS parameters in nasal epithelial cells. Therefore, given the importance of these cells in different respiratory pathologies and the important role of OS in their development, we present a new method based on flow cytometry to assess the oxidative profile of human nasal epithelial cells, which could be very useful in the future research of several respiratory diseases.

2. Experimental Section

2.1. Biological Samples

Nasal epithelial cells were obtained from six healthy donors (3 males and 3 females; ages (mean ± Standard Deviation) 27 ± 1.5 and 28 ± 2.3, respectively) at the Hospital Clínico Universitario de Valencia (HCUV) and Hospital General Universitario de Valencia (HGUV) (Valencia, Spain). A cytology brush (Covaca SA CE2005, Madrid, Spain) was inserted into the patient's nostril, and the nasal epithelium of the middle meatus was gently brushed, yielding strips of ciliated nasal epithelium. Samples were transported using Medium199 supplemented with Hanks' salts, L-glutamine, 25 mM HEPES, and 1% penicillin/streptomycin. Before labelling, samples were filtered using 50 μm CellTrics® filters (Sysmex; Sant Just Desvern; Barcelona, Spain) (25004-0042-2317 Sysmex) to isolate cells from cell debris and aggregates. Participants were healthy, non-smoking individuals without respiratory bronchial disease, local or systemic disease, allergies, rhinosinusitis, or upper respiratory tract infection for at least one month before sampling. The study protocol was approved by the Ethics Committees of the HCUV and HGUV and followed the ethical guidelines of the 1975 Declaration of Helsinki [23]. All the participating individuals gave their written informed consent. Samples were analysed in the Cytometry Service of the Unidad Central de Investigación Medicina (UCIM) of Instituto de Investigación Sanitaria INCLIVA.

2.2. Reagents

The probes used in this study are detailed, including global distributors, in the Supplementary Materials (Reagents). Flow cytometry methods, including reagent concentrations; storage temperature; species studied; incubation protocols in basal tubes; and positive controls, cytometers, and lasers used for each measurement are summarized in Tables 1 and 2. Additionally, a step-by-step protocol is available in the Supplementary Materials section.

2.3. Determination of Dead and Live Cells

Dead cells may compromise flow cytometric data analysis, especially when studying physiological conditions, such as OS. As cellular viability is usually determined by measuring cells' capacity to exclude vital dyes, we excluded dead cells from our analysis by adding a DNA-binding dye. 4′,6-diamidino-2-phenylindole (DAPI) was added into tubes with dihydroethidium (HE), 2′-7′dichlorofluorescin diacetate (DCFH), Dihydrorhodamine 123 (DHR1,2,3), Diaminofluorescein-FM diacetate (DAF-FM DA), 5-chloromethylfluorescein diacetate (CMFDA), Tetramethylrhodamine, methyl ester (TMRM), MitoTracker Green, MitoSOX, MitoPY 1, FLUO-4, BODIPY 665 (B665), and FTC, whereas propidium iodide (PI) was used with Bis(1,3-dibutylbarbituric acid)trimethine oxonol (DIBAC). PI is widely used with Annexin V to determine if cells are viable, apoptotic, or necrotic through differences in plasma membrane integrity and permeability. PI does not stain live or early apoptotic cells due to the presence of an intact plasma membrane, but in late apoptotic and necrotic cells the integrity of the plasma and nuclear membranes decreases, allowing PI to cross the cell membrane, intercalate into nucleic acids, and display red fluorescence [24,25].

2.4. Reactive Oxygen Species and Reactive Nitrogen Species Assessment

Superoxide anion (O_2^-) is detected by HE, a fluorescent probe selectively oxidised and hydroxylated by O_2^- to 2-OH-ethidium, emitting fluorescence when bound to DNA [26,27]. Hydrogen peroxide (H_2O_2) detection was based on DCFH oxidation, which generally exhibits a low basal fluorescence, but is converted to highly fluorescent DCF when oxidised by H_2O_2 in the presence of peroxidase [27,28]. Peroxynitrite ($ONOO^-$) production was assessed using DHR1,2,3, an uncharged, nonfluorescent ROS indicator that passively diffuses across membranes where it is oxidised to cationic rhodamine 123, exhibiting green fluorescence [29,30]. Nitric oxide (NO) production was assessed using DAF-FM DA, an otherwise nonfluorescent probe that forms a fluorescent benzotriazole when it reacts with NO, thereby acting as a specific NO detector [31,32]. Intracellular thiol-reduced status, including reduced glutathione (GSH), was measured using CMFDA [33,34]. For each measurement, cells were incubated with the appropriate probe in individual tubes—i.e., HE (2.5 ug/mL), DCFH (2.5 μg/mL), DHR1,2,3 (100 μM), DAF-FM DA (1 μM), or CMFDA (25 nM)—for 20 min at 37 °C. Fluorescence was measured by flow cytometry with the appropriate settings.

2.5. Plasmatic Membrane Potential Assessment

Plasma membrane potential was evaluated using DIBAC, a potential-sensitive fluorescent probe that can enter depolarised cells and bind to intracellular proteins or membranes. Increased depolarisation results in an additional influx in the anionic dye and increases fluorescence. Conversely, hyperpolarisation results in a decrease in fluorescence. DIBAC dyes are excluded from mitochondria because of their negative charge, making them suitable for measuring plasma membrane potentials [35,36]. Cells were incubated with DIBAC (1.2 μM) for 20 min at 37 °C, and fluorescence was measured by flow cytometry with the appropriate settings.

Table 1. Summary of the flow cytometry methods.

Reactive Species	Measurement	Stock Concentration	Storage Temperature	Final Concentration	Flow Cytometer	Excitation Laser	Detector	Cell Number	Total Volume	Incubation Time	Incubation Temperature
DIBAC	Plasma membrane potential	100 µM	−20 °C	1.2 µM	FACS Verse	Blue (488 nm)	527/32507 LP	8.000	250 µL	20 min	37 °C
FLUO-4	Intracellular Ca^{2+}	50 µM	−20 °C	0.5 µM	LSR Fortessa X-20	Blue (488 nm)	530/30505LP	8.000	250 µL	20 min	37 °C
CMFDA	Reduced thiols (GSH)	10 µM	−20 °C	25 nM	FACS Verse	Blue (488 nm)	527/32507 LP	8.000	250 µL	20 min	37 °C
DAF-FMDA	NO	1.25 mM	−20 °C	1 µM	LSR Fortessa X-20	Blue (488 nm)	530/30505LP	8.000	250 µL	20 min	37 °C
DCF	Intracellular peroxides	1 mg/mL	−20 °C	2.5 µg/mL	FACS Verse	Blue (488 nm)	527/32507 LP	8.000	250 µL	20 min	37 °C
MitoSOX	Mitochondrial O$_2^-$	0.5 mM	−20 °C	640 nM	FACS Verse	Blue (488 nm)	700/54665LP	8.000	250 µL	20 min	37 °C
Mitotracker Green	Mitochondrial mass	10 µM	−20 °C	78 nM	FACS Verse	Blue (488 nm)	527/32507 LP	8.000	250 µL	20 min	37 °C
BODIPY 665/676	Oxidized/reduced lipid ratio	1 mM	−20 °C	800 nM	FACS Aria III	Blue (488 nm) Red (635 nm)	586/42556LP and 780/60735LP	12.000	250 µL	30 min	37 °C
TMRM	Mitochondrial Ψm	240 µM	−20 °C	600 nM	FACS Verse	Blue (488 nm)	586/42560LP	8.000	250 µL	20 min	37 °C
DHR 123	ONOO$^-$	5 mM	−20 °C	100 µM	LSR Fortessa X-20	Blue (488 nm)	530/30505LP	12.000	250 µL	20 min	37 °C
HE	O$_2^-$	1 mg/mL	−20 °C	2.5 µg/mL	FACS Verse	Blue (488 nm)	700/54665LP	8.000	250 µL	20 min	37 °C
FTC	Protein carbonylation	1 mM	−20 °C	800 nM	FACS Verse	Blue (488 nm)	527/32507 LP	8.000	250 µL	20 min	37 °C
MitoPY	Mitochondrial H$_2$O$_2$	1 mM	−20 °C	4 µM	FACS Verse	Blue (488 nm)	527/32507 LP	8.000	250 µL	20 min	37 °C
DAPI	Cell death	1 mg/mL	−20 °C	800 ng/mL	FACS Verse	Violet (405 nm)	448/45	8.000	250 µL	20 min	37 °C
PI	Cell death	1 mg/mL	4 °C	8 µg/mL	FACS Verse	Blue (488 nm)	586/42560LP	12.000	100 µL	15 min	RT
Annexin V	Apoptosis	-	4 °C	-	FACS Verse	Blue (488 nm)	527/32507 LP	12.000	100 µL	15 min	RT

Table 2. Summary of cytometry methods for positive controls.

Reactive Species	Measurement	Inductor	Stock Concentration	Final Concentration	Storage Temperature	Inductor Incubation Time	Inductor Incubation Temperature	Reactive Incubation Time	Reactive Incubation Temperature
DIBAC	Plasmatic membrane potential	t-BHP	7.7 mM	100 µM	4 °C	15 min	37 °C	30 min	37 °C
FLUO-4	Intracellular Ca^{2+}	Ionomycin	1.338 mM	50 µM	−20 °C	Kynetics		Kynetics	
CMFDA	Reduced thiols	DEM	-	20 mM	−20 °C	90 min	37 °C	30 min	37 °C
DAF-FM DA	NO	NOR-1	1 mg/mL	16 µg/mL	−20 °C	Kynetics		Kynetics	
DCF	Intracellular peroxides	t-BHP	7.7 mM	100 µM	4 °C	15 min	37 °C	30 min	37 °C
MitoSOX	Mitochondrial O_2^-	PB	2.8 mg/mL	2.24 µg/mL	−20 °C	15 min	37 °C	30 min	37 °C
BODIPY 665/676	Oxidized/reduced lipids ratio	t-BHP	7.7 mM	100 µM	4 °C	15 min	37 °C	30 min	37 °C
TMRM	Mitochondrial Ψ_m	FCCP	10 mM	52 µM	−20 °C	15 min	37 °C	30 min	37 °C
DHR 123	$ONOO^-$	NOR-1 and PB	1 mg/mL and 2.8 mg/mL	16 µg/mL and 2.24 µg/mL	−20 °C	Kynetics		Kynetics	
HE	O_2^-	PB	2.8 mg/mL	2.24 µg/mL	−20 °C	15 min	37 °C	30 min	37 °C
FTC	Protein carbonylation	Menadione	10 mg/mL	1 mM	−20 °C	60 min	37 °C	30 min	37 °C
MitoPY	Mitochondrial H_2O_2	t-BHP	7.7 mM	100 µM	4 °C	15 min	37 °C	30 min	37 °C

2.6. Mitochondrial Assessment

Mitochondrial membrane potential (Ψ_m) was analysed using TMRM, a fluorescent probe that accumulates inside mitochondria directly proportional to their membrane potential [37,38]. Mitochondrial mass was determined using MitoTracker Green, a fluorescent dye that locates mitochondria independently to Ψ_m [39,40]. Mitochondrial O_2^- (mtO_2^-) was measured using MitoSOX, which enters live cells, specifically the mitochondria, where it is rapidly oxidised by O_2^- [30,41]. Mitochondrial H_2O_2 (mtH_2O_2) was measured using mitoPY 1, a cell-permeable fluorescent probe that selectively tracks the mitochondria of living cells by selectively binding to mtH_2O_2 [30,42]. For each measurement, cells were incubated with the appropriate probe in individual tubes—i.e., TMRM (600 nM), MitoTracker Green (78 nM), MitoSOX (640 nM), or MitoPY 1 (4 µM)—for 20 min at 37 °C. Fluorescence was measured by flow cytometry with the appropriate settings.

2.7. Intracellular Calcium Assessment

Intracellular calcium (Ca^{2+}) was measured using FLUO-4, a fluorogenic probe that detects intracellular Ca^{2+} [43,44]. Cells were incubated with FLUO-4 (0.5 µM) for 20 min at 37 °C, and fluorescence was measured by flow cytometry with the appropriate settings.

2.8. Oxidative Damage to Biomolecules

Lipid peroxidation was detected using the lipophilic probe BODIPY 665/676 dye, which exhibits a change in fluorescence emission after interaction with peroxyl radicals [45,46]. Cells were incubated with B665 (800 nM) for 30 min at 37 °C, and fluorescence was measured by flow cytometry with the appropriate settings.

Protein oxidation (carbonylation) levels were measured using FTC, a molecule that emits green fluorescence when it interacts with carbonyl groups of proteins [26,47]. Cells were incubated with FTC (800 nM) for 20 min at 37 °C, and fluorescence was measured by flow cytometry with the appropriate settings.

2.9. Apoptosis Assay

Apoptosis status was determined using Annexin V, a 35–36 kDa Ca^{2+}-dependent phospholipid-binding protein with a high affinity for phosphatidylserine (PS), which binds to PS on exposed apoptotic cell surfaces [48]. Cells were incubated in the dark for 15 min at room temperature with Annexin V, PI, and Annexin V-binding buffer (previously diluted to 1/10 in PBS). After incubation, 300 µL of the 1/10 Annexin V-binding buffer was added to the dilution. Samples were analysed by flow cytometry with the appropriate settings.

2.10. Positive Control Incubations

As controls, appropriate fluorochromes were added to each tube after previous incubation with their respective inducers. An H_2O_2 generator, t-BHP (100 µM) [49,50], was used for the B665, DCFH, MitoPY 1, and DIBAC tubes. PB (2.24 µg/mL), an O_2^- generator [50,51], was used for HE and MitoSOX tubes. DEM (20 mM), which produces GSH depletion [33,50], was used for CMFDA. Menadione (1 mM) was used for FTC to increase the carbonylated protein levels [50,52], and FCCP (52 µM), a mitochondrial uncoupler that decreases Ψ_m [50,53], was used for TMRM. Each tube was incubated in the dark for 15 min (except menadione, which was incubated for an hour, and DEM, which was incubated for 90 min) at 37 °C with their respective inducers. Next, each tube was incubated in the dark for 30 min at 37 °C. Samples were run on the flow cytometer with the appropriate settings.

A kinetic strategy was designed for the real-time follow-up of intracellular NO, $ONOO^-$, and Ca^{2+} generation. Cells were previously incubated with their respective fluorochromes—i.e., DAF (1 µM), DHR1,2,3 (100 µM), or FLUO-4 (0.5 µM), and DAPI. Each tube was incubated in the dark for 20 min at 37 °C. Afterwards, the acquisition process was paused to add the inducers. In the NO-positive control, two doses of NOR-1 (16 µg/mL), a nitric oxide generator [35], were added, and the acquisition process was continued until 300 s. In the $ONOO^-$-positive control, PB (2.24 µg/mL) and NOR-1 (16 µg/mL) were added, and the acquisition was continued until 200 s. In the Ca^{2+}-positive control, the ionophore ionomycin (50 µM) was added to stimulate Ca^{2+} influx, and acquisition was continued until 600 s.

2.11. Cytometer Settings and Data Analysis

All flow cytometry assays were carried out using the FACSVerse cytometer (BD Biosciences, San Jose, CA, USA), except the lipid oxidised/lipid reduced ratio, which was carried out using the FacsAria III cytometer (BD Biosciences), and kinetic analyses of NO, ONOO, and Ca^{2+} generation, which were carried out using the LSR Fortessa X-20 (BD Biosciences) (Table 1).

Blue (488 nm), violet (405 nm), and red (635 nm) lasers were used. The fluorescence results of DCFH, CMFDA, FTC, Mitotracker Green, Annexin, DIBAC, and MitoPY 1 were collected using a 527/32 507LP filter. Fluorescence results of MitoSOX and HE were collected using a 700/54 665LP filter, and TMRM and PI fluorescence results were collected using a 586/42 560LP filter. The fluorescence of DAPI was collected using a 448/45 filter. The fluorescence of B665 was detected using 586/42 556LP and 780/60 735LP filters. The DAF-FM DA, DHR1,2,3, and FLUO-4 fluorescence were gathered using a 530/30 505LP filter.

BD FACSSuite software was used for data acquisition with the FACSVerse cytometer, and the FACSDiva 4.0 software was used for FACSAriaIII and LSR Fortessa X-20 cytometer data acquisition. Offline data analysis was performed using the FLOWJO V.10.1 software (FlowJo™ Software Version 10.1. Becton, Dickinson and Company, 2019; Ashland, OR, USA).

3. Results

Due to the lack of previous research regarding the OS profile of the human nasal epithelial cells, a complex experimental design was needed. Besides cell quantity adjustment, reactive concentration, and voltage, positive controls were used to ensure that each parameter was correctly determined, as explained below. Basal labelling, the positive control and the corresponding graphics for each parameter from the six healthy individuals included in the study are shown in the Supplementary Materials section.

3.1. Gating Strategy

Figure 1 shows the population gating strategy used for each parameter. Nasal epithelial cells were selected by morphology, as measured by forward scatter (FSC), a cell size indicator, and side scatter (SSC), which estimates the internal complexity of the cells (1A). After this, individual cells were selected from all nasal epithelial cells through height confrontation (high-FSC) in front of the FSC area (area-FSC), disregarding doublets (1B). Dead cells were excluded using DAPI or PI (1C).

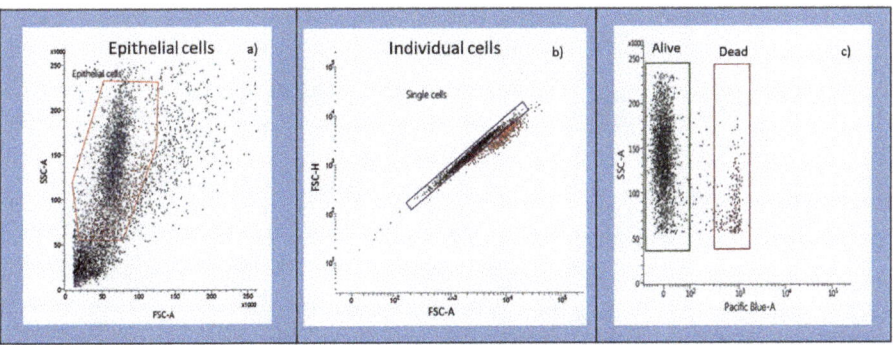

Figure 1. Gating strategy used to select the population of interest using a FACS Verse cytometer. (a) Nasal epithelial cells were selected by side scatter characteristic (SSC) and forward scatter characteristic (FSC) density plots. (b) A gate was applied to identify specific populations of individual cells. Each dot represents one nasal epithelial cell that passed through the cytometer laser. (c) Dead cells were identified and excluded from further analysis using either DAPI or PI.

3.2. ROS and RNS Generation

Supplementary Tables S1 and S2 show an example of intracellular peroxides and total O_2^- levels detected after incubating the nasal epithelial cells with the respective fluorescent probes and inductors in positive controls. The gating strategy shown in Figure 1 was used, and dead cells were discarded using DAPI.

A kinetic strategy was designed for the real-time follow-up of intracellular NO (Supplementary Table S3) and $ONOO^-$ generation (Supplementary Table S4). Single human nasal epithelial cells were selected based on morphology and DAPI exclusion. The strategies for the sequential gating of NO and $ONOO^-$ generation are shown in Figures 2 and 3, respectively.

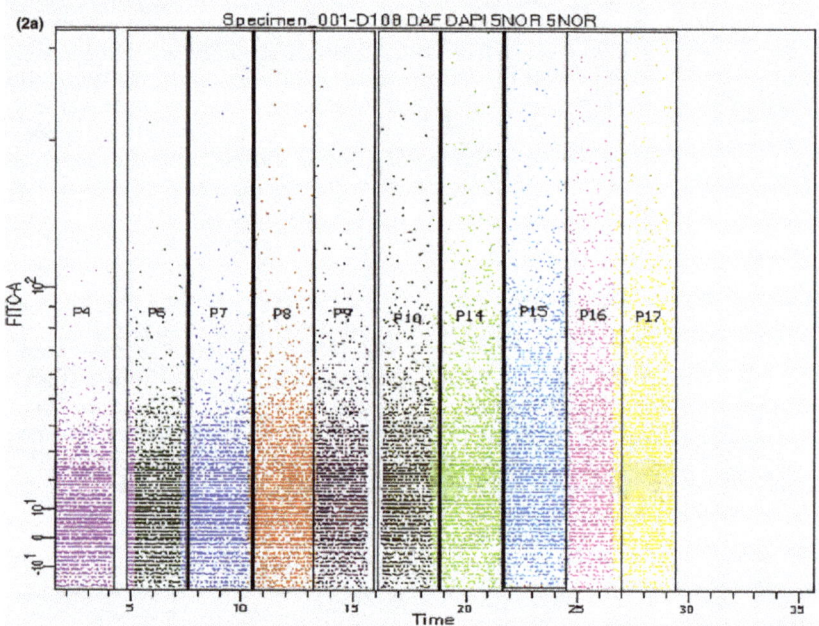

Population	#Events	%Parent	FITC-A Mean	Time Mean
All Events	29,381	####	20	14,105
P4	4,082	13.9	9	2,911
P6	3,245	11.0	13	6,628
P7	4,192	14.3	15	9,199
P8	4,162	14.2	18	12,303
P9	3,769	12.8	19	15,345
P10	3,122	10.6	23	17,845
P14	3,827	13.0	29	20,475
P15	3,766	12.8	34	23,552
P16	2,807	9.6	37	26,095
P17	2,407	8.2	38	27,964

Figure 2. Kinetic measurements of nitric oxide (NO) assays using flow cytometry. (**a**) Dot blot acquired from kinetic measurements. Live nasal epithelial cells were gated according to FSC and SSC, and the gated events were plotted against a FITC-A channel (in this case, DAF-FM DA) and time. (**b**) Table showing gating percentages and fluorescence levels increasing over time.

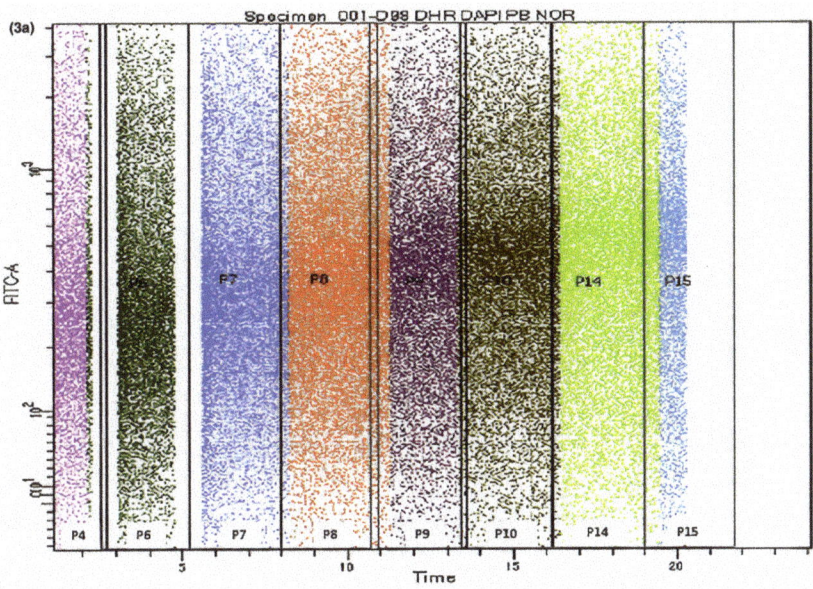

Figure 3. Flow cytometric analysis of peroxynitrite generation kinetics in nasal epithelial cells. (**a**) Dot blot acquired from kinetic measurements. Live nasal epithelial cells were gated according to FSC and SSC, and the gated events were plotted against a FITC-A channel (in this case DHR123) and time. Acquisition was paused at two points to add plumbagin (PB) (an O_2^- provider) and NOR-1 (a NO inductor). (**b**) Table showing gating percentages and fluorescence levels increasing over time.

3.3. GSH Detection

Supplementary Table S5 shows an example of total GSH levels after incubating the nasal epithelial cells with CMF and DEM as a positive control. The gating strategy shown in Figure 1 was used, and DAPI was used to identify dead cells.

3.4. Intracellular Ca^{2+} and Plasma Membrane Potential Detection

A kinetic strategy was designed for the real-time follow-up of intracellular Ca^{2+} generation. Human nasal epithelial cells were selected based on morphology. After that, single cells were selected, and dead cells were discarded using DAPI. Gating percentages and fluorescence values for FLUO-4 are shown in Figure 4 and Supplementary Table S6.

Population	#Events	%Parent	FITC-A Mean	Time Mean
All Events	23,369	####	223	41,268
P4	1,133	4.8	163	2,755
P6	1,356	5.8	258	6,207
P7	1,142	4.9	274	9,212
P8	1,065	4.6	268	12,297
P9	1,111	4.8	245	15,352
P10	806	3.4	285	17,963
P14	1,108	4.7	234	20,431
P15	1,117	4.8	240	23,576
P16	859	3.7	272	26,128

Figure 4. Flow cytometric analysis of intracellular calcium (iCa2+) generation kinetics in nasal epithelial cells. Intracellular calcium was measured using FLUO-4. Human nasal cells were gated accordingly to SSC and FSC. Dead cells were excluded using DAPI. Gating percentages and iCa2+ levels are shown.

Plasmatic membrane potential levels detected after incubating the nasal epithelial cells with DIBAC and t-BHP (positive controls) are shown in Supplementary Table S7. The gating strategy shown in Figure 1 was used, with PI used to identify any dead cells.

3.5. Mitochondrial Function

Supplementary Tables S8–S11 show the levels of mitochondrial membrane potential, mitochondrial mass, and mitochondrial H_2O_2 and O_2^- detected after incubating the nasal epithelial cells with their respective fluorochromes and inductors for positive controls. The gating strategy in Figure 1 was used, and DAPI was used to identify dead cells.

3.6. Oxidative Damage in Lipids and Proteins Analysis

Supplementary Table S12 shows the carbonylated protein levels after incubating the nasal epithelial cells with FTC and menadione in the positive controls. The gating strategy in Figure 1 was used, and DAPI was used to identify dead cells.

Figure 5 shows the detection and gating strategy and the corresponding fluorescence values of the lipidic peroxidation levels in the human nasal epithelial cells after incubation with BODIPY665. Nasal epithelial cells were selected based on morphology after eliminating doublets, and fluorescence levels were determined for BODIPY665. Supplementary Table S13 shows the basal sample results and the control, which were previously incubated with t-BHP and then with BODIPY665.

3.7. Apoptosis and Cell Death Detection

Figure 6 shows the levels of apoptosis and cell death of human nasal epithelial cells after Annexin V and PI staining. Nasal epithelial cells were selected based on morphology after eliminating doublets. Gating for Annexin V−/PI− (live), Annexin V+/PI− (early apoptosis), Annexin V−/PI+ (necrosis), and Annexin V+/PI+ (late apoptosis) populations are demonstrated.

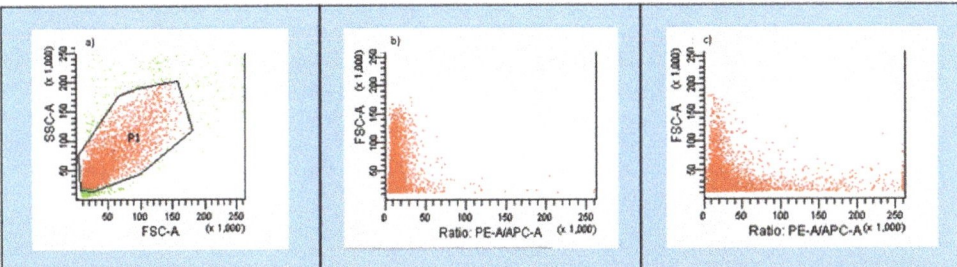

Figure 5. Evaluation of lipid peroxidation using BODIPY 665/676 C11. (**a**) Nasal epithelial cells were selected based on morphology and PI staining to exclude dead cells. (**b**) and (**c**) show the ratios of oxidised vs. reduced lipids.

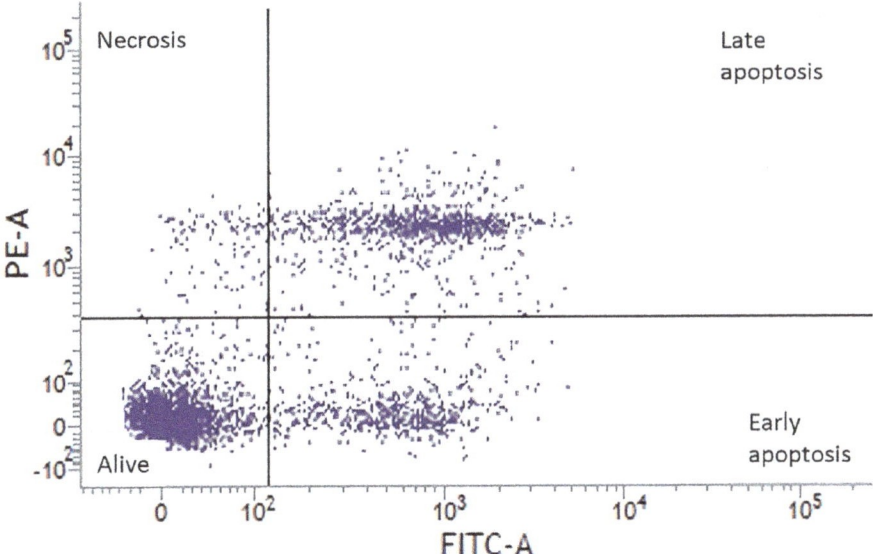

Figure 6. Apoptosis and cell death determination using Annexin V and propidium iodide (PI) staining. Nasal epithelial cells were selected based on morphology. Apoptosis status was determined by Annexin V staining. Cell death was determined by PI staining. Gating methods for Annexin V−/PI− (live), Annexin V+/PI− (early apoptosis), Annexin V−/PI+ (necrosis), and Annexin V+/PI+ (late apoptosis) are shown.

4. Discussion

Numerous studies have shown the importance of OS in the physiopathology of diseases. Therefore, detailed knowledge of the association between OS and pathogenesis could be used to deepen the understanding of the disease's pathophysiology and the discovery of new therapeutic targets that will allow the development of new drugs with clinical utility. Three approaches are used to measure OS: (i) the direct determination of ROS/RNS; (ii) the determination of oxidative damage to biomolecules (lipids, proteins, and nucleic acids); and (iii) the determination of enzymatic and non-enzymatic antioxidant systems [54]. Whichever method is used, OS is difficult to measure for several reasons. Firstly, sampling itself is a source of OS and must be carried out carefully to avoid OS artificial generation that could oxidise the biomolecules, giving rise to false results. The addition of a control group whose samples are manipulated in the same way as those of the patients would partially solve this problem, since the differences between groups could be attributed to changes related to the disease's physiopathology. Secondly, many of the techniques used have a low sensitivity, which implies that a large number of cells must be used to obtain reliable results. This is a significant problem, mainly when often limited clinical samples are used. Thirdly, ROS/RNS have a very short half-life and it is therefore difficult to determine them accurately and precisely. To solve this problem, the indirect measurement of ROS/RNS was used by assessing the oxidative damage that these radicals cause in biomolecules [55,56].

Although many analytical techniques have been developed to measure OS over the years, there is still no gold standard. Methods such as electron spin resonance or nuclear magnetic resonance lack sensitivity and are unfeasible due to the short half-life of some ROS/RNS. Other methods, such as gas chromatography/mass spectrometry or high-performance liquid chromatography, require highly trained personnel. Recently, techniques based on spectrophotometry and enzyme assays have been developed. These methods have several advantages, such as being easy to perform, quantitative, and high-throughput and having a high sensitivity and the ability to be used with a wide variety of biological samples (serum, plasma, saliva, etc.). However, when analysing heterogeneous populations (e.g., blood), all these methods can lead to biased results as they are not able to separate the different cell populations, and therefore only overall results are obtained [55–58].

Flow cytometry has several advantages over previous methods in determining OS. It can measure OS in a large number of individual cells quickly and identify subpopulations within heterogeneous samples, providing qualitative results from a high number of individual cells from a particular subpopulation, instead of measuring the average of the total population. It also allows the analysis of multiple parameters from the same biological sample in a single experiment. Besides, sorting of subpopulations is possible, allowing further analysis by other methods of these sorted subpopulations. Our group aims to characterise the role of OS in rare respiratory diseases, such as PCD, to study its potential implication in disease pathophysiology. As sample yield obtained from biopsies is often a limiting factor when studying the affected tissue in respiratory diseases, we developed a novel method based on flow cytometry to determine fourteen parameters related to cell metabolism using a small amount of sample. To our knowledge, this is the first use of flow cytometry to assess OS levels in human nasal epithelial cells and could represent a new procedure for the study of respiratory diseases in which nasal epithelial cells are the affected tissue.

It has been described that mitochondria, which are the main cellular organelles involved in the production of ROS/RNS, are affected in some respiratory diseases [59]. Therefore, a new protocol to study the mitochondrial mass, mitochondrial membrane potential, and mitochondrial production of H_2O_2 and O_2^- in human nasal epithelial cell samples was set up. Moreover, a method to measure the general oxidative status of these cells and their ROS and RNS production, including intracellular peroxides, O_2^-, and $ONOO^-$, was developed. As some respiratory diseases are related to inflammation, which is also related to OS, this methodology allowing us to study reactive species production in affected tissues could be advantageous [1,11]. In addition, the study of intracellular Ca^{2+} and plasma membrane potential provides investigators with necessary information regarding cell metabolism, which could provide insight into various diseases. In our study, Fluo-4 has been used to measure intracellular Ca^{2+} levels. Single-wavelength dyes, such as Fluo-4, cannot provide quantitative data as the variability of dye concentration and/or photobleaching influence the emission intensities. Consequently, using Fluo-4 only the presence/absence of intracellular Ca^{2+} can be determined, and the use of dual-wavelength dyes, such as Fura-2 AM, that allows for accurate quantification of intracellular Ca^{2+} concentration, is only limited by the C^{2+} response of Fura-2 [60]. Finally, mitochondrial GSH, one of the most important non-enzymatic defences against OS, can be studied relatively quickly and cheaply using this protocol [9].

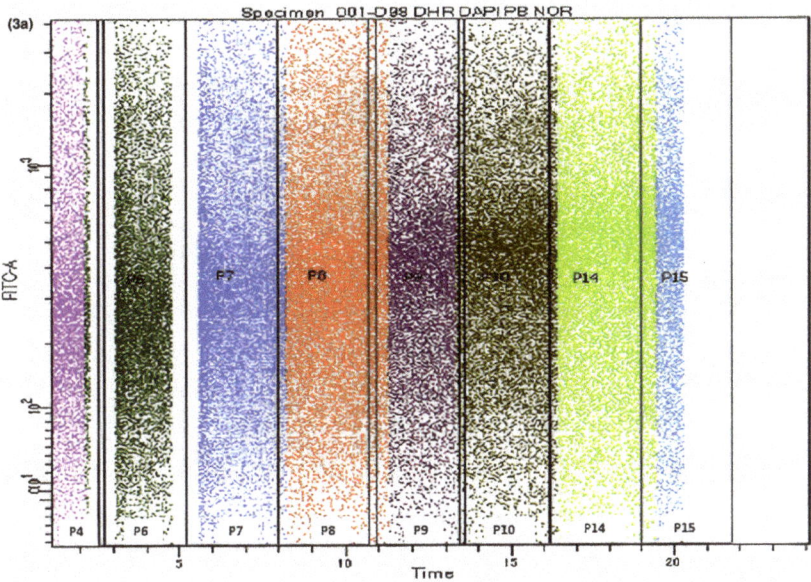

Figure 3. Flow cytometric analysis of peroxynitrite generation kinetics in nasal epithelial cells. (**a**) Dot blot acquired from kinetic measurements. Live nasal epithelial cells were gated according to FSC and SSC, and the gated events were plotted against a FITC-A channel (in this case DHR123) and time. Acquisition was paused at two points to add plumbagin (PB) (an O_2^- provider) and NOR-1 (a NO inductor). (**b**) Table showing gating percentages and fluorescence levels increasing over time.

3.3. GSH Detection

Supplementary Table S5 shows an example of total GSH levels after incubating the nasal epithelial cells with CMF and DEM as a positive control. The gating strategy shown in Figure 1 was used, and DAPI was used to identify dead cells.

3.4. Intracellular Ca^{2+} and Plasma Membrane Potential Detection

A kinetic strategy was designed for the real-time follow-up of intracellular Ca^{2+} generation. Human nasal epithelial cells were selected based on morphology. After that, single cells were selected, and dead cells were discarded using DAPI. Gating percentages and fluorescence values for FLUO-4 are shown in Figure 4 and Supplementary Table S6.

Population	#Events	%Parent	FITC-A Mean	Time Mean
All Events	23,369	####	223	41,268
P4	1,133	4.8	163	2,755
P6	1,356	5.8	258	6,207
P7	1,142	4.9	274	9,212
P8	1,065	4.6	268	12,297
P9	1,111	4.8	245	15,352
P10	806	3.4	285	17,963
P14	1,108	4.7	234	20,431
P15	1,117	4.8	240	23,576
P16	859	3.7	272	26,128

Figure 4. Flow cytometric analysis of intracellular calcium (iCa2+) generation kinetics in nasal epithelial cells. Intracellular calcium was measured using FLUO-4. Human nasal cells were gated accordingly to SSC and FSC. Dead cells were excluded using DAPI. Gating percentages and iCa2+ levels are shown.

Plasmatic membrane potential levels detected after incubating the nasal epithelial cells with DIBAC and t-BHP (positive controls) are shown in Supplementary Table S7. The gating strategy shown in Figure 1 was used, with PI used to identify any dead cells.

3.5. Mitochondrial Function

Supplementary Tables S8–S11 show the levels of mitochondrial membrane potential, mitochondrial mass, and mitochondrial H_2O_2 and O_2^- detected after incubating the nasal epithelial cells with their respective fluorochromes and inductors for positive controls. The gating strategy in Figure 1 was used, and DAPI was used to identify dead cells.

3.6. Oxidative Damage in Lipids and Proteins Analysis

Supplementary Table S12 shows the carbonylated protein levels after incubating the nasal epithelial cells with FTC and menadione in the positive controls. The gating strategy in Figure 1 was used, and DAPI was used to identify dead cells.

Figure 5 shows the detection and gating strategy and the corresponding fluorescence values of the lipidic peroxidation levels in the human nasal epithelial cells after incubation with BODIPY665. Nasal epithelial cells were selected based on morphology after eliminating doublets, and fluorescence levels were determined for BODIPY665. Supplementary Table S13 shows the basal sample results and the control, which were previously incubated with t-BHP and then with BODIPY665.

3.7. Apoptosis and Cell Death Detection

Figure 6 shows the levels of apoptosis and cell death of human nasal epithelial cells after Annexin V and PI staining. Nasal epithelial cells were selected based on morphology after eliminating doublets. Gating for Annexin V−/PI− (live), Annexin V+/PI− (early apoptosis), Annexin V−/PI+ (necrosis), and Annexin V+/PI+ (late apoptosis) populations are demonstrated.

Additionally, this work allows the study of OS damage in biomolecules, such as proteins and lipids [1] [10]. Combined with the study of apoptosis and cellular death, this provides a complete profile of the effect of oxidative stress on human nasal epithelial cells, which make up part of the affected tissues in some respiratory diseases, such as PCD [61]. Finally, a great advantage of this method is that a comprehensive set of OS parameters regarding different respiratory diseases could be studied in future research using tiny samples and non-invasive sampling techniques.

5. Limitations

This article was written to show a laboratory protocol to measure OS parameters in nasal epithelial cells. The study was performed using samples from a small number of healthy individuals, so it is not intended to draw conclusions on OS status, which should be done in future research. As an example, the fluorescence values obtained in the samples (Supplementary Tables S1–S13) are shown.

6. Conclusions

We have established a method based on flow cytometry to study a comprehensive set of OS parameters in nasal epithelial cells that could be useful in research on respiratory diseases. This method has the additional advantage of using small amounts of sample and a non-invasive sampling technique.

Supplementary Materials: The following are available online at https://www.mdpi.com/2077-0383/10/6/1172/s1, Table S1: Basal labeling and the corresponding positive control for intracellular H_2O_2 from six healthy individuals; Table S2: Basal labeling and the corresponding positive control for O_2^- from six healthy individuals; Table S3: Basal labeling and the corresponding positive control for nitric oxide (NO) from six healthy individuals; Table S4: Basal labeling and the corresponding positive control for peroxynitrite ($ONOO^-$) from six healthy individuals; Table S5: Basal labeling and the corresponding positive control for GSH from six healthy individuals; Table S6: Basal labeling and the corresponding positive control for intracellular Calcium (iCa_2^+) from six healthy individuals; Table S7: Basal labeling and the corresponding positive control for plasmatic membrane potential (PMP) from six healthy individuals; Table S8: Basal labeling and the corresponding positive control for mitochondrial membrane potential ($\Delta\psi m$) from six healthy individuals; Table S9: Basal labeling and the corresponding positive control for mitochondrial H_2O_2 (mt H_2O_2) from six healthy individual; Table S10: Basal labeling and the corresponding positive control for mitochondrial O_2^- (mtO_2^-) from six healthy individuals; Table S11: Labeling for mitochondrial mass from six healthy individuals; Table S12: Basal labeling and the corresponding positive control for carbonylated proteins from six healthy individuals; Table S13: Basal labeling and the corresponding positive control for the oxidized/reduced lipid ratio (ox/red lipid) from six healthy individuals.

Author Contributions: Conceptualisation, A.R., D.P., S.C., M.M., M.A., G.H., J.-E.O., L.B., M.M.N.-G., A.E. and F.D.; methodology, A.R., G.H.; formal analysis, A.R.; investigation, A.R.; resources, S.C., M.A., F.D.; data curation, A.R.; writing—original draft preparation, F.D.; writing—review and editing, M.M.N.-G.; visualisation, M.M.N.-G.; supervision, F.D.; project administration, F.D.; funding acquisition, A.E. and F.D. All authors have read and agreed to the published version of the manuscript.

Funding: The present work was funded by grants from the Spanish Paediatric Pneumology Society 2014, and Valencia Pneumology Society 2015. Some equipment employed in this work was funded by Generalitat Valenciana and co-financed with European Regional Development funds (OP ERDF of Comunitat Valenciana 2014–2020). L.B. is funded by GVA grant number ACIF/2019/231.

Institutional Review Board Statement: The study was conducted according to the guidelines of the Declaration of Helsinki, and approved by the Ethics Committee of the Hospital Clínico Universitario Valencia (date of approval: 29 January 2015) and the Hospital General Universitario de Valencia (date of approval: 10 March 2015).

Informed Consent Statement: Informed consent was obtained from all subjects involved in the study.

Data Availability Statement: The data presented in this study are available on request from the corresponding author. The data are not publicly available due to privacy/ethical restrictions.

Acknowledgments: We would like to thank the Spanish association of patients with alpha-1 antitrypsin deficiency for donations of research funds to our research group on rare respiratory diseases at IIS INCLIVA/UVEG.

Conflicts of Interest: The authors declare no conflict of interest.

References

1. Finkel, T.; Holbrook, N.J. Oxidants, oxidative stress and the biology of ageing. *Nature* **2000**, *408*, 239–247. [CrossRef] [PubMed]
2. Le Bras, M.; Clément, M.-V.; Pervaiz, S.; Brenner, C. Reactive oxygen species and the mitochondrial signaling pathway of cell death. *Histol. Histopathol.* **2005**, *20*, 205–219.
3. Weidinger, A.; Kozlov, A.V. Biological activities of reactive oxygen and nitrogen species: Oxidative stress versus signal transduction. *Biomolecules* **2015**, *5*, 472–484. [CrossRef]
4. Figueira, T.R.; Barros, M.H.; Camargo, A.A.; Castilho, R.F.; Ferreira, J.C.; Kowaltowski, A.J.; Sluse, F.E.; Souza-Pinto, N.C.; Vercesi, A.E. Mitochondria as a source of reactive oxygen and nitrogen species: From molecular mechanisms to human health. *Antioxid. Redox Signal.* **2013**, *18*, 2029–2074. [CrossRef] [PubMed]
5. Schroder, P.; Krutmann, J. Environmental oxidative stress—Environmental sources of ROS. *Handb. Environ. Chem.* **2005**, *2*, 19–31. [CrossRef]
6. Gupta, R.K.; Patel, A.K.; Shah, N.; Choudhary, A.K.; Jha, U.K.; Yadav, U.C.; Gupta, P.K.; Pakuwal, U. Oxidative stress and antioxidants in disease and cancer: A review. *Asian Pac. J. Cancer Prev.* **2014**, *15*, 4405–4409. [CrossRef]
7. Sies, H.; Berndt, C.; Jones, D.P. Oxidative stress. *Annu. Rev. Biochem.* **2017**, *86*, 715–748. [CrossRef]
8. Pamplona, R.; Costantini, D. Molecular and structural antioxidant defenses against oxidative stress in animals. *Am. J. Physiol. Integr. Comp. Physiol.* **2011**, *301*, R843–R863. [CrossRef]
9. Alfadda, A.A.; Sallam, R.M. Reactive oxygen species in health and disease. *J. Biomed. Biotechnol.* **2012**, *2012*, 936486. [CrossRef]
10. Evans, M.D.; Cooke, M.S. Factors contributing to the outcome of oxidative damage to nucleic acids. *BioEssays* **2004**, *26*, 533–542. [CrossRef]
11. Rahman, T.; Hosen, I.; Islam, M.M.T.; Shekhar, H.U. Oxidative stress and human health. *Adv. Biosci. Biotechnol.* **2012**, *3*, 997–1019. [CrossRef]
12. Guerra, J.I.E. Oxidative stress, diseases and antioxidant treatment. *An. Med. Interna* **2001**, *18*, 326–335.
13. Günther, J.; Seyfert, H.-M. The first line of defence: Insights into mechanisms and relevance of phagocytosis in epithelial cells. *Semin. Immunopathol.* **2018**, *40*, 555–565. [CrossRef] [PubMed]
14. Müller, L.; Brighton, L.E.; Carson, J.L.; Ii, W.A.F.; Jaspers, I. Culturing of human nasal epithelial cells at the air liquid interface. *J. Vis. Exp.* **2013**, e50646. [CrossRef]
15. Thavagnanam, S.; Parker, J.C.; McBrien, M.E.; Skibinski, G.; Shields, M.D.; Heaney, L.G. Nasal epithelial cells can act as a physiological surrogate for paediatric asthma studies. *PLoS ONE* **2014**, *9*, e85802. [CrossRef]
16. Domej, W.; Oetll, K.; Renner, W. Oxidative stress and free radicals in COPD—Implications and relevance for treatment. *Int. J. Chronic Obs. Pulm. Dis.* **2014**, *9*, 1207–1224. [CrossRef]
17. Mishra, V.; Banga, J.; Silveyra, P. Oxidative stress and cellular pathways of asthma and inflammation: Therapeutic strategies and pharmacological targets. *Pharm. Ther.* **2017**, *181*, 169–182. [CrossRef] [PubMed]
18. Escribano, A.; Pastor, S.; Reula, A.; Castillo, S.; Vicente, S.; Sanz, F.; Casas, F.; Torres, M.; Fernández-Fabrellas, E.; Codoñer-Franch, P.; et al. Accelerated telomere attrition in children and teenagers with α1-antitrypsin deficiency. *Eur. Respir. J.* **2016**, *48*, 350–358. [CrossRef]
19. Torres-Durán, M.; Lopez-Campos, J.L.; Barrecheguren, M.; Miravitlles, M.; Martinez-Delgado, B.; Castillo, S.; Escribano, A.; Baloira, A.; Navarro-Garcia, M.M.; Pellicer, D.; et al. Alpha-1 antitrypsin deficiency: Outstanding questions and future directions. *Orphanet J. Rare Dis.* **2018**, *13*, 114. [CrossRef]
20. Escribano, A.; Amor, M.; Pastor, S.; Castillo, S.; Sanz, F.; Codoñer-Franch, P.; Dasí, F. Decreased glutathione and low catalase activity contribute to oxidative stress in children with α-1 antitrypsin deficiency: Table 1. *Thorax* **2014**, *70*, 82–83. [CrossRef] [PubMed]
21. Magallón, M.; Navarro-García, M.M.; Dasí, F. Oxidative Stress in COPD. *J. Clin. Med.* **2019**, *8*, 1953. [CrossRef]
22. Zihlif, N.; Paraskakis, E.; Tripoli, C.; Lex, C.; Bush, A. Markers of airway inflammation in primary ciliary dyskinesia studied using exhaled breath condensate. *Pediatr. Pulmonol.* **2006**, *41*, 509–514. [CrossRef]
23. Rickham, P.P. Human experimentation: Code of ethics of W.M.A. *BMJ* **1964**, *2*, 177. [CrossRef]
24. Wallberg, F.; Tenev, T.; Meier, P. Analysis of apoptosis and necroptosis by fluorescence-activated cell sorting. *Cold Spring Harb. Protoc.* **2016**, *2016*, 087387. [CrossRef] [PubMed]
25. Zhang, G.; Gurtu, V.; Kain, S.R.; Yan, G. Early detection of apoptosis using a fluorescent conjugate of annexin V. *Biotechniques* **1997**, *23*, 525–531. [CrossRef]
26. Kalyanaraman, B. Oxidative chemistry of fluorescent dyes: Implications in the detection of reactive oxygen and nitrogen species. *Biochem. Soc. Trans.* **2011**, *39*, 1221–1225. [CrossRef] [PubMed]
27. Kalyanaraman, B.; Hardy, M.; Podsiadly, R.; Cheng, G.; Zielonka, J. Recent developments in detection of superoxide radical anion and hydrogen peroxide: Opportunities, challenges, and implications in redox signaling. *Arch. Biochem. Biophys.* **2017**, *617*, 38–47. [CrossRef] [PubMed]

28. Eruslanov, E.; Kusmartsev, S. Identification of ROS using oxidized DCFDA and flow-cytometry. *Methods Mol. Biol.* **2010**, *594*, 57–72. [CrossRef]
29. Crow, J.P. Dichlorodihydrofluorescein and Dihydrorhodamine 123 are sensitive indicators of Peroxynitritein Vitro: Implications for intracellular measurement of reactive nitrogen and oxygen species. *Nitric Oxide* **1997**, *1*, 145–157. [CrossRef]
30. Dikalov, S.I.; Harrison, D.G. Methods for detection of mitochondrial and cellular reactive oxygen species. *Antioxid. Redox Signal.* **2014**, *20*, 372–382. [CrossRef]
31. Díez, I.; Calatayud, S.; Hernandez, C.; Quintana, E.; O'Connor, J.; Esplugues, J.; Barrachina, M.D. Nitric oxide, derived from inducible nitric oxide synthase, decreases hypoxia inducible factor-1α in macrophages during aspirin-induced mesenteric inflammation. *Br. J. Pharm.* **2010**, *159*, 1636–1645. [CrossRef]
32. Namin, S.M.; Nofallah, S.; Joshi, M.S.; Kavallieratos, K.; Tsoukias, N.M. Kinetic analysis of DAF-FM activation by NO: Toward calibration of a NO-sensitive fluorescent dye. *Nitric Oxide* **2013**, *28*, 39–46. [CrossRef] [PubMed]
33. Hedley, D.W.; Chow, S. Evaluation of methods for measuring cellular glutathione content using flow cytometry. *Cytometry* **1994**, *15*, 349–358. [CrossRef]
34. Sebastià, J.; Cristòfol, R.; Martin, M.; Rodríguez-Farré, E.; Sanfeliu, C. Evaluation of fluorescent dyes for measuring intracellular glutathione content in primary cultures of human neurons and neuroblastoma SH-SY5Y. *Cytom. Part A* **2002**, *51*, 16–25. [CrossRef]
35. Evans, J.A.; Darlington, D.N.; Gann, D.S. A circulating factor(s) mediates cell depolarization in hemorrhagic shock. *Ann. Surg.* **1991**, *213*, 549–557. [CrossRef]
36. Perry, S.W.; Norman, J.P.; Barbieri, J.; Brown, E.B.; Gelbard, H.A. Mitochondrial membrane potential probes and the proton gradient: A practical usage guide. *Biotechnique* **2011**, *50*, 98–115. [CrossRef]
37. Petrat, F.; Pindiur, S.; Kirsch, M.; De Groot, H. "Mitochondrial" photochemical drugs do not release toxic amounts of 1O2 within the mitochondrial matrix space. *Arch. Biochem. Biophys.* **2003**, *412*, 207–215. [CrossRef]
38. Scaduto, R.C.; Grotyohann, L.W. Measurement of mitochondrial membrane potential using fluorescent rhodamine derivatives. *Biophys. J.* **1999**, *76*, 469–477. [CrossRef]
39. Presley, A.D.; Fuller, K.M.; Arriaga, E.A. MitoTracker Green labeling of mitochondrial proteins and their subsequent analysis by capillary electrophoresis with laser-induced fluorescence detection. *J. Chromatogr. B* **2003**, *793*, 141–150. [CrossRef]
40. Doherty, E.; Perl, A. Measurement of mitochondrial mass by flow cytometry during oxidative stress. *React. Oxyg. Species* **2017**, *4*, 275–283. [CrossRef]
41. Mukhopadhyay, P.; Rajesh, M.; Yoshihiro, K.; Haskó, G.; Pacher, P. Simple quantitative detection of mitochondrial superoxide production in live cells. *Biochem. Biophys. Res. Commun.* **2007**, *358*, 203–208. [CrossRef]
42. Dickinson, B.C.; Lin, V.S.; Chang, C.J. Preparation and use of MitoPY1 for imaging hydrogen peroxide in mitochondria of live cells. *Nat. Protoc.* **2013**, *8*, 1249–1259. [CrossRef]
43. Gee, K.; Brown, K.; Chen, W.-N.; Bishop-Stewart, J.; Gray, D.; Johnson, I. Chemical and physiological characterization of fluo-4 Ca^{2+}-indicator dyes. *Cell Calcium* **2000**, *27*, 97–106. [CrossRef] [PubMed]
44. Wesseling, M.C.; Wagner-Britz, L.; Boukhdoud, F.; Asanidze, S.; Nguyen, D.B.; Kaestner, L.; Bernhardt, I. Measurements of intracellular Ca^{2+} content and phosphatidylserine exposure in human red blood cells: Methodological issues. *Cell. Physiol. Biochem.* **2016**, *38*, 2414–2425. [CrossRef] [PubMed]
45. Naguib, Y.M.A. Antioxidant Activities of Astaxanthin and Related Carotenoids. *J. Agric. Food Chem.* **2000**, *48*, 1150–1154. [CrossRef] [PubMed]
46. Raudsepp, P.; Brüggemann, D.A.; Andersen, M.L. Detection of radicals in single droplets of oil-in-water emulsions with the lipophilic fluorescent probe BODIPY665/676 and confocal laser scanning microscopy. *Free Radic. Biol. Med.* **2014**, *70*, 233–240. [CrossRef]
47. Chaudhuri, A.R.; De Waal, E.M.; Pierce, A.; Van Remmen, H.; Ward, W.F.; Richardson, A. Detection of protein carbonyls in aging liver tissue: A fluorescence-based proteomic approach. *Mech. Ageing Dev.* **2006**, *127*, 849–861. [CrossRef] [PubMed]
48. Perumalsamy, H.; Sankarapandian, K.; Kandaswamy, N.; Balusamy, S.R.; Periyathambi, D.; Raveendiran, N. Cellular effect of styrene substituted biscoumarin caused cellular apoptosis and cell cycle arrest in human breast cancer cells. *Int. J. Biochem. Cell Biol.* **2017**, *92*, 104–114. [CrossRef]
49. Akasaki, Y.; Alvarez-Garcia, O.; Saito, M.; Caramés, B.; Iwamoto, Y.; Lotz, M.K. FoxO transcription factors support oxidative stress resistance in human chondrocytes. *Arthritis Rheumatol.* **2014**, *66*, 3349–3358. [CrossRef]
50. Beltrán, B.; Nos, P.; Dasí, F.; Iborra, M.; Bastida, G.; Martínez, M.; O'connor, J.-E.; Sáez, G.; Moret, I.; Ponce, J. Mitochondrial dysfunction, persistent oxidative damage, and catalase inhibition in immune cells of naïve and treated Crohn's disease. *Inflamm. Bowel Dis.* **2010**, *16*, 76–86. [CrossRef] [PubMed]
51. Herrera, G.; Martínez, A.; O'Cornor, J.; Blanco, M. Functional assays of oxidative stress using genetically engineered *Escherichia coli* Strains. *Curr. Protoc. Cytom.* **2003**, *24*, 11–16. [CrossRef]
52. Thor, H.; Smith, M.T.; Hartzell, P.; Bellomo, G.; Jewell, S.A.; Orrenius, S. The metabolism of menadione (2-methyl-1,4-naphthoquinone) by isolated hepatocytes. A study of the implications of oxidative stress in intact cells. *J. Biol. Chem.* **1982**, *257*, 12419–12425. [CrossRef]
53. Khailova, L.S.; Rokitskaya, T.I.; Kotova, E.A.; Antonenko, Y.N. Effect of cyanide on mitochondrial membrane depolarization induced by uncouplers. *Biochemistry* **2017**, *82*, 1140–1146. [CrossRef]

54. Katerji, M.; Filippova, M.; Duerksen-Hughes, P. Approaches and methods to measure oxidative stress in clinical samples: Research applications in the cancer field. *Oxidative Med. Cell. Longev.* **2019**, *2019*, 1279250. [CrossRef]
55. Palmieri, B.; Sblendorio, V. Oxidative stress tests: Overview on reliability and use. Part II. *Eur. Rev. Med Pharm. Sci.* **2008**, *11*, 383–399.
56. Palmieri, B.; Sblendorio, V. Oxidative stress tests: Overview on reliability and use. Part I. *Eur. Rev. Med. Pharm. Sci.* **2007**, *11*, 309–342.
57. Palmieri, B.; Sblendorio, V. Current status of measuring oxidative stress. *Methods Mol. Biol.* **2009**, *594*, 3–17. [CrossRef]
58. Rahman, I.; Biswas, S.K. Non-invasive biomarkers of oxidative stress: Reproducibility and methodological issues. *Redox Rep.* **2004**, *9*, 125–143. [CrossRef]
59. Bhatti, J.S.; Bhatti, G.K.; Reddy, P.H. Mitochondrial dysfunction and oxidative stress in metabolic disorders—A step towards mitochondria based therapeutic strategies. *Biochim. Biophys. Acta Basis Dis.* **2017**, *1863*, 1066–1077. [CrossRef]
60. Tinning, P.W.; Franssen, A.J.P.M.; Hridi, S.U.; Bushell, T.J.; McConnell, G. A 340/380 Nm Light Emitting Diode Illuminator for Fura-2 AM Ratiometric Ca^{2+} imaging of live cells with better than 5 NM Precision. *J Microsc.* **2018**, *269*, 212–220. [CrossRef] [PubMed]
61. Reula, A.; Lucas, J.S.; Moreno-Galdó, A.; Romero, T.; Milara, X.; Carda, C.; Mata-Roig, M.; Escribano, A.; Dasi, F.; Armengot-Carceller, M. New insights in primary ciliary dyskinesia. *Expert Opin. Orphan Drugs* **2017**, *5*, 537–548. [CrossRef]

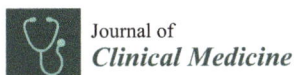

Review

Oxidative Stress and Endoplasmic Reticulum Stress in Rare Respiratory Diseases

María Magallón [1,2], Ana Esther Carrión [1,2], Lucía Bañuls [1,2], Daniel Pellicer [1,2], Silvia Castillo [2,3], Sergio Bondía [2], María Mercedes Navarro-García [2], Cruz González [2,4] and Francisco Dasí [1,2,*]

1. Research Group on Rare Respiratory Diseases (ERR), Department of Physiology, School of Medicine, University of Valencia, Avda. Blasco Ibáñez, 15, 46010 Valencia, Spain; mariamagallon94@gmail.com (M.M.); carrionanaesther@gmail.com (A.E.C.); lucia.banyuls.soto@gmail.com (L.B.); dpellicerroig@gmail.com (D.P.)
2. Research Group on Rare Respiratory Diseases (ERR), Instituto de Investigación Sanitaria INCLIVA, Fundación Investigación Hospital Clínico Valencia, Avda. Menéndez y Pelayo, 4, 46010 Valencia, Spain; sccorullon@gmail.com (S.C.); sergibondia@gmail.com (S.B.); mer_navarro2002@yahoo.es (M.M.N.-G.); cruz.gonzalez@uv.es (C.G.)
3. Paediatrics Unit, Hospital Clínico Universitario de Valencia, Avda. Blasco Ibáñez, 17, 46010 Valencia, Spain
4. Pneumology Unit, Hospital Clínico Universitario de Valencia, Avda. Blasco Ibáñez, 17, 46010 Valencia, Spain
* Correspondence: Francisco.Dasi@uv.es; Tel.: +34-67-651-5598

Abstract: Several studies have shown that some rare respiratory diseases, such as alpha-1 antitrypsin deficiency (AATD), idiopathic pulmonary fibrosis (IPF), cystic fibrosis (CF), and primary ciliary dyskinesia (PCD) present oxidative stress (OS) and endoplasmic reticulum (ER) stress. Their involvement in these pathologies and the use of antioxidants as therapeutic agents to minimize the effects of OS are discussed in this review.

Keywords: oxidative stress; endoplasmic reticulum stress; antioxidant therapies; rare respiratory diseases; Alpha-1 antitrypsin deficiency; idiopathic pulmonary fibrosis; cystic fibrosis; primary ciliary dyskinesia

1. Introduction

Oxidative stress (OS) is defined as an imbalance between pro-oxidant and anti-oxidant substances favouring the former [1]. In the physiological state, Reactive Oxygen Species (ROS) are necessary to neutralise pathogens that may attack the organism. One of their functions is to activate inflammatory intracellular signalling pathways, leading to the immune system activation [2]. However, when ROS appear in excess and accumulate within the cells, they create a highly oxidative state that can cause severe and irreparable damage to the tissues either directly or through altering signaling pathways [3]. Endoplasmic reticulum (ER) stress is the consequence of the accumulation of misfolded proteins in the ER lumen. Consequently, the ER activates the unfolded protein response (UPR), which leads to the elimination or repair of these proteins [4].

Considerable evidence has shown that oxidative and ER stress play an essential role in the pathophysiology of multiple disorders, including rare respiratory diseases, a group of hereditary disorders affecting the respiratory tract, characterized by low incidence and very heterogeneous symptoms [5].

In this review, we summarize the implications of ER and OS in the pathophysiology of four of the most common rare respiratory diseases: alpha-1 antitrypsin deficiency (AATD), idiopathic pulmonary fibrosis (IPF), cystic fibrosis (CF), and primary ciliary dyskinesia (PCD), for which there is no definitive treatment. In addition, since considerable evidence indicates that OS and ER stress could be potential therapeutic targets for these conditions, the current status of antioxidant therapies for treating these diseases will be discussed.

2. What Is Oxidative Stress?

Free radicals are molecules with an unpaired electron in their outer orbital; therefore, they are prone to react with other molecules to obtain the electron they need to reach their electrochemical stability [6]. Thus, free radicals can react with DNA, lipids, and proteins, leading to oxidation and, generally, to the loss of these biomolecules' activity [7].

As a product of aerobic cell metabolism, two basic types of free radicals are generated in cells. Reactive oxygen species (ROS) include the hydroxyl radical (OH.), the superoxide anion (O_2^-), the hypochlorite ion (OCl^-), and hydrogen peroxide (H_2O_2); as well as reactive nitrogen species (RNS) such as nitric oxide (NO) and peroxynitrite ($ONOO^-$) [8]. The main sources of intracellular ROS and/or RNS generation are mitochondria, lysosomes, peroxisomes, xanthine oxidase, cytochrome P450, and the ER. Free radicals are also generated by exposure to external factors such as cigarette smoke, ionizing radiation, UV radiation, or environmental toxins [9,10].

Eukaryotic cells possess some mechanisms that diminish oxidative damage caused by ROS. The most straightforward defence mechanism involves small molecules such as reduced glutathione (GSH) and dietary components (i.e., vitamins, lipoic acid, and carotene), which oxidate themselves, thereby protecting the biomolecules. A more complex defence mechanism involving enzymes such as superoxide dismutase (SOD), catalase (CAT), glutathione peroxidase (GPx), and glutathione reductase (GR), has evolved to reduce ROS levels [7,11,12].

Under physiological conditions, a balance exists between production and degradation of ROS. When the balance between pro- and anti-oxidants shifts in favour of the former, a condition known as OS is produced, linked to the development of numerous diseases. Overproduction of ROS, induced by various exogenous and endogenous cellular sources, depletes antioxidant capacity and contributes to developing several disease-related processes. When the defence mechanisms cannot prevent ROS accumulation, the activation of specific signalling pathways causes changes in gene expression and protein synthesis. All these effects led to the hypothesis that increased free radicals and oxidative damage cause an increase in cell damage, which leads to the development of various pathological conditions, such as carcinogenesis [13], chronic inflammation [14], ageing [15], autoimmunity [16], cardiovascular diseases [17], neurodegenerative diseases [18], and respiratory diseases [3], among others.

However, OS cannot be only defined by a quantitative disbalance between reactive species and antioxidant defence mechanisms. OS is a more complex concept, besides the increment of ROS, other features such as their cellular, subcellular, or tissue location, chemical nature, the kinetics of formation and degradation, and time of exposure should be considered. Moreover, even in the absence of OS, basal levels of ROS exist in the cells. ROS act as regulatory and signalling molecules and are essential to proper cell function in a system known as REDOX regulation [19], participating in cell division, differentiation, and death. Consequently, OS also produces dysregulation of the redox signalling, and therefore, an alteration in cellular homeostasis [20,21].

Specific cell mechanisms remove oxidized lipids and oxidized proteins. However, oxidised DNA cannot be replaced and has to be repaired [22]. In response to the oxidative DNA damage, the cell reacts through several mechanisms, such as repairing these lesions; activation of control points of the cell cycle, which produces cell cycle arrest and prevents the transmission of damaged chromosomes; and apoptosis [23].

As a result of the various molecular oxidation processes, some products are produced and released to the extracellular media and can be used to measure the redox state. Three approaches are used to measure OS. The first approach involves determining oxidative damage to biomolecules, including lipids, proteins and nucleic acids. The most representative markers of lipid peroxidation include isoprostanes and malondialdehyde (MDA) [24], while carbonyl groups reflect the oxidative modification of proteins [25], and mutagenic and modified base 8-hydroxy-2′-deoxyguanosine (8-OHdG) reflecting DNA oxidation [26] products, which can be either nuclear or mitochondrial. A second approach involves the direct determination of ROS/RNS. Finally, a third approach involves measuring the enzymatic and non-enzymatic antioxidant systems (oxidized glutathione/reduced glutathione, dietary vitamins, and oligo-elements).

3. Clinical Relevance of Oxidative Stress

Redox homeostasis involves a wide range of substances. As mentioned above, the balance of pro-oxidant and anti-oxidant substances is conditioned by many variables, which are complex to understand. Oxidative damage is the endpoint in which the cells' biomolecules are oxidized and lose their functionality (Figure 1) [27].

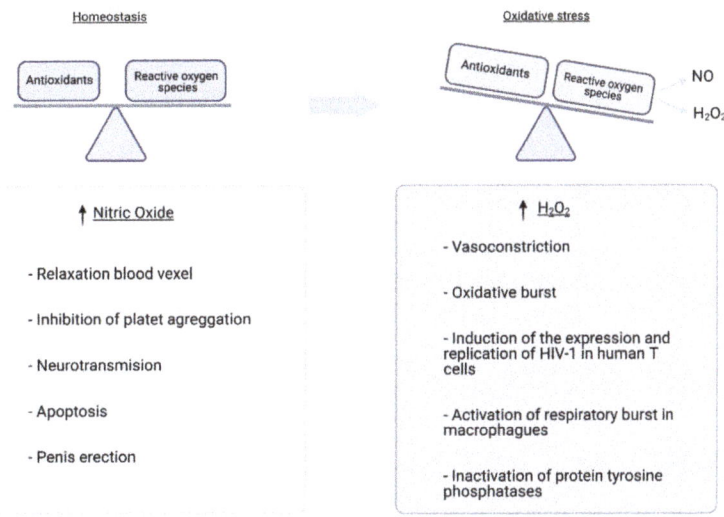

Figure 1. Clinical relevance of reactive oxygen species. Reactive oxygen species (ROS) have numerous functions involved in maintaining cellular homeostasis, such as those shown in the figure. However, when ROS levels increase, these functions are altered by dysregulation of signalling pathways.

Given the complexity of the oxidant-antioxidant pathways and their relationships, it is essential from a clinical perspective to understand the cause of the OS and its source because various free radicals act differently, causing different cell responses. It was initially thought that all free radicals could act as second messengers. However, further research showed that only H_2O_2 and other hydroperoxides fit the requirements to be considered as second messengers [28]. Among the RNS, NO is a well-known second messenger [29]. Other free radicals are not second messengers, although they trigger adaptive cell responses [28].

Second messengers are the intracellular component through which cells or organs interact with each other [30]. They should have a significant specificity with effectors from signalling pathways, and the reaction should be fast enough to not react with other molecules [28]. The hydroxyl radical does not fit the specificity requirement because it can oxidize any organic molecule [31], nor does the superoxide radical because the reduction of O_2^- to H_2O_2 by SOD [32] occurs in the cell more rapidly than the interaction with the signalling pathways effectors [28]. When O_2^- has been produced extracellularly (as in NADPH oxidases (NOX)), it can move into the cell and alter signalling pathways [33]. Even though O_2^- cannot be considered a second messenger, it oxidizes GSH and other thiols, but it only produces a physiological effect when there is little SOD present, such as in phagosomes or endosomes [34]. GSH can scavenge O_2^-, but it generates thiol radicals, which further react to generate O_2^- and subsequently H_2O_2 [34]. Therefore, O_2^- might be considered as an H_2O_2 precursor [28,31].

H_2O_2 oxidizing potential can occur in two different ways. The first one is a one-electron reduction reaction, where a transition metal reduces H_2O_2. For instance, in the Fenton reaction, Fe^{2+} reduces the H_2O_2, forming a hydroxyl radical plus Fe^{3+}. As stated above, the hydroxyl radical is not a second messenger because it can react with any organic molecule, so it is not specific enough to be involved in controlled cell signalling [28]. Conversely, H_2O_2 can be reduced through another mechanism, the two-electron nucleophilic substitution reaction, where a thiol is converted to a thiolate anion, which reacts with the neighbouring cysteine residues of proteins such as peroxiredoxins. This reaction allows H_2O_2 or any peroxide to act as a second messenger [19].

Depending on the cell type targeted by H_2O_2, different cell responses can be achieved. It was demonstrated that exogenous addition of H_2O_2 in T cells activates the nuclear factor-κB (NF-κB) transcription factor [35], as does endogenous production [36]; a protein kinase C (PKC) is upstream of this signalling pathway [37]. In addition, hydroperoxides and H_2O_2 are linked with the respiratory burst in macrophages. At high concentrations, hydroperoxides inhibit the respiratory burst without killing the cells [38], but low concentrations stimulate it [39] by increasing intracellular Ca^{2+} levels [40] and activating the phosphatidylcholine specific to phospholipase C [41]. The oxidative burst activation in the extracellular-regulated kinase (ERK) pathway is also H_2O_2-dependent [42]. Likewise, the increase in the endogenous production of H_2O_2 causes a transitory inactivation of the protein tyrosine phosphatase 1B (PTP1B). PTP1B inhibits the activation of the ERK signalling pathway, dephosphorylating Raf1 [43]. This inactivation is reversible [44].

NO is a second messenger because it can pass across plasma membranes to exert its action in adjacent cells in a paracrine way. The NO mechanism of action consists of activation of guanylyl cyclase, which rapidly increases cyclic guanosine monophosphate (cGMP) concentration, leading to the phosphorylation of other proteins kinases that become involved in diverse cell functions such as relaxation of blood vessels, apoptosis, or penile erection [45].

OS parameters can be used as non-invasive diagnostic [46] or prognostic biomarkers because, as previously stated, in different diseases, free radicals have different effects. Although numerous studies have attempted to achieve this, limitations in the sample size or the fact that the study was a meta-analysis with a high heterogeneity among the studies have not allowed the establishment of a cut-off point for the use of OS parameters in rapid molecular risk stratification and outcome prediction. To overcome these limitations, extensive multicentric longitudinal studies with a larger sample size should be performed.

4. Endoplasmic Reticulum Stress

ER stress is the consequence of a mismatch between the load of unfolded and misfolded proteins in the ER and the cellular machinery's capacity to cope with that load [4].

Protein folding occurs in the ER lumen, and its efficiency depends on several intrinsic and extrinsic factors, such as the ER environment, gene mutations, or altered posttranscriptional modifications. Every protein, before being secreted, must pass a quality control to check that it is correctly folded. Misfolded proteins are retained in the ER lumen to be correctly folded or degraded. Accumulation of unfolded/misfolded proteins leads to ER stress. This complex situation activates the UPR using three main approaches: increased ER capacity to fold and modify proteins, decreased global mRNA translation, and activated ER-associated degradation (ERAD) and autophagy. When UPR cannot solve the problem, it becomes chronic, and cell death is promoted by the activation of the pro-apoptotic signalling machinery.

ER stress activates three different signalling pathways of the UPR: inositol-requiring protein-1 (IRE1), activating transcription factor-6 (ATF6), or protein kinase R-like endoplasmic reticulum kinase (PERK) (Figure 2).

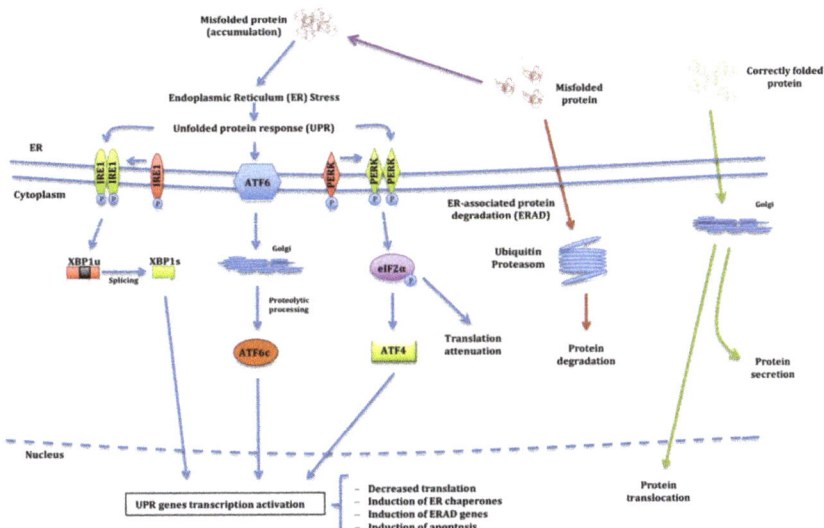

Figure 2. Signalling pathways of the Unfolded Protein Response (UPR). In a normal situation inside the endoplasmic reticulum, proteins are folded and taken to the places where they carry out their function (green arrows). When proteins are not folded correctly, they are stored in the lumen of the endoplasmic reticulum (ER), and the ER-associated protein degradation machinery (ERAD) is activated (red arrows). Occasionally, the ER shows dysfunctions that cause malformed proteins not to be degraded by ERAD and the proteins associate with each other creating aggregates, producing what is known as ER stress (blue arrows). When this occurs, the cell activates the UPR, which might mean that accumulated misfolded proteins can be detected by inositol-requiring enzyme 1 (IRE1), which activates transcription factor 6 (ATF6) and protein kinase R-like endoplasmic reticulum kinase (PERK) proteins.

Consequently, IRE1 dimerises and autophosphorylates, activating its endoribonuclease activity, removing an intron of the transcription factor X-box-binding protein 1 (XBP1u) converting it into XBP1s, which activates transcription of UPR target genes. On the other hand, and as a consequence of the accumulation of these unfolded proteins, the ER can also activate ATF6, which splits and activates the transcription factor ATF6c, which travels to the nucleus and activates UPR genes. Finally, another option for UPR pathway activation is PERK activation. PERK dimerises and phosphorylates eukaryotic initiation factor 2α (eIF2α), which activates the transcription factor ATF4 that, like the previous ones, targets the nucleus to activate UPR gene transcription. Nevertheless, UPR genes can also decrease translation by preventing the accumulation of more misfolded proteins. They can also induce activation of ER chaperones to increase protein folding capacity, induce transcription of ERAD genes to increase degradation capacity, and activate apoptosis of ER-presenting cells if needed. Reproduced with permission from Torres-Durán et al. [47] under the terms of the Creative Commons Attribution 4.0 International License (http://creativecommons.org/licenses/by/4.0/ (accessed on 17 March 2021)).

The ATF6 pathway is activated by unfolded/misfolded proteins sequestering the immunoglobulin heavy chain binding protein (BiP). BiP was previously attached to ATF6, and the sequestration of BiP triggers that signalling pathway [48]. IRE1 and PERK have related and interchangeable sensing domains when activating homodimerize, although the activation mechanism is not fully understood. Three different hypotheses have been proposed [4]: direct recognition, where the luminal domain directly binds the unfolded proteins [49]; indirect recognition, in which BiP is attached to IRE1 and PERK [50], and finally the hybrid recognition model, where both BiP dissociation and unfolded protein binding cause the activation of the signalling pathways [51].

4.1. ATF6

ATF6 is a regulatory protein that binds to ER stress-response elements (ERSE), a consensus sequence (CCAAT-N9-CCACG) that promotes UPR responsive genes. It has two homologous proteins: ATF6α (90 kDa) and ATF6β (110 kDa); both are synthesized in all cell types as ER transmembrane proteins [52]. In normal conditions, ATF6 is attached to the ER membrane-bound to BiP, but when the unfolded proteins accumulate, BiP dissociates from ATF6, and ATF6 goes to the Golgi complex, where it is cleaved by two proteases [48]. Serine protease site-1 (S1P) cleaves ATF6 in the luminal domain, whereas metalloprotease site-2 (S2P) cleaves the N-terminal portion within the phospholipid bilayer [53]. These reactions release the basic leucine zipper (bZIP) domain, which translocates to the nucleus to activate transcription. ATF6 binds to ATF/cAMP response element (CRE) and ERSE [54] to upregulate the expression of refolding genes [55].

4.2. IRE1

IRE1 was the first-identified component of the UPR, and it is an atypical type I protein kinase endoribonuclease, with a luminal dimerization, a cytosolic kinase, and an endonuclease domain [56–58]. When unfolded proteins are detected, IRE1 homodimerizes and trans-autophosphorylates to activate its RNAse domain. The IRE1p endonuclease substrate was first discovered in yeast. It is an mRNA that encodes bZIP, containing the transcription factor Hac1p [56]. The homologue in mammals is X-box binding protein (XBP1) [59,60], which is cleaved by IRE1 to remove an intron that causes frameshift. This splicing causes a change in the C-terminal region of XBP1, and only the spliced form of XBP1, XBP1(S), is a transcriptional factor involved in a variety of UPR target genes [61], both refolding and degrading genes [55].

4.3. PERK

PERK is a type I transmembrane protein with a kinase domain. During ER stress, PERK homodimerizes and trans-autophosphorylates (same way as IRE1). The C-terminal cytoplasmic domain of activated PERK directly phosphorylates the Ser51 of eukaryotic initiation factor 2 (eIF2α), attenuating global protein synthesis, thereby reducing the ER protein-folding burden. PERK activation occurs within minutes after developing ER stress [62]. Phosphorylated eIF2 α is required for selective translation of a subset of mRNAs. One important transcription factor activated by eIF2 α is transcription factor 4 (ATF4), which promotes the transcription of genes involved in amino acid biosynthesis, antioxidant responses, ER chaperones, growth arrest, DNA damage 34 (GADD34), and CAAT/enhancer-binding protein (C/REB) homologous protein (CHOP).

5. Endoplasmic Reticulum Stress and Oxidative Stress

Several studies have shown a link between ER and OS together (Table 1), but this relationship's mechanism is still not completely understood. For clarity, we have separate it into three sections: (i) ER oxidative environment for disulfide-bond-forming; (ii) crosstalk between ER, mitochondria, and UPR, and (iii) activation of antioxidant genes (*Nrf2*) (Figure 3).

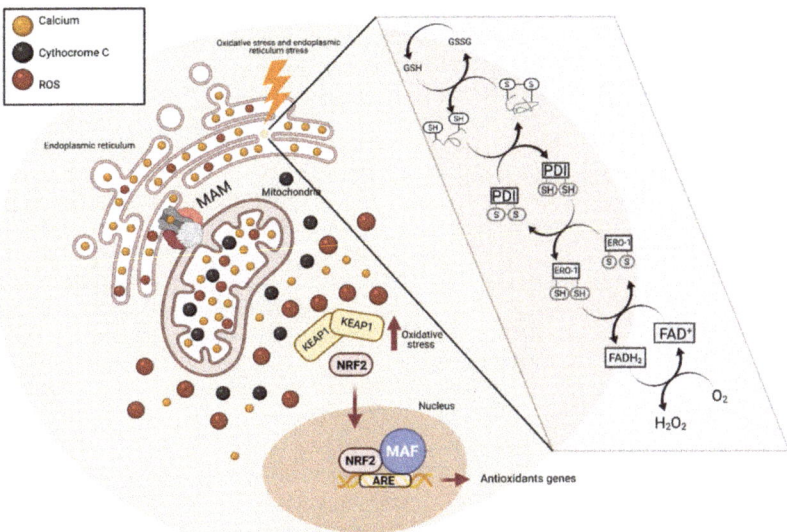

Figure 3. The connection between oxidative stress and endoplasmic reticulum stress. The presence of reactive species inside the endoplasmic reticulum favours the formation of the disulphide bonds in the protein folding. When this occurs, two electrons are released and accepted by protein disulphide isomerase (PDI), which loses its original conformation, accumulating inside the endoplasmic reticulum (ER) and triggering ER stress. PDI then releases two more electrons that are accepted by ER oxidoreductase (ERO1). Finally, the electrons are accepted by O_2, leading to the production of H_2O_2. An increase in H_2O_2 causes Ca^{2+} levels in the ER to increase. The ER and mitochondria are linked by channels called MAM. When Ca^{2+} increases in the ER, it moves to the mitochondria. Elevated Ca^{2+} levels in the mitochondria stimulate mitochondrial metabolism, producing even more ROS. Ca^{2+} also increases the permeability of the mitochondrial membrane, allowing cytochrome C to be released and activate cellular apoptosis pathways. The increased ROS levels induce the release of *Nrf2* from Keap1, translocates to the nucleus where it binds to an accessory protein, Maf. The complex formed by *Nrf2* and Maf leads to the activation of antioxidant genes, interacting with an antioxidant response element (ARE).

In physiological conditions, the ER environment is between 10 and 100 times more oxidative than the cytosolic compartment [63]. This oxidative environment of the ER favours protein folding, particularly forming disulfide bonds between two cysteine residues with the generation of H_2O_2. Disulfide bond formation is a reversible process achieved by a thiol-disulfide exchange reaction; this stabilizes the tertiary and quaternary protein structures [64]. It has been suggested that increased H_2O_2 levels oxidize and inactivate ER-resident proteins, such as protein disulfide isomerases (PDI), contributing to unfolded protein accumulation [65]. During disulfide bond formation, PDI accepts two electrons from the cysteine residues in polypeptide substrates, leading to the reduction of PDI and oxidation of the protein substrate. Then, PDI transfers the electrons to another acceptor, ER oxidoreductase 1 (ERO1), starting another cycle of disulfide bond formation. Then, ERO1 transfers the electrons to molecular oxygen (O_2) to produce H_2O_2, the major ROS produced in the ER lumen [61,64]. It was calculated that 25% of the cellular ROS is the H_2O_2 produced in the ER by ERO1 folding activity [66].

The ER is the principal intracellular reservoir of calcium that controls Ca^{2+} homeostasis. However, more actors directly or indirectly play this role, such as mitochondria, pyruvate, isocitrate, and α-ketoglutarate dehydrogenases [67]. The ER and mitochondria are physically connected by mitochondrial-associated membranes (MAM), where membrane and luminal components can be exchanged [68]. The MAM composition depends on internal and external stimuli. The formation and destruction of mitochondrial associated membranes (MAMs) depend on changes in organelle dynamics [69]. Under ER stress conditions, CHOP expression increases in the ER's cytosolic membrane, favouring the formation of a complex between CHOP and the mitochondrial translocase, translocase of outer mitochondrial membrane 22 (Tom22), either directly or through steroidogenic acute regulatory protein (StAR). The formation of this complex allows a stronger interaction between Tom22 and 3β-hydroxysteroid dehydrogenase type 2 (3βHSD2) increasing steroid metabolism [70,71]. Moreover, the inositol 1,4,5-trisphosphate receptor (IP3R), the voltage-dependent anion channel (VDAC), and the chaperon glucose-regulated protein 75 (GRP75) form a complex that provides the main Ca^{2+} transfer channel in MAMs [72]. Verfaille et al. suggested PERK as a novel component of MAMs in the ER surface. The perturbations of the ER/mitochondria contact sites reduce the propagation of ROS signals to the surrounding mitochondrion, attenuating the onset of apoptosis provoked by ROS-based ER stress [73]. This structure has lipids and proteins that suggest a two-way supply of fundamental metabolites and messengers that control mitochondrial function, thereby controlling the bioenergetics rate [69].

Bravo et al. showed that in early ER stress stages, MAMs increase, so the Ca^{2+} transfer increases from ER to mitochondria, thus enhancing mitochondrial respiration, reductive power, and ATP production [74]. Moreover, mitochondrial Ca^{2+} uptake stimulates the activity of some Krebs cycle enzymes both directly (isocitrate and α-ketoglutarate dehydrogenases) and indirectly (pyruvate dehydrogenase) [75], which, in time, increases O_2 consumption, resulting in an ROS increase [61]. Ca^{2+} opens the permeability transition pore so that cytochrome c can be released, blocking the respiratory chain complex III, which increases O_2^- production [76]. Wang et al. showed that chronic ER stress oppositely modulates cellular metabolism, decreasing the mitochondrial metabolism, lowering the mitochondrial membrane potential and the mitochondrial mass [77].

The nuclear factor erythroid-derive-2 (*Nrf2*) protein is a bZIP transcription factor characterized by its conserved structural domain, referred to as the cap'n'collar (CNC) domain. These CNC transcription factors function as heterodimers, binding to accessory proteins such as Mafs to activate gene expression [78]. *Nrf2* binds an antioxidant response element (ARE), a cis-element in the promoters of many anti-oxidative genes that is crucial to their inducible activation [79]. Under non-stressed conditions, *Nrf2* persists at low levels in the cytoplasm, where it is bound to its inhibitor, Keap1 [80]. Keap1 serves to anchor *Nrf2* in the cytoplasm and signal its ubiquitination and subsequent proteasomal degradation, resulting in low baseline expression of the *Nrf2*-dependent genes. However, the disulfide bonds in Keap1 are susceptible to OS, and exposure to a wide variety of electrophiles/oxidants triggers a conformational change in Keap1, caused by the modification of thiol residues, releasing *Nrf2*. Other post-translational modifications also facilitate this dissociation, including phosphorylation of *Nrf2* and S-nitrosylation of Keap1.

Upon dissociation from Keap1, *Nrf2* translocates to the nucleus, heterodimerizes with Maf proteins, binds ARE, and activates the coordinate expression of hundreds of genes. The net result is an adaptive cytoprotective response that detoxifies stressors.

PERK-dependent phosphorylation triggers the dissociation of *Nrf2*/Keap1 complexes and inhibits the reassociation of *Nrf2*/Keap1 complexes in vitro. Activation of PERK via agents that trigger the UPR is necessary and sufficient for the dissociation of cytoplasmic *Nrf2*/Keap1 and the subsequent *Nrf2* nuclear import [81]. *Nrf2* activation contributes to the maintenance of GSH levels, which functions as a buffer of ROS accumulation during the UPR. The nocive effects of *Nrf2* or PERK deficiencies could be attenuated by the restoration of cellular GSH levels or *Nrf2* activity. The inhibition of ROS production attenuates apoptotic induction following ER stress. These data suggest that perturbations in cellular redox status sensitize cells to the harmful effects of ER stress [82].

Table 1. Summary of some studies where endoplasmic reticulum (ER) stress and oxidative stress (OS) are present simultaneously.

Cell Type	Stimulus	ER Stress Measurement	OS Measurement	ER-OS Branch	Observation	Ref
PERK-/- and PERK+/+ MEFs	Phox-ER stress	CHOP and Chaperones ↑	DiOC6 ↓ (Ψm) NAO ↑ (oxidized cardiolipin)	Cross-talk ER-mitochondria	PERK is a component of MAMs.	[73]
Bax-/- haemopoietic cells	Tunicamycin	CHOP ↑ BiP/GRP78 ↑	Mitotracker Red ↓ (Ψm) → ↑mitochondrial O_2^-	Cross-talk ER-mitochondria	Mitochondrial mass, O2 consumption & ATP production ↓.	[77]
S. cerevisiae Hip deficient cells (erv29Δ)	CPY (a misfolded mutant form of protein carboxypeptidase)	IRE1 ↑	DHR-123 ↑ (General ROS)	Antioxidant genes	GSH suppress ROS and cell death but not ER stress.	[83]
CHO cells	Misfolded factor VIII expression	BiP ↑ eIF2α-P ↑ CHOP ↑	DCF ↑ (peroxides), DHE ↑ (superoxide), MDA ↑, GSH ↓, GSSG ↑, HODE ↑ (hydroxioctadecaidienoic acid) Prot. Carbonyls ↓	Antioxidant genes	BHA (butylated hydroxyanisole) antioxidant ↓apoptosis, ↓intracellular accumulation of misfolded proteins and ↑secretion of properly folded proteins.	[84]
PERK-/- and ATF4-/- fibroblast and C. elegans PERK -/-	Tunicamycin	Several genes	DCF ↑ (peroxides)	ER oxidative environment for disulfide bond forming	ATF4-/- cells are impaired in expressing genes involved in aa import, GSH synthesis, and OS resistance. PERK-/- cells accumulate endogenous peroxides during ER stress, whereas interference with the ER oxidase ERO1 abrogates such accumulation. eIF2α phosphorylation protects cells against metabolic consequences of ER oxidation by promoting the linked processed of sufficiency and resistance to OS.	[85]
Left ventricle cells form five-month-old Lee-Sung (Met-S) and Lanyu (MHO) obese minipig	High-fat diet	CHOP ↑ (Met S & MHO) PERK ↑ (Met S & MHO) IRE1α = (Met S & MHO) ATF6 ↑ (Met S & = MHO)	TBARS (Thiobarbituric acid reactive substances) (↑ Met S & ↑ MHO)			[86]
Primary murine brain endothelial cells from 2 month-old BL/6 mice	T-BHP (Tert-butyl hydroperoxide)	XBP1-S ↓ CHOP ↑	DCF ↑ (peroxides) MDA ↑ 4-HNE ↑ CAT = SOD = GPx = RH ↑ (Ψm)	Cross-talk ER-mitochondria	Down-regulation of Homer1 protects against t-BHP-induced endothelial injury. Down-regulation of Homer1 reduces t-BHP-induced OS. Down-regulation of Homer1 preserves Ca²⁺ homeostasis in mBECs. Down-regulation of Homer1 attenuates t-BHP-induced ER stress.	[87]
Human PBMCs cognitive impairment. PBMCs and brain cortex cells from a transgenic mouse with Alzheimer's disease	Thapsigargin	GRP78 ↑ XBP1 ↑	DCF ↑ (peroxides) Nrf2 ↑ GCLc	Antioxidant genes		[88]
MIA PaCa-2 human pancreatic cells	Piperlongumine	ATF4 ↑ IRE1α ↑ XBP1 ↑	OSGIN1 ↑ ABCB10 ↓			[89]
Hepatopancreas from Litopenaeus vannamei	Ammonia nitrogen	BiP ↑ eIF2α ↑ ATF4 ↑ IRE1 ↑ XBP1-S ↑	SOD ↓ MDA ↑			[90]

↑: Indicates increased expression or production; ↓: Indicates decreased expression or production; =: Expression or production are not modified

Malhotra et al. showed both in vivo (mice) and in vitro (CHO-H9 cells) that antioxidant treatment reduced ER stress and the associated OS, and protein secretion was improved [84]. Therefore, even though it is unknown how the misfolded proteins accumulated in the ER produce ROS, these authors demonstrated that accumulated unfolded proteins are sufficient to produce ROS and that both unfolded proteins and ROS are required to activate UPR [84].

6. Endoplasmic Reticulum and Oxidative Stress in Rare Respiratory Diseases

6.1. Serpinopathies, Endoplasmic Reticulum, and Oxidative Stress

Serpins are a protein superfamily of around 350–500 amino acids distributed in the metazoan, plantae, and certain viruses [91]. They have a similar structure with a high homology in sequence and alike structures. Their primary function is to inhibit proteases, but studies using model organisms have shown that serpins also control proteolysis in molecular pathways associated with cell survival, development, and host defence. Non-inhibitory serpins are described as essential elements with diverse biological systems serving as chaperones, hormone transporters, or anti-angiogenic factors [92]. Serpins are vulnerable to mutations that lead to protein misfolding and polymerization of mutant proteins frequently occurs, reducing the number of active inhibitors and leading to the accumulation of polymers, causing cell death and organ failure [93]. These diseases are called serpinopathies.

The most studied serpinopathy is AATD (ORPHA:60), a rare genetic disease with a prevalence of 1–5/10,000. In this case, the serine protease inhibitor is alpha-1 antitrypsin (AAT), which is mainly synthesized and secreted by hepatocytes. AAT's main function is to protect lung tissues from neutrophil elastase [94]. Z-AAT is the deficient variant with the most clinical relevance leading to the formation of polymers that accumulate in the hepatocytes, producing severe liver disease in some patients. The lack of circulating AAT predisposes to emphysema.

There are some AATD studies related to ER stress, and it is unclear if Z polymers activate the UPR. Some studies showed that Z polymers do not cause UPR, nor in CHO-K1 expressing human Z-AAT [95], nor in HeLa cells [96] or rat liver [96,97], but they do in human peripheral blood monocytes [98] and HepG2 cells [99], which could be explained by the UPR needing secondary stress to activate the UPR. Lawless et al. reported that in CHO cells, the expression of the Z-AAT polymer alone does not lead to UPR, but when they added thapsigargin (an ER stressor) or heat stress, UPR was triggered [100]. Ordóñez et al. supported the theory of the second stressor to activate the UPR. They observed that polymer-forming mutants of AAT (Z-AAT) only activate the ER overload response (EOR), whereas truncated AAT mutants only activate the UPR. These two pathways usually occur together. Their data revealed that polymers of AAT that accumulate in a spheric manner produce a loss of the normal tubule ER network, forming a vesiculated ER, which leads to impairment of luminal protein mobility [87]. ER vesiculation is associated with other cellular stresses, including mechanical injury and elevated cytosolic calcium concentration [101,102]. The truncated polymers cause classical ER stress (UPR) and are efficiently degraded by the proteasome, showing a different ultrastructural change characterized by gross expansion of ER cisternae. Z-AAT activate chaperones. The observation of enhanced sensitivity to ER stress following Z-AAT expression correlates with marked changes in the ER's biophysical features. In cells experiencing ER overload, misfolded proteins cannot diffuse freely, decreasing their accessibility to the quality control required for folding and transportation. Conversely, in cells with reticular and highly interconnected ER, chaperones can diffuse to misfolded proteins' sites. Therefore, a model is proposed in which decreased mobility or availability of ER chaperones due to changes in the diffusive features or/and obstruction caused by protein overload sensitizes the cell to subsequent activation of the UPR [96].

A study conducted in mice carrying the human mutant *Z-AAT* gene showed that protein aggregation does not trigger the elevation of the major stress proteins in UPR (calnexin, Gpr78, Gpr94, and PDI). The most abundant disulfide isomerase and chaperone in the ER, PDI, was found attached to the Z-AAT protein. Protein disulfide reductase (PDR) activity is predominantly performed in the ER by PDI, which is decreased in these transgenic mice, probably because of PDI sequestration in PiZ aggregates. PiZ mice were found to have more reduced ER, with a more considerable amount of reduced protein thiol groups, GSH, and GSH/GSSH ratio. The redox status in the cytoplasmic fraction was a little more oxidized, with the same amount of protein thiol groups and GSH but a slightly lower GSH/GSSG [97], which is consistent with our study, where we found that children with AATD have systemic OS, in part, through a decrease in GSH [103]. Thus, the shift in ER redox potential toward a reduced state promotes PDI acting as a chaperone rather than a disulfide isomerase [104]. The reduction of PDI disulfides and PDI's decreased availability could explain the PDR deficiency of PiZ transgenic mice [97], which can be an adaptation of the ER, as found in other long-term stress models, such as diabetes [105]. Altogether, these data reveal a rescuing mechanism activated in long-term, nonlethal stress, during which a less productive, but more protective, steady-state of the ER is maintained, in which a more reducing environment protects the ER from OS and apoptosis and regulates PDI to act as a chaperone rather than an oxidoreductase [88]. To conclude, the study suggested a model for chronic ER stress, where different protective pathways are activated in contrast to short-term ER stress. The reduced ER environment, the change in PDI function, decreases in PDR activity, and the differences in chaperone complexes in the ER and chaperone and antioxidant enzyme induction in the cytoplasm, suggest a long-term adaptive response, which sacrifices efficient protein folding for long-term survival [97].

Some studies have linked OS and AATD. The first, performed in the PiZ mouse liver model, showed that Z transgenic mice experience oxidative was damage by increasing protein carbonylation, MDA, and 8-OHdG levels. This study also found that ageing liver tissue from older PiZ mice had elevated ROS and generally lower antioxidant enzyme levels than younger mice [106]. Another study showed that healthy children with AATD experienced increased oxidative damage caused by decreased GSH levels, decreased GSH/GSSG ratio and diminished CAT activity. Oxidative damage in lipids (MDA), DNA (8-OHdG), and carbonyl proteins was also observed [103]. Along this line, a report showed two PiZZ patients with severe emphysema and extremely high urine levels of 8-OHdG. The patient with the highest 8-OHdG also had a mutation in glutathione S-transferase pi 1(GSTP1) [107], an enzyme that plays an important role in detoxification by catalyzing the conjugation of many hydrophobic and electrophilic compounds with GSH [108]. A recent study showed that AATD patients with an intermediate and high risk of developing lung and/or liver disease were observed to have significantly shorter telomeres and increased oxidative damage than control individuals [109], indicating an association between telomere length and OS markers in AATD patients.

AAT is a protein that acts as an antioxidant because it has nine methionine residues, which may protect proteins from oxidative damage [110]. These methionines can be oxidized, but mainly two (351 and 358) are prone to it. The oxidation of these two methionines results in the loss of antielastase activity [111]. Another study showed that exogenous AAT increases the antioxidant defence (SOD and GPx) and prevents preeclampsia development [112]. Then, deficient patients have less serum AAT and increased OS, which oxidizes the AAT and inactivates it, so the antielastase activity is even lower, increasing lung disease risk. Altogether, these findings suggest that OS is associated with AATD-related lung disease [103,107].

6.2. Interstitial Lung Diseases, Endoplasmic Reticulum, and Oxidative Stress

IPF is an interstitial lung disease (ILDs), a heterogeneous group of lung diseases characterized by inflammation and fibrosis. ILDs can be produced by exposure to environmental and pharmacological agents or sarcoidosis. Some patients have no identifiable cause, and the disease is classified as idiopathic interstitial pneumonia (IIPs). IPF is the most common form of ILD and one of the most aggressive forms of IIP [113].

The global IPF incidence ranges from 0.2 to 9.4 per 100,000 per year. The prevalence was estimated to be higher in men than in women (ORPHA:2032). IPF is a chronic disorder characterized by progressive fibrosis that leads to a severe decline in lung function, progressive respiratory failure, and high mortality [113]. The aetiology of IPF remains unknown; however, some pathogenic factors have been proposed: aberrant wound healing, profibrotic proteins (i.e., TGFβ), OS, and inflammation [114].

Recent studies have suggested that ER stress could also be involved in the pathogenesis of IPF. Various ER stress markers (i.e., ATF4, ATF6, CHOP BiP, EDEM, and XBP1) were found to be increased in alveolar epithelial cells (AECs) from IPF patients [115,116]. Fibroblasts in lung tissue from IPF patients show upregulated expression of BiP [117]. Alveolar macrophages from mice with asbestos-induced lung fibrosis and bronchoalveolar macrophages from asbestosis patients also showed increased BiP expression [118]. M2 macrophages from IPF patients were reported to express CHOP [119].

Based on the available data, ER stress could modulate several key components of lung fibrosis such as AEC apoptosis, myofibroblast differentiation, epithelial-mesenchymal transition (EMT), and M2 macrophage polarization [120]. Kamp et al. provided evidence that asbestos-induced ER stress can induce AEC apoptosis through IRE1 expression and ER Ca^{2+} release [121]. There is evidence of the influence of ER stress in cell differentiation. Baek et al. suggested that ER stress through UPR could induce differentiation of fibroblasts to myofibroblasts [117]. Other studies have reported that ER stress induces EMT in epithelial cells [122,123]. In a recent report using macrophages, Yao et al. showed that the ER stress might be able to induce M2 (pro-fibrotic phenotype) polarization through Jun N-terminal kinase (JNK) or CHOP in IPF [119].

Several studies have provided evidence of augmented OS in biological fluids and lung tissue from IPF patients. Oxidized proteins have been identified in the bronchoalveolar lavages (BAL) of IPF patients. Oxidation may lead to dysfunctional proteins, suggesting a pathological role of OS in IPF [124,125]. A remarkable increase in serum isoprostane levels was observed in IPF patients [126]. These findings suggest that increased OS and could be negatively correlated with the disease's severity [127].

Additional studies showed higher ROS levels in IPF patients compared to healthy controls. In exhaled breath condensates (EBCs) from IPF patients, higher levels of H_2O_2 were determined [128]; pulmonary inflammatory cells were obtained from epithelial lining fluid (ELF) of IPF patients showed increased levels of ROS [129]. NOX, a family of pro-oxidant enzymes, was found to be upregulated in the lungs of IPF patients, and several studies have reported an increase in mitochondrial ROS generation [130,131].

The role of nitrosative stress in IPF has also been studied; NO seems to induce TGFβ- and ECM-degrading enzymes in fibroblasts in animal models of lung fibrosis [114,132]. Upregulated expression of inducible NO synthase (iNOS) was demonstrated in IPF epithelial cells, macrophages, and fibroblasts, which can provoke abnormal nitrosative stress, contributing to fibrogenesis [133].

The antioxidant defence is also altered in IPF patients. GSH is decreased in the alveolar ELF of the lower respiratory tract of IPF patients [134]. Several antioxidant enzymes, including SOD, are lower in fibroblast foci from IPF patients [135].

Increasing the expression of *Nrf2* in fibrotic lungs was not able to counteract the OS [136]. It has also been suggested that polymorphisms in *Nrf2* may participate in IPF susceptibility [137].

These alterations in redox signalling can affect the development of disease through different processes. ROS-induced DNA damage can lead to apoptosis of airway epithelial cells; ROS can increase the production of cytokines and TGFβ, which favours chronic inflammation, leading to progressive fibrosis [138].

6.3. Cystic Fibrosis, Endoplasmic Reticulum, and Oxidative Stress

CF is a rare autosomal recessive disease (ORPHA:586). The incidence of CF is currently 1:3500 [139]. It is a monogenic disease affecting the *CFTR* gene, located on chromosome

7 [140]. This gene codes for a type of ATP-binding cassette (ABC) transporter, whose function is to transport chloride and sodium ions and other anions such as GSH or bicarbonate (H_3CO_3). Located mainly in the apical membranes of epithelial cells in many tissues [141], CFTR can be affected by numerous types of mutations; more than 2000 variants of the *CFTR* gene are currently described [142]. Malfunctioning CFTR often affects ion conductance efficiency through the membrane pores [143], which changes the characteristics and composition of cellular secretions by changing the composition of the extracellular milieu. This accumulation of events causes organs to become gradually obstructed, eventually leading to fibrosis [140].

One of the main causes of CF is a mutation in the *CFTR* gene. The most common mutation is the loss of a phenylalanine at position 508, ΔF508 [144]. This sequence defect renders the protein unable to properly perform its transporter function, so it should be tagged by Hsc70-CHIP ubiquitin ligase and taken to the proteasome for degradation [145]. However, numerous studies have shown that the ER can fail in this process and produce an unwanted accumulation of CFTR protein, leading the cell to experience ER stress [144,146]. As discussed above, an accumulation of misshaped proteins leads to the activation of the UPR, which consists of three different but complementary signalling pathways: IRE1, ATF6, and PERK.

Kerbiriou et al. studied the relationship of CF pathogenesis in the activation of UPR pathways [147]. These researchers analyzed the presence of markers, showing that UPR signalling pathways were activated and studied ATF6, a bZIP transcription factor synthesized in the reticulum membrane that, during UPR activation, binds to the Golgi apparatus, converting itself into an active form and migrates to the nucleus, where it acts as a transcription factor generating a stress response [148]. Another marker they studied was Grp78, a glucose-regulated protein. Grp78 binds to the hydrophobic part of unfolded proteins and is related to the activation of ATF6, IRE1, and PERK, which makes it an exciting marker for studying UPR activation [149]. Finally, they showed that, as proposed, ATF6 and Grp78 levels were elevated in cells with mutated CFTR [147]. This could confirm the existence of ER stress in CF.

In another study, Tang et al. [150] aimed to find a relationship between the worsening of inflammation in CF patients and the activation of UPR pathways to find a therapeutic pathway involving ER stress in CF. They proposed that UPR signalling cascades lead to stimulation of the IκB kinase (IKK) through the interaction of tumour necrosis factor (TNFα) and IRE1α, leading to the activation of NF-κB. Nevertheless, they were unable to find such a relationship.

A CTFR abnormality in bronchial epithelial and ciliated cells leads to alteration of the pulmonary extracellular medium due to poor conduction of Na^+, Cl^- ions, or GSH, resulting in excessive O_2 consumption [151], causing hypoxia, among other effects [152] making the airways of CF patients a niche for bacterial infections [140]. This situation results in the activation of inflammatory MAPK pathways [140], leading to stimulation of NF-kB [153], which targets the nucleus and activates the cytokines IL-8 and IL-6 and TNFα [154]. These biomolecules attract the polymorphonuclear (PMN) cells of the immune system, the neutrophils, to the airway surface liquid (ASL). The primary function of neutrophils is to kill bacteria by phagocytosis. For the destruction of ingested material, neutrophils release ROS, such as O_2^-, H_2O_2, or free OH. resulting from NADPH's oxidation [155]. Although neutrophil activation is a defence mechanism of the body, if ROS are not neutralized or controlled, they can cause irreparable damage in CF patients. Therefore, neutrophils are a significant ROS source in the ASL of children with CF [156,157].

Bronchial ciliated and type II AECs are the second source of oxidants in CF lungs through DUOX1 and DUOX2, two isoforms of the NOX family found in epithelial cells [158].

One of the main mechanisms of ROS neutralization is GSH. In 1993, Roum et al. demonstrated that GSH levels in CF patients are below those of healthy controls [159]. Years later, in 1998, Lindsell et al. studied the relationship of the CFTR channel to these decreased values, then demonstrated that CFTR, along with its chloride and sodium transport function, is also actively involved in the transfer of GSH from the intracellular to the extracellular environment [160] indicating that an alteration in the CFTR gene could lead to a decrease in GSH levels in the ASL, producing an oxidative imbalance. This hypothesis is now accepted and is proposed as one of the main reasons for OS in CF.

Other factors contributing to this OS, such as NO and H_2O_2, are currently being studied. It was shown that NO is decreased in CF patients' bronchial airways, allowing an abnormal interaction of its mediator species with the surrounding environment, which would produce harmful effects [161]. Asymmetric dimethylarginine, an endogenous NOS inhibitor, is increased in CF airways [162], contributing to the reduced levels of NO in CF airways. Conversely, increased H_2O_2 levels have been found in different cultured epithelial cell models of CF, which are related to the elevated IL-6 and IL-8 production in CF epithelia [163]. These augmented H_2O_2 levels are associated with a lack of expression of regulatory agents due to the poor interaction between CFTR and *Nrf2*, a factor responsible for activating H_2O_2 regulatory mechanisms [163]. According to this finding, differential expression of antioxidant proteins was reported in cultured CF models compared with normal controls, such as TRX-1, GSTP1, peroxiredoxin (PRDX) 6, TRX-dependent peroxide reductase (PRDX-1), and CAT [163].

Biomarkers of oxidative damage have been reported in lipids and proteins from CF patients. Variations in lipid peroxidation have been found: MDA was demonstrated to be increased in plasma or serum from patients with CF [164] and 8-isoprostane was also found elevated in CF plasma [165], buccal mucosal cells [166], and breath condensate [167]. Oxysterols, a biomarker of cholesterol oxidation, are also increased in CF plasma [168]. Moreover, oxidative damage in proteins was observed in the airways of children with CF [157].

6.4. Primary Ciliary Dyskinesia and Oxidative Stress

PCD is a rare disease, with an estimated incidence of 1:20,000 live births (ORPHA:244). PCD is a genetically heterogeneous disorder. Disease-causing mutations in at least 40 genes have already been reported [169]. It is characterized by structural and/or functional alteration in motile cilia, which causes a deficit in the mucociliary clearance of the respiratory secretions [170] leading to chronic respiratory infections and chronic inflammation of the airways. An inefficient inflammatory process increases the number of neutrophils, increasing ROS and RNS, as explained above [171].

OS has rarely been studied in PCD. Altered RNS has been reported in PCD. Nasal NO (nNO) measurement is recommended as the initial test in patients with clinical suspicion of PCD since diminished nNO values are characteristic of patients with PCD [172]. However, despite its good sensitivity, there are cases of PCD with normal values of nNO, so even if the nNO is normal—if the symptoms are consistent—the disease should not be ruled out [173,174].

Patients with PCD suffer from oxidative damage, and increased levels of the OS marker, 8-isoprostane, has been observed in the exhaled breath condensate (EBC) of children with PCD compared to healthy controls [175].

A study of nasal epithelium cells from patients with PCD showed an alteration in the OS state compared to cells from healthy volunteers. Patients with PCD have lower apoptosis levels, NO, $ONOO^-$, O_2^-, H_2O_2, and mitochondrial O_2^- in nasal epithelium cells compared to healthy individuals [176]. Nevertheless, no significant differences were observed in the oxidative damage in lipids and proteins [176].

More studies are needed to determine the role that OS plays in the pathophysiology of the disease.

7. Antioxidants Therapies in Rare Respiratory Diseases

Due to the extensive evidence of oxidant/antioxidant imbalance and the role of OS in the pathogenesis of disease, several research groups have proposed antioxidants as promising therapeutic agents in AATD [177], IPF [178], and FQ [179].

7.1. Alpha-1 Antitrypsin Deficiency and Antioxidant Therapy

The only currently available specific treatment for AATD that currently exists is augmentation therapy, which consists of the intravenous administration of AAT purified from the plasma of healthy human donors [47]. This treatment has proved its clinical efficacy by delaying emphysema progression, protecting the lungs from excessive neutrophil elastase [47]. However, there had been controversy regarding the use of augmentation therapy and its efficacy [180] until the appearance of randomized, placebo-controlled trials, such as the RAPID trial [181]. Augmentation therapy requires regular intravenous infusion of AAT, which depends on the protein's availability from donors. Therefore, to overcome these problems, other strategies are currently being investigated.

More than 5% of patients diagnosed with chronic obstructive disease (COPD) are also diagnosed with AATD, and more than 40% of AATD patients develop COPD [47]. OS is one of the pathogenic mechanisms in COPD, as well as in AATD. OS enhances chronic inflammation and favours the appearance of emphysema. These findings have provided the possibility to study antioxidant therapies. Various studies have been conducted using GSH generating antioxidants, which have been observed to reduce exacerbations in COPD patients, although it has not been confirmed whether the benefit is due to their antioxidant or mucolytic properties. Various research groups are currently looking for more effective antioxidants; along this line, studies have been conducted using different types of antioxidants such as SOD mimetics, NOX inhibitors, mitochondria-directed antioxidants, or *Nrf2* activators [182]. The last one shows promise as a therapeutic target for COPD patients since it was observed that it is not increased in response to ROS as it does in normal cells. However, an antioxidant has yet to be found that demonstrates a clinical benefit for patients, so further studies evaluating the OS in lung tissue are required to identify more effective antioxidant therapies for COPD and, consequently, for AATD patients.

There is no specific treatment for AATD-related liver disease, other than liver transplantation, which has high associated risks [183]. Several studies have suggested that antioxidant therapy may modulate the secretion of AAT polymers into the bloodstream from hepatocytes. Ronzoni et al. suggested that the redox state in the ER could contribute to the retention of AAT, since the formation of disulfide bonds favours the accumulation of Z-AAT and other variants inside hepatocytes, being, therefore, OS, an AATD-modifying factor and a possible therapeutic target [184]. Studies reported that tobacco smoke induces the oxidation and polymerization of Z-AAT, which would explain emphysema's premature appearance in smoking ZZ individuals. Using the antioxidant N-acetyl cysteine, the same authors managed to avoid the oxidation induced by tobacco extract in vitro and by the polymerization of Z-AAT [185].

7.2. Idiopathic Pulmonary Fibrosis and Antioxidant Therapy

ROS scavengers and drugs targeting redox imbalances might be promising strategies in treating IPF, among other targets such as senescence or the immune response. N-acetylcysteine (NAC) is a precursor to GSH and a free radical scavenger widely tested in the treatment of IPF. Various studies in animal models have proven the efficacy of this exogenous scavenger in mitigating bleomycin-induced fibrosis [186–188]. However, NAC did not show clear evidence of benefit in IPF patients [189]. Interestingly, specific patient subpopulations with the TOLLIP TT genotype show different responses, suggesting the need for personalized medicine in IPF [190].

Another therapeutic target studied for IPF is SOD, which is decreased in patients. A study on mice showed decreased bleomycin-induced fibrosis after intravenous administration of lecithinized SOD, a more biologically stable form of SOD [191]. However, in humans, a randomized controlled trial using lecithinized SOD in IPF patients showed no lung function improvement [192].

Novel targets for IPF have been investigated, targeting the redox imbalance. Hecker et al. suggested that GKT137831, a dual inhibitor of both NOX1 and NOX4, could be a promising therapeutic strategy in age-associated fibrotic disorders, able to reverse bleomycin-induced fibrosis in mice [193]. The anti-fibrotic role of metformin was also examined in a bleomycin-induced lung fibrosis model, being found to inhibit TGFβ1-induced NOX4 expression [194]. Azithromycin was found to enhance the proteasome degradation of NOX4 [195], and in another study in mice models, this compound was able to reduce bleomycin-induced fibrosis [196]. A single-centre, retrospective, observational study, carried out in IPF patients with acute exacerbation treat with azithromycin, indicated a possible improvement in mortality [197].

Activators of *Nrf2* might be promising as an IPF treatment as they are supported by several studies in animal models. Rapamycin seems to protect against paraquat-induced pulmonary fibrosis [198]. The ability of several substances, such as sulforaphane, pirfenidone, salidroside, and salvianolic acid B, to attenuate bleomycin-induced pulmonary fibrosis has been examined [199–202]. However, human trials are needed to evaluate the utility of *Nrf2* activators in IPF.

Another possible approach to IPF treatment is targeting ER stress. An example could be phenylbutyric acid (PBA), a chemical chaperone, which was found to inhibit EMT in the lungs, reduce the expression of pulmonary TGFβ1, and attenuate bleomycin-induced pulmonary fibrosis [203].

7.3. Cystic Fibrosis and Antioxidant Therapy

Antioxidants proposed as possible therapies include vitamin E, β-carotene, vitamin C, selenium supplements, and GSH or NAC [140,179].

GSH, both inhaled and orally, has been examined in numerous studies. Griese et al. showed that inhalation of GSH does not reduce inflammation nor OS [204]. Regarding the use of oral GSH, some controversy exists since some studies showed a reduction in OS [179], while others suggested the incompatibility that may exist between this treatment and those patients who have absorption difficulties, which is quite common in CF patients, opening up the possibility for further research with targeted therapies [140,205].

However, some of these studies suggested that it is difficult to obtain accurate results due to the effects of the treatment to which the patient is subjected, so repeating GSH and NAC treatments is proposed in children for a prolonged time [179].

Another common strategy in antioxidant research is the administration of NAC. Conrad et al. showed that NAC oral administration could, if not improve lung capacity, at least slow the process [206].

The use of vitamin E, vitamin C, or β-carotene, has also been extensively studied. These biomolecules have a great capacity as radical-scavenging antioxidants and could be used as neutralizers of free radicals [140,179,207]. However, no studies have analyzed their effects on redox imbalance in FC, leaving an open door for research with these substances.

Although still in the study phase, for selenium supplements, it has been observed that, together with other antioxidants such as vitamin E or β-carotene, they can improve lung function in CF patients [208].

8. Conclusions

The presence of increased OS and elevated biomarkers of oxidation damage on biomolecules implies that AATD, IPF, and CF patients have a higher demand for antioxidant defence mechanisms. Therefore, targeting OS with antioxidant therapies is a logical approach in these three conditions to delay disease progression and improve patient quality of life. For PCD, the available data are limited, and further studies are required to determine the pathological role of OS in the disease and, therefore, the possibility of antioxidant supplementation.

As discussed above, several approaches to reduce OS have been explored in animal models or cultured cells in rare respiratory diseases, but few have been tested clinically. Basic research is needed to improve our knowledge of the underlying effects of OS in the lungs to develop more effective antioxidant therapies. Some authors have suggested that antioxidants with relevant therapeutic benefits are molecules that increase the physiological antioxidant response, such as the *Nrf2* activators, and not the antioxidant molecules, which is a promising area for drug development in the future.

As for ER stress-targeting therapy, PERK [209], IRE1 [210], or XBP1 [211,212] knockout mice have lethal consequences. Therefore, blocking primary UPR components is unlikely to be a suitable solution. Nevertheless, some studies suggested the use of drugs that improve the chaperone functions, such as a chemical chaperon 4-phenylbutyrate (4-PBA) [213] and tauroursodeoxycholic acid (TUDCA) [214,215], as an alternative to reduce the consequences of ER stress.

Author Contributions: Conceptualization, F.D.; S.C.; and C.G.; Methodology, M.M.; A.E.C.; F.D.; Writing—Original draft preparation, M.M., A.E.C., L.B., D.P.; Writing—Figure drawing and preparation, S.B., M.M.N.-G.; Writing—Review and editing, F.D.; Project administration, M.M.N.-G.; Funding acquisition, F.D., S.C., C.G. All authors have read and agreed to the published version of the manuscript.

Funding: This research was funded by Sociedad Valenciana de Neumología 2015 and 2017 grants and ISCIII PI17/01250 grant and European Regional Development Funds. S.B. is funded by FP Dual GVA Program. L.B. is funded by GVA grant number ACIF/2019/231.

Institutional Review Board Statement: Not applicable.

Informed Consent Statement: Not applicable.

Data Availability Statement: Not applicable.

Acknowledgments: We would like to thank the Spanish association of patients with alpha-1 antitrypsin deficiency for donations of research funds to our research group on rare respiratory diseases at IIS INCLIVA/UVEG.

Conflicts of Interest: The authors declare no conflict of interest.

References

1. Slimen, I.B.; Najar, T.; Ghram, A.; Dabbebi, H.; Ben Mrad, M.; Abdrabbah, M. Reactive Oxygen Species, Heat Stress and Oxidative-Induced Mitochondrial Damage. A Review. *Int. J. Hyperth.* **2014**, *30*, 513–523. [CrossRef] [PubMed]
2. McGuinness, A.; Sapey, E. Oxidative Stress in COPD: Sources, Markers, and Potential Mechanisms. *J. Clin. Med.* **2017**, *6*, 21. [CrossRef]
3. Magallón, M.; Navarro-García, M.M.; Dasí, F. Oxidative Stress in COPD. *J. Clin. Med.* **2019**, *8*, 1953. [CrossRef] [PubMed]
4. Ron, D.; Walter, P. Signal Integration in the Endoplasmic Reticulum Unfolded Protein Response. *Nat. Rev. Mol. Cell Biol.* **2007**, *8*, 519–529. [CrossRef]
5. Blanco, I.; Lara, B. *Déficit de alfa1-Antitripsina: Fisiopatología, Enfermedades Relacionadas, Diagnóstico y Tratamiento*, 2nd ed.; Editorial Respira: Barcelona, Spain, 2016.
6. Rahman, K. Studies on Free Radicals, Antioxidants, and Co-Factors. *Clin. Interv. Aging* **2007**, *2*, 219–236. [PubMed]
7. Finkel, T.; Holbrook, N.J. Oxidants, Oxidative Stress and the Biology of Ageing. *Nature* **2000**, *408*, 239–247. [CrossRef]
8. Dröge, W. Free Radicals in the Physiological Control of Cell Function. *Physiol. Rev.* **2002**, *82*, 47–95. [CrossRef] [PubMed]
9. Sauer, H.; Wartenberg, M.; Hescheler, J. Reactive Oxygen Species as Intracellular Messengers during Cell Growth and Differentiation. *Cell. Physiol. Biochem.* **2001**, *11*, 173–186. [CrossRef] [PubMed]
10. Schröder, P.; Krutmann, J. Environmental Oxidative Stress—Environmental Sources of ROS. *Handb. Environ. Chem.* **2005**, *2*, 19–31. [CrossRef]
11. Wang, X.; Hai, C. Novel Insights into Redox System and the Mechanism of Redox Regulation. *Mol. Biol. Rep.* **2016**, *43*, 607–628. [CrossRef]
12. Sies, H. Oxidative Stress: Oxidants and Antioxidants. *Exp. Physiol.* **1997**, *82*, 291–295. [CrossRef]
13. Ohnishi, S.; Ma, N.; Thanan, R.; Pinlaor, S.; Hammam, O.; Murata, M.; Kawanishi, S. DNA Damage in Inflammation-Related Carcinogenesis and Cancer Stem Cells. *Oxid. Med. Cell. Longev.* **2013**, *2013*, 387014. [CrossRef]
14. Baierle, M.; Nascimento, S.N.; Moro, A.M.; Brucker, N.; Freitas, F.; Gauer, B.; Durgante, J.; Bordignon, S.; Zibetti, M.; Trentini, C.M.; et al. Relationship between Inflammation and Oxidative Stress and Cognitive Decline in the Institutionalized Elderly. *Oxid. Med. Cell. Longev.* **2015**, *2015*, 804198. [CrossRef] [PubMed]
15. Vitale, G.; Salvioli, S.; Franceschi, C. Oxidative Stress and the Ageing Endocrine System. *Nat. Rev. Endocrinol.* **2013**, *9*, 228–240. [CrossRef] [PubMed]
16. Laddha, N.C.; Dwivedi, M.; Mansuri, M.S.; Singh, M.; Gani, A.R.; Yeola, A.P.; Panchal, V.N.; Khan, F.; Dave, D.J.; Patel, A.; et al. Role of Oxidative Stress and Autoimmunity in Onset and Progression of Vitiligo. *Exp. Dermatol.* **2014**, *23*, 352–353. [CrossRef] [PubMed]

17. Assies, J.; Mocking, R.J.T.; Lok, A.; Ruhé, H.G.; Pouwer, F.; Schene, A.H. Effects of Oxidative Stress on Fatty Acid- and One-Carbon-Metabolism in Psychiatric and Cardiovascular Disease Comorbidity. *Acta Psychiatr. Scand.* **2014**, *130*, 163–180. [CrossRef] [PubMed]
18. Kim, G.H.; Kim, J.E.; Rhie, S.J.; Yoon, S. The Role of Oxidative Stress in Neurodegenerative Diseases. *Exp. Neurobiol.* **2015**, *24*, 325–340. [CrossRef]
19. Ray, P.D.; Huang, B.W.; Tsuji, Y. Reactive Oxygen Species (ROS) Homeostasis and Redox Regulation in Cellular Signaling. *Cell. Signal.* **2012**, *24*, 981–990. [CrossRef]
20. Schmidt, H.H.; Stocker, R.; Vollbracht, C.; Paulsen, G.; Riley, D.; Daiber, A.; Cuadrado, A. Antioxidants in Translational Medicine. *Antioxid. Redox Signal.* **2015**, *23*, 1130–1143. [CrossRef] [PubMed]
21. Scialo, F.; Sanz, A. Coenzyme Q Redox Signalling and Longevity. *Free Radic. Biol. Med.* **2021**, *164*, 187–205. [CrossRef]
22. Evans, M.D.; Dizdaroglu, M.; Cooke, M.S. Oxidative DNA Damage and Disease: Induction, Repair and Significance. *Mutat. Res. Rev. Mutat. Res.* **2004**, *567*, 1–61. [CrossRef]
23. Evans, M.D.; Cooke, M.S. Factors Contributing to the Outcome of Oxidative Damage to Nucleic Acids. *BioEssays* **2004**, *26*, 533–542. [CrossRef]
24. Tsikas, D. Assessment of Lipid Peroxidation by Measuring Malondialdehyde (MDA) and Relatives in Biological Samples: Analytical and Biological Challenges. *Anal. Biochem.* **2017**, *524*, 13–30. [CrossRef]
25. Dalle-Donne, I.; Rossi, R.; Giustarini, D.; Milzani, A.; Colombo, R. Protein Carbonyl Groups as Biomarkers of Oxidative Stress. *Clin. Chim. Acta* **2003**, *329*, 23–38. [CrossRef]
26. Valavanidis, A.; Vlachogianni, T.; Fiotakis, C. 8-Hydroxy-2′-Deoxyguanosine (8-OHdG): A Critical Biomarker of Oxidative Stress and Carcinogenesis. *J. Environ. Sci. Health Part C Environ. Carcinog. Ecotoxicol. Rev.* **2009**, *27*, 120–139. [CrossRef]
27. Ott, M.; Gogvadze, V.; Orrenius, S.; Zhivotovsky, B. Mitochondria, Oxidative Stress and Cell Death. *Apoptosis* **2007**, *12*, 913–922. [CrossRef]
28. Forman, H.J.; Maiorino, M.; Ursini, F. Signaling Functions of Reactive Oxygen Species. *Biochemistry* **2010**, *49*, 835–842. [CrossRef] [PubMed]
29. Bohme, E.; Schmidt, H.H.H.W. Nitric Oxide and Cytosolic Guanylate Cyclase: Components of an Intercellular Signalling System. *Z. Kardiol.* **1989**, *78*, 75–79.
30. McIlwain, H. Extended Roles in the Brain for Second-Messenger Systems. *Neuroscience* **1977**, *2*, 357–372. [CrossRef]
31. Forman, H.J.; Ursini, F.; Maiorino, M. An Overview of Mechanisms of Redox Signaling. *J. Mol. Cell. Cardiol.* **2014**, *73*, 2–9. [CrossRef] [PubMed]
32. McCord, J.M.; Fridovich, I. Superoxide Dismutase. An Enzymic Function for Erythrocuprein (Hemocuprein). *J. Biol. Chem.* **1969**, *244*, 6049–6055. [CrossRef]
33. Hawkins, B.J.; Madesh, M.; Kirkpatrick, C.J.; Fisher, A.B. Superoxide Flux in Endothelial Cells via the Chloride Channel-3 Mediates Intracellular Signaling. *Mol. Biol. Cell* **2007**, *18*, 2002–2012. [CrossRef] [PubMed]
34. Winterbourn, C.C. Revisiting the Reactions of Superoxide with Glutathione and Other Thiols. *Arch. Biochem. Biophys.* **2016**, *595*, 68–71. [CrossRef]
35. Schreck, R.; Rieber, P.; Baeuerle, P.A. Reactive Oxygen Intermediates as Apparently Widely Used Messengers in the Activation of the NF-Kappa B Transcription Factor and HIV-1. *EMBO J.* **1991**, *10*, 2247–2258. [CrossRef] [PubMed]
36. Kaul, N.; Forman, H.J. Activation of NFκB by the Respiratory Burst of Macrophages. *Free Radic. Biol. Med.* **1996**, *21*, 401–405. [CrossRef]
37. Kaul, N.; Gopalakrishna, R.; Gundimeda, U.; Choi, J.; Forman, H.J. Role of Protein Kinase C in Basal and Hydrogen Peroxide-Stimulated NF-KB Activation in the Murine Macrophage J774A.1 Cell Line. *Arch. Biochem. Biophys.* **1998**, *350*, 79–86. [CrossRef] [PubMed]
38. Hoyal, C.R.; Gozal, E.; Zhou, H.; Foldenauer, K.; Forman, H.J. Modulation of the Rat Alveolar Macrophage Respiratory Burst by Hydroperoxides Is Calcium Dependent. *Arch. Biochem. Biophys.* **1996**, *326*, 166–171. [CrossRef]
39. Murphy, J.K.; Livingston, F.R.; Gozal, E.; Torres, M.; Forman, H.J. Stimulation of the Rat Alveolar Macrophage Respiratory Burst by Extracellular Adenine Nucleotides. *Am. J. Respir. Cell Mol. Biol.* **1993**, *9*, 505–510. [CrossRef]
40. Hoyal, C.R.; Thomas, A.P.; Forman, H.J. Hydroperoxide-Induced Increases in Intracellular Calcium Due to Annexin VI Translocation and Inactivation of Plasma Membrane Ca 2+-ATPase. *J. Biol. Chem.* **1996**, *271*, 29205–29210. [CrossRef]
41. Girón-Calle, J.; Srivatsa, K.; Forman, H.J. Priming of Alveolar Macrophage Respiratory Burst by H2O2 Is Prevented by Phosphatidylcholine-Specific Phospholipase C Inhibitor Tricyclodecan-9-Yl-Xanthate (D609). *J. Pharmacol. Exp. Ther.* **2002**, *301*, 87–94. [CrossRef]
42. Torres, M.; Forman, H.J. Activation of Several MAP Kinases upon Stimulation of Rat Alveolar Macrophages: Role of the NADPH Oxidase. *Arch. Biochem. Biophys.* **1999**, *366*, 231–239. [CrossRef]
43. Rinna, A.; Torres, M.; Forman, H.J. Stimulation of the Alveolar Macrophage Respiratory Burst by ADP Causes Selective Glutathionylation of Protein Tyrosine Phosphatase 1B. *Free Radic. Biol. Med.* **2006**, *41*, 86–91. [CrossRef]
44. Denu, J.M.; Tanner, K.G. Specific and Reversible Inactivation of Protein Tyrosine Phosphatases by Hydrogen Peroxide: Evidence for a Sulfenic Acid Intermediate and Implications for Redox Regulation. *Biochemistry* **1998**, *37*, 5633–5642. [CrossRef] [PubMed]
45. Murad, F. Nitric Oxide: The Coming of the Second Messenger. *Rambam Maimonides Med. J.* **2011**, *2*, e0038. [CrossRef] [PubMed]

46. Reis, G.S.; Augusto, V.S.; Silveira, A.P.C.; Jordão, A.A.; Baddini-Martinez, J.; Poli Neto, O.; Rodrigues, A.J.; Evora, P.R.B. Oxidative-Stress Biomarkers in Patients with Pulmonary Hypertension. *Pulm. Circ.* **2013**, *3*, 856–861. [CrossRef] [PubMed]
47. Torres-Durán, M.; Lopez-Campos, J.L.; Barrecheguren, M.; Miravitlles, M.; Martinez-Delgado, B.; Castillo, S.; Escribano, A.; Baloira, A.; Navarro-Garcia, M.M.; Pellicer, D.; et al. Alpha-1 Antitrypsin Deficiency: Outstanding Questions and Future Directions. *Orphanet J. Rare Dis.* **2018**, *13*, 114. [CrossRef] [PubMed]
48. Chen, X.; Shen, J.; Prywes, R. The Luminal Domain of ATF6 Senses Endoplasmic Reticulum (ER) Stress and Causes Translocation of ATF6 from the Er to the Golgi. *J. Biol. Chem.* **2002**, *277*, 13045–13052. [CrossRef]
49. Credle, J.J.; Finer-Moore, J.S.; Papa, F.R.; Stroud, R.M.; Walter, P. On the Mechanism of Sensing Unfolded Protein in the Endoplasmic Reticulum. *Proc. Natl. Acad. Sci. USA* **2005**, *102*, 18773–18784. [CrossRef]
50. Bertolotti, A.; Zhang, Y.; Hendershot, L.M.; Harding, H.P.; Ron, D. Dynamic Interaction of BiP and ER Stress Transducers in the Unfolded-Protein Response. *Nat. Cell Biol.* **2000**, *2*, 326–332. [CrossRef] [PubMed]
51. Kimata, Y.; Oikawa, D.; Shimizu, Y.; Ishiwata-Kimata, Y.; Kohno, K. A Role for BiP as an Adjustor for the Endoplasmic Reticulum Stress-Sensing Protein Ire1. *J. Cell Biol.* **2004**, *167*, 445–456. [CrossRef] [PubMed]
52. Yoshida, H.; Haze, K.; Yanagi, H.; Yura, T.; Mori, K. Identification of the Cis-Acting Endoplasmic Reticulum Stress Response Element Responsible for Transcriptional Induction of Mammalian Glucose- Regulated Proteins: Involvement of Basic Leucine Zipper Transcription Factors. *J. Biol. Chem.* **1998**, *273*, 33741–33749. [CrossRef]
53. Ye, J.; Rawson, R.B.; Komuro, R.; Chen, X.; Dave, U.P.; Prywes, R.; Brown, M.S.; Goldstein, J.L. Of Membrane-Bound ATF6 by the Same Proteases That Process SREBPs. *Mol. Cell* **2000**, *6*, 1355–1364. [CrossRef]
54. Yoshida, H.; Okada, T.; Haze, K.; Yanagi, H.; Yura, T.; Negishi, M.; Mori, K. Endoplasmic Reticulum Stress-Induced Formation of Transcription Factor Complex ERSF Including NF-Y (CBF) and Activating Transcription Factors 6α and 6β That Activates the Mammalian Unfolded Protein Response. *Mol. Cell. Biol.* **2001**, *21*, 1239–1248. [CrossRef]
55. Yoshida, H.; Matsui, T.; Hosokawa, N.; Kaufman, R.J.; Nagata, K.; Mori, K. A Time-Dependent Phase Shift in the Mammalian Unfolded Protein Response. *Dev. Cell* **2003**, *4*, 265–271. [CrossRef]
56. Cox, J.S.; Walter, P. A Novel Mechanism for Regulating Activity of a Transcription Factor That Controls the Unfolded Protein Response. *Cell* **1996**, *87*, 391–404. [CrossRef]
57. Morl, K.; Ma, W.; Gething, M.J.; Sambrook, J. A Transmembrane Protein with a Cdc2+ CDC28-Related Kinase Activity Is Required for Signaling from the ER to the Nucleus. *Cell* **1993**, *74*, 743–756. [CrossRef]
58. Cox, J.S.; Shamu, C.E.; Walter, P. Transcriptional Induction of Genes Encoding Endoplasmic Reticulum Resident Proteins Requires a Transmembrane Protein Kinase. *Cell* **1993**, *73*, 1197–1206. [CrossRef]
59. Yoshida, H.; Matsui, T.; Yamamoto, A.; Okada, T.; Mori, K. XBP1 MRNA Is Induced by ATF6 and Spliced by IRE1 in Response to ER Stress to Produce a Highly Active Transcription Factor. *Cell* **2001**, *107*, 881–891. [CrossRef]
60. Calfon, M.; Zeng, H.; Urano, F.; Till, J.H.; Hubbard, S.R.; Harding, H.P.; Clark, S.G.; Ron, D. IRE1 Couples Endoplasmic Reticulum Load to Secretory Capacity by Processing the XBP-1 MRNA. *Nature* **2002**, *415*, 92–96. [CrossRef] [PubMed]
61. Malhotra, J.D.; Kaufman, R.J. Endoplasmic Reticulum Stress and Oxidative Stress: A Vicious Cycle or a Double-Edged Sword? *Antioxid. Redox Signal.* **2007**, *9*, 2277–2293. [CrossRef] [PubMed]
62. Harding, H.P.; Zhang, Y.; Ron, D. Protein Translation and Folding Are Coupled by an Endoplasmic- Reticulum-Resident Kinase. *Nature* **1999**, *397*, 271–274. [CrossRef]
63. Hwang, C.; Sinskey, A.J.; Lodish, H.F. Oxidized Redox State of Glutathione in the Endoplasmic Reticulum. *Science* **1992**, *257*, 1496–1502. [CrossRef]
64. Cao, S.S.; Kaufman, R.J. Endoplasmic Reticulum Stress and Oxidative Stress in Cell Fate Decision and Human Disease. *Antioxid. Redox Signal.* **2014**, *21*, 396–413. [CrossRef]
65. Van der Vlies, D.; Makkinje, M.; Jansens, A.; Braakman, I.; Verkleij, A.J.; Wirtz, K.W.A.; Post, J.A. Oxidation of ER Resident Proteins upon Oxidative Stress: Effects of Altering Cellular Redox/Antioxidant Status and Implications for Protein Maturation. *Antioxid. Redox Signal.* **2003**, *5*, 381–387. [CrossRef]
66. Tu, B.P.; Weissman, J.S. Oxidative Protein Folding in Eukaryotes: Mechanisms and Consequences. *J. Cell Biol.* **2004**, *164*, 341–346. [CrossRef]
67. Bravo, R.; Parra, V.; Gatica, D.; Rodriguez, A.E.; Torrealba, N.; Paredes, F.; Wang, Z.V.; Zorzano, A.; Hill, J.A.; Jaimovich, E.; et al. Endoplasmic Reticulum and the Unfolded Protein Response. Dynamics and Metabolic Integration. *Int. Rev. Cell Mol. Biol.* **2013**, *301*, 215–290. [CrossRef]
68. Vance, J.E. Phospholipid Synthesis in a Membrane Fraction Associated with Mitochondria. *J. Biol. Chem.* **1990**, *265*, 7248–7256. [CrossRef]
69. Bravo, R.; Gutierrez, T.; Paredes, F.; Gatica, D.; Rodriguez, A.E.; Pedrozo, Z.; Chiong, M.; Parra, V.; Quest, A.F.G.; Rothermel, B.A.; et al. Endoplasmic Reticulum: ER Stress Regulates Mitochondrial Bioenergetics. *Int. J. Biochem. Cell Biol.* **2012**, *44*, 16–20. [CrossRef] [PubMed]
70. Prasad, M.; Walker, A.N.; Kaur, J.; Thomas, J.L.; Powell, S.A.; Pandey, A.V.; Whittal, R.M.; Burak, W.E.; Petruzzelli, G.; Bose, H.S. Endoplasmic Reticulum Stress Enhances Mitochondrial Metabolic Activity in Mammalian Adrenals and Gonads. *Mol. Cell. Biol.* **2016**, *36*, 3058–3074. [CrossRef] [PubMed]
71. Kim, S.R.; Lee, Y.C. Endoplasmic Reticulum Stress and the Related Signaling Networks in Severe Asthma. *Allergy Asthma Immunol. Res.* **2015**, *7*, 106–117. [CrossRef]

72. Szabadkai, G.; Bianchi, K.; Várnai, P.; De Stefani, D.; Wieckowski, M.R.; Cavagna, D.; Nagy, A.I.; Balla, T.; Rizzuto, R. Chaperone-Mediated Coupling of Endoplasmic Reticulum and Mitochondrial Ca^{2+} Channels. *J. Cell Biol.* **2006**, *175*, 901–911. [CrossRef]
73. Verfaillie, T.; Rubio, N.; Garg, A.D.; Bultynck, G.; Rizzuto, R.; Decuypere, J.P.; Piette, J.; Linehan, C.; Gupta, S.; Samali, A.; et al. PERK Is Required at the ER-Mitochondrial Contact Sites to Convey Apoptosis after ROS-Based ER Stress. *Cell Death Differ.* **2012**, *19*, 1880–1891. [CrossRef]
74. Bravo, R.; Vicencio, J.M.; Parra, V.; Troncoso, R.; Munoz, J.P.; Bui, M.; Quiroga, C.; Rodriguez, A.E.; Verdejo, H.E.; Ferreira, J.; et al. Increased ER-Mitochondrial Coupling Promotes Mitochondrial Respiration and Bioenergetics during Early Phases of ER Stress. *J. Cell Sci.* **2011**, *124*, 2143–2152. [CrossRef]
75. Decuypere, J.P.; Monaco, G.; Bultynck, G.; Missiaen, L.; De Smedt, H.; Parys, J.B. The IP3 Receptor-Mitochondria Connection in Apoptosis and Autophagy. *Biochim. Biophys. Acta* **2011**, *1813*, 1003–1013. [CrossRef] [PubMed]
76. St-Pierre, J.; Buckingham, J.A.; Roebuck, S.J.; Brand, M.D. Topology of Superoxide Production from Different Sites in the Mitochondrial Electron Transport Chain. *J. Biol. Chem.* **2002**, *277*, 44784–44790. [CrossRef] [PubMed]
77. Wang, X.; Eno, C.O.; Altman, B.J.; Zhu, Y.; Zhao, G.; Olberding, K.E.; Rathmell, J.C.; Li, C. ER Stress Modulates Cellular Metabolism. *Biochem. J.* **2011**, *435*, 285–296. [CrossRef]
78. Itoh, K.; Chiba, T.; Takahashi, S.; Ishii, T.; Igarashi, K.; Katoh, Y.; Oyake, T.; Hayashi, N.; Satoh, K.; Hatayama, I.; et al. An Nrf2/Small Maf Heterodimer Mediates the Induction of Phase II Detoxifying Enzyme Genes through Antioxidant Response Elements. *Biochem. Biophys. Res. Commun.* **1997**, *236*, 313–322. [CrossRef] [PubMed]
79. Venugopal, R.; Jaiswal, A.K. Nrf1 and Nrf2 Positively and C-Fos and Fra1 Negatively Regulate the Human Antioxidant Response Element-Mediated Expression of NAD(P)H:Quinone Oxidoreductase1 Gene. *Proc. Natl. Acad. Sci. USA* **1996**, *93*, 14960–14965. [CrossRef] [PubMed]
80. Itoh, K.; Wakabayashi, N.; Katoh, Y.; Ishii, T.; Igarashi, K.; Engel, J.D.; Yamamoto, M. Keap1 Represses Nuclear Activation of Antioxidant Responsive Elements by Nrf2 through Binding to the Amino-Terminal Neh2 Domain. *Genes Dev.* **1999**, *13*, 76–86. [CrossRef]
81. Cullinan, S.B.; Zhang, D.; Hannink, M.; Arvisais, E.; Kaufman, R.J.; Diehl, J.A. Nrf2 Is a Direct PERK Substrate and Effector of PERK-Dependent Cell Survival. *Mol. Cell. Biol.* **2003**, *23*, 7198–7209. [CrossRef]
82. Cullinan, S.B.; Diehl, J.A. PERK-Dependent Activation of Nrf2 Contributes to Redox Homeostasis and Cell Survival Following Endoplasmic Reticulum Stress. *J. Biol. Chem.* **2004**, *279*, 20108–20117. [CrossRef]
83. Haynes, C.M.; Titus, E.A.; Cooper, A.A. Degradation of Misfolded Proteins Prevents ER-Derived Oxidative Stress and Cell Death. *Mol. Cell* **2004**, *15*, 767–776. [CrossRef]
84. Malhotra, J.D.; Miao, H.; Zhang, K.; Wolfson, A.; Pennathur, S.; Pipe, S.W.; Kaufman, R.J. Antioxidants Reduce Endoplasmic Reticulum Stress and Improve Protein Secretion. *Proc. Natl. Acad. Sci. USA* **2008**, *105*, 18525–18530. [CrossRef] [PubMed]
85. Harding, H.P.; Zhang, Y.; Zeng, H.; Novoa, I.; Lu, P.D.; Calfon, M.; Sadri, N.; Yun, C.; Popko, B.; Paules, R.; et al. An Integrated Stress Response Regulates Amino Acid Metabolism and Resistance to Oxidative Stress. *Mol. Cell* **2003**, *11*, 619–633. [CrossRef]
86. Li, S.J.; Liu, C.H.; Chu, H.P.; Mersmann, H.J.; Ding, S.T.; Chu, C.H.; Wang, C.Y.; Chen, C.Y. The High-Fat Diet Induces Myocardial Fibrosis in the Metabolically Healthy Obese Minipigs—The Role of ER Stress and Oxidative Stress. *Clin. Nutr.* **2017**, *36*, 760–767. [CrossRef] [PubMed]
87. Guo, Z.Y.; Zhang, Y.H.; Xie, G.Q.; Liu, C.X.; Zhou, R.; Shi, W. Down-Regulation of Homer1 Attenuates t-BHP-Induced Oxidative Stress through Regulating Calcium Homeostasis and ER Stress in Brain Endothelial Cells. *Biochem. Biophys. Res. Commun.* **2016**, *477*, 970–976. [CrossRef] [PubMed]
88. Mota, S.I.; Costa, R.O.; Ferreira, I.L.; Santana, I.; Caldeira, G.L.; Padovano, C.; Fonseca, A.C.; Baldeiras, I.; Cunha, C.; Letra, L.; et al. Oxidative Stress Involving Changes in Nrf2 and ER Stress in Early Stages of Alzheimer's Disease. *Biochim. Biophys. Acta Mol. Basis Dis.* **2015**, *1852*, 1428–1441. [CrossRef]
89. Dhillon, H.; Mamidi, S.; Mcclean, P.; Reindl, K.M. Transcriptome Analysis of Piperlongumine-Treated Human Pancreatic Cancer Cells Reveals Involvement of Oxidative Stress and Endoplasmic Reticulum Stress Pathways. *J. Med. Food* **2016**, *19*, 578–585. [CrossRef]
90. Liang, Z.; Liu, R.; Zhao, D.; Wang, L.; Sun, M.; Wang, M.; Song, L. Ammonia Exposure Induces Oxidative Stress, Endoplasmic Reticulum Stress and Apoptosis in Hepatopancreas of Pacific White Shrimp (Litopenaeus Vannamei). *Fish Shellfish Immunol.* **2016**, *54*, 523–528. [CrossRef]
91. Silverman, G.A.; Bird, P.I.; Carrell, R.W.; Church, F.C.; Coughlin, P.B.; Gettins, P.G.W.; Irving, J.A.; Lomas, D.A.; Luke, C.J.; Moyer, R.W.; et al. The Serpins Are an Expanding Superfamily of Structurally Similar but Functionally Diverse Proteins. *J. Biol. Chem.* **2001**, *276*, 33293–33296. [CrossRef]
92. Silverman, G.A.; Whisstock, J.C.; Bottomley, S.P.; Huntington, J.A.; Kaiserman, D.; Luke, C.J.; Pak, S.C.; Reichhart, J.-M.; Bird, P.I. Serpins Flex Their Muscle. *J. Biol. Chem.* **2010**, *285*, 24299–24305. [CrossRef]
93. Stein, P.E.; Carrell, R.W. What Do Dysfunctional Serpins Tell Us about Molecular Mobility and Disease? *Nat. Struct. Biol.* **1995**, *2*, 96–113. [CrossRef] [PubMed]
94. Janoff, A. Inhibition of Human Granulocyte Elastase by Serum Alpha-1-Antitrypsin. *Am. Rev. Respir. Dis.* **1972**, *105*, 121–122. [CrossRef] [PubMed]
95. Ordóñez, A.; Snapp, E.L.; Tan, L.; Miranda, E.; Marciniak, S.J.; Lomas, D.A. Endoplasmic Reticulum Polymers Impair Luminal Protein Mobility and Sensitize to Cellular Stress in Alpha1-Antitrypsin Deficiency. *Hepatology* **2013**, *57*, 2049–2060. [CrossRef]

96. Hidvegi, T.; Schmidt, B.Z.; Hale, P.; Perlmutter, D.H. Accumulation of Mutant A1-Antitrypsin Z in the Endoplasmic Reticulum Activities Caspases-4 and -12, NFκB, and BAP31 but Not the Unfolded Protein Response. *J. Biol. Chem.* **2005**, *280*, 39002–39015. [CrossRef] [PubMed]
97. Papp, E.; Száiraz, P.; Korcsmáiros, T.; Csermely, P.; Papp, E.; Száiraz, P.; Korcsmáiros, T.; Csermely, P. Changes of Endoplasmic Reticulum Chaperone Complexes, Redox State, and Impaired Protein Disulfide Reductase Activity in Misfolding Ai-antitrypsin Transgenic Mice. *FASEB J.* **2006**, *20*, 1018–1020. [CrossRef]
98. Carroll, T.P.; Greene, C.M.; O'Connor, C.A.; Nolan, Á.M.; O'Neill, S.J.; McElvaney, N.G. Evidence for Unfolded Protein Response Activation in Monocytes from Individuals with α-1 Antitrypsin Deficiency. *J. Immunol.* **2010**, *184*, 4538–4546. [CrossRef] [PubMed]
99. Kelly, E.; Greene, C.M.; Carroll, T.P.; McElvaney, N.G.; O'Neill, S.J. Selenoprotein S/SEPS1 Modifies Endoplasmic Reticulum Stress in Z Variant A1-Antitrypsin Deficiency. *J. Biol. Chem.* **2009**, *284*, 16891–16897. [CrossRef]
100. Lawless, M.W.; Greene, C.M.; Mulgrew, A.; Taggart, C.C.; O'Neill, S.J.; McElvaney, N.G. Activation of Endoplasmic Reticulum-Specific Stress Responses Associated with the Conformational Disease Z A1-Antitrypsin Deficiency. *J. Immunol.* **2004**, *172*, 5722–5726. [CrossRef]
101. Raeymaekers, L.; Larivière, E. Vesicularization of the Endoplasmic Reticulum Is a Fast Response to Plasma Membrane Injury. *Biochem. Biophys. Res. Commun.* **2011**, *414*, 246–251. [CrossRef]
102. Subramanian, K.; Meyer, T. Calcium-Induced Restructuring of Nuclear Envelope and Endoplasmic Reticulum Calcium Stores. *Cell* **1997**, *89*, 963–971. [CrossRef]
103. Escribano, A.; Amor, M.; Pastor, S.; Castillo, S.; Sanz, F.; Codoñer-Franch, P.; Dasí, F. Decreased Glutathione and Low Catalase Activity Contribute to Oxidative Stress in Children with α-1 Antitrypsin Deficiency. *Thorax* **2015**, *70*, 82–83. [CrossRef]
104. Sitia, R.; Molteni, S.N. Stress, Protein (Mis)Folding, and Signaling: The Redox Connection. *Sci. STKE* **2004**, *2004*, e27. [CrossRef]
105. Nardai, G.; Stadler, K.; Papp, E.; Korcsmáros, T.; Jakus, J.; Csermely, P. Diabetic Changes in the Redox Status of the Microsomal Protein Folding Machinery. *Biochem. Biophys. Res. Commun.* **2005**, *334*, 787–795. [CrossRef]
106. Marcus, N.Y.; Blomenkamp, K.; Ahmad, M.; Teckman, J.H. Oxidative Stress Contributes to Liver Damage in a Murine Model of Alpha-1-Antitrypsin Deficiency. *Exp. Biol. Med.* **2012**, *237*, 1163–1172. [CrossRef]
107. Topic, A.; Nagorni-Obradovic, L.; Francuski, D.; Ljujic, M.; Malic, Z.; Radojkovic, D. Oxidative Stress and Polymorphism of Xenobiotic-Metabolizing Enzymes in Two Patients with Severe Alpha-1-Antitrypsin Deficiency. *Biochem. Genet.* **2016**, *54*, 746–752. [CrossRef] [PubMed]
108. GSTP1 Glutathione S-Transferase Pi 1 [Homo Sapiens (Human)]-Gene-NCBI. Available online: https://www.ncbi.nlm.nih.gov/gene?Cmd=DetailsSearch&Term=2950 (accessed on 28 January 2020).
109. Escribano, A.; Pastor, S.; Reula, A.; Castillo, S.; Vicente, S.; Sanz, F.; Casas, F.; Torres, M.; Fernández-Fabrellas, E.; Codoñer-Franch, P.; et al. Accelerated Telomere Attrition in Children and Teenagers with A1-Antitrypsin Deficiency. *Eur. Respir. J.* **2016**, *48*, 350–358. [CrossRef] [PubMed]
110. Levine, R.L.; Berlett, B.S.; Moskovitz, J.; Mosoni, L.; Stadtman, E.R. Methionine Residues May Protect Proteins from Critical Oxidative Damage. *Mech. Ageing Dev.* **1999**, *107*, 323–332. [CrossRef]
111. Taggart, C.; Cervantes-Laurean, D.; Kim, G.; McElvaney, N.G.; Wehr, N.; Moss, J.; Levine, R.L. Oxidation of Either Methionine 351 or Methionine 358 in A1-Antitrypsin Causes Loss of Anti-Neutrophil Elastase Activity. *J. Biol. Chem.* **2000**, *275*, 27258–27265. [CrossRef]
112. Feng, Y.; Xu, J.; Zhou, Q.; Wang, R.; Liu, N.; Wu, Y.; Yuan, H.; Che, H. Alpha-1 Antitrypsin Prevents the Development of Preeclampsia through Suppression of Oxidative Stress. *Front. Physiol.* **2016**, *7*, 176. [CrossRef]
113. Barratt, S.; Creamer, A.; Hayton, C.; Chaudhuri, N. Idiopathic Pulmonary Fibrosis (IPF): An Overview. *J. Clin. Med.* **2018**, *7*, 201. [CrossRef] [PubMed]
114. Kliment, C.R.; Oury, T.D. Oxidative Stress, Extracellular Matrix Targets, and Idiopathic Pulmonary Fibrosis. *Free Radic. Biol. Med.* **2010**, *49*, 707–717. [CrossRef] [PubMed]
115. Korfei, M.; Ruppert, C.; Mahavadi, P.; Henneke, I.; Markart, P.; Koch, M.; Lang, G.; Fink, L.; Bohle, R.M.; Seeger, W.; et al. Epithelial Endoplasmic Reticulum Stress and Apoptosis in Sporadic Idiopathic Pulmonary Fibrosis. *Am. J. Respir. Crit. Care Med.* **2008**, *178*, 838–846. [CrossRef] [PubMed]
116. Lawson, W.E.; Crossno, P.F.; Polosukhin, V.V.; Roldan, J.; Cheng, D.S.; Lane, K.B.; Blackwell, T.R.; Xu, C.; Markin, C.; Ware, L.B.; et al. Endoplasmic Reticulum Stress in Alveolar Epithelial Cells Is Prominent in IPF: Association with Altered Surfactant Protein Processing and Herpesvirus Infection. *Am. J. Physiol.-Lung Cell. Mol. Physiol.* **2008**, *294*, 1119–1126. [CrossRef] [PubMed]
117. Baek, H.A.; Kim, D.S.; Park, H.S.; Jang, K.Y.; Kang, M.J.; Lee, D.G.; Moon, W.S.; Chae, H.J.; Chung, M.J. Involvement of Endoplasmic Reticulum Stress in Myofibroblastic Differentiation of Lung Fibroblasts. *Am. J. Respir. Cell Mol. Biol.* **2012**, *46*, 731–739. [CrossRef] [PubMed]
118. Ryan, A.J.; Larson-Casey, J.L.; He, C.; Murthy, S.; Brent Carter, A. 3 Asbestos-Induced Disruption of Calcium Homeostasis Induces Endoplasmic Reticulum Stress in Macrophages. *J. Biol. Chem.* **2014**, *289*, 33391–33403. [CrossRef]
119. Yao, Y.; Wang, Y.; Zhang, Z.; He, L.; Zhu, J.; Zhang, M.; He, X.; Cheng, Z.; Ao, Q.; Cao, Y.; et al. Chop Deficiency Protects Mice against Bleomycin-Induced Pulmonary Fibrosis by Attenuating M2 Macrophage Production. *Mol. Ther.* **2016**, *24*, 915–925. [CrossRef]
120. Burman, A.; Tanjore, H.; Blackwell, T.S. Endoplasmic Reticulum Stress in Pulmonary Fibrosis. *Matrix Biol.* **2018**, *68–69*, 355–365. [CrossRef]

121. Kamp, D.W.; Liu, G.; Cheresh, P.; Kim, S.J.; Mueller, A.; Lam, A.P.; Trejo, H.; Williams, D.; Tulasiram, S.; Baker, M.; et al. Asbestos-Induced Alveolar Epithelial Cell Apoptosis: The Role of Endoplasmic Reticulum Stress Response. *Am. J. Respir. Cell Mol. Biol.* **2013**, *49*, 892–901. [CrossRef]
122. Zhong, Q.; Zhou, B.; Ann, D.K.; Minoo, P.; Liu, Y.; Banfalvi, A.; Krishnaveni, M.S.; Dubourd, M.; Demaio, L.; Willis, B.C.; et al. Role of Endoplasmic Reticulum Stress in Epithelial-Mesenchymal Transition of Alveolar Epithelial Cells: Effects of Misfolded Surfactant Protein. *Am. J. Respir. Cell Mol. Biol.* **2011**, *45*, 498–509. [CrossRef]
123. Tanjore, H.; Cheng, D.S.; Degryse, A.L.; Zoz, D.F.; Abdolrasulnia, R.; Lawson, W.E.; Blackwell, T.S. Alveolar Epithelial Cells Undergo Epithelial-to-Mesenchymal Transition in Response to Endoplasmic Reticulum Stress. *J. Biol. Chem.* **2011**, *286*, 30972–30980. [CrossRef] [PubMed]
124. Bargagli, E.; Penza, F.; Vagaggini, C.; Magi, B.; Perari, M.G.; Rottoli, P. Analysis of Carbonylated Proteins in Bronchoalveolar Lavage of Patients with Diffuse Lung Diseases. *Lung* **2007**, *185*, 139–144. [CrossRef] [PubMed]
125. Rottoli, P.; Magi, B.; Cianti, R.; Bargagli, E.; Vagaggini, C.; Nikiforakis, N.; Pallini, V.; Bini, L. Carbonylated Proteins in Bronchoalveolar Lavage of Patients with Sarcoidosis, Pulmonary Fibrosis Associated with Systemic Sclerosis and Idiopathic Pulmonary Fibrosis. *Proteomics* **2005**, *5*, 2612–2618. [CrossRef] [PubMed]
126. Malli, F.; Bardaka, F.; Tsilioni, I.; Karetsi, E.; Gourgoulianis, K.I.; Daniil, Z. 8-Isoprostane Levels in Serum and Bronchoalveolar Lavage in Idiopathic Pulmonary Fibrosis and Sarcoidosis. *Food Chem. Toxicol.* **2013**, *61*, 160–163. [CrossRef]
127. Daniil, Z.D.; Papageorgiou, E.; Koutsokera, A.; Kostikas, K.; Kiropoulos, T.; Papaioannou, A.I.; Gourgoulianis, K.I. Serum Levels of Oxidative Stress as a Marker of Disease Severity in Idiopathic Pulmonary Fibrosis. *Pulm. Pharmacol. Ther.* **2008**, *21*, 26–31. [CrossRef]
128. Psathakis, K.; Mermigkis, D.; Papatheodorou, G.; Loukides, S.; Panagou, P.; Polychronopoulos, V.; Siafakas, N.M.; Bouros, D. Exhaled Markers of Oxidative Stress in Idiopathic Pulmonary Fibrosis. *Eur. J. Clin. Investig.* **2006**, *36*, 362–367. [CrossRef]
129. Cantin, A.M.; North, S.L.; Fells, G.A.; Hubbard, R.C.; Crystal, R.G. Oxidant-Mediated Epithelial Cell Injury in Idiopathic Pulmonary Fibrosis. *J. Clin. Investig.* **1987**, *79*, 1665–1673. [CrossRef]
130. Hecker, L.; Vittal, R.; Jones, T.; Jagirdar, R.; Luckhardt, T.R.; Horowitz, J.C.; Pennathur, S.; Martinez, F.J.; Thannickal, V.J. NADPH Oxidase-4 Mediates Myofibroblast Activation and Fibrogenic Responses to Lung Injury. *Nat. Med.* **2009**, *15*, 1077–1081. [CrossRef]
131. Veith, C.; Boots, A.W.; Idris, M.; Van Schooten, F.J.; Van Der Vliet, A. Redox Imbalance in Idiopathic Pulmonary Fibrosis: A Role for Oxidant Cross-Talk between NADPH Oxidase Enzymes and Mitochondria. *Antioxid. Redox Signal.* **2019**, *31*, 1092–1115. [CrossRef]
132. Zeidler, P.C.; Hubbs, A.; Battelli, L.; Castranova, V. Role of Inducible Nitric Oxide Synthase-Derived Nitric Oxide in Silica-Induced Pulmonary Inflammation and Fibrosis. *J. Toxicol. Environ. Health Part A* **2004**, *67*, 1001–1026. [CrossRef]
133. Saleh, D.; Barnes, P.J.; Giaid, A. Increased Production of the Potent Oxidant Peroxynitrite in the Lungs of Patients with Idiopathic Pulmonary Fibrosis. *Am. J. Respir. Crit. Care Med.* **1997**, *155*, 1763–1769. [CrossRef]
134. Cantin, A.M.; Hubbard, R.C.; Crystal, R.G. Glutathione Deficiency in the Epithelial Lining Fluid of the Lower Respiratory Tract in Idiopathic Pulmonary Fibrosis. *Am. Rev. Respir. Dis.* **1989**, *139*, 370–372. [CrossRef]
135. Mazur, W.; Lindholm, P.; Vuorinen, K.; Myllärniemi, M.; Salmenkivi, K.; Kinnula, V.L. Cell-Specific Elevation of NRF2 and Sulfiredoxin-1 as Markers of Oxidative Stress in the Lungs of Idiopathic Pulmonary Fibrosis and Non-Specific Interstitial Pneumonia. *APMIS* **2010**, *118*, 703–712. [CrossRef]
136. Markart, P.; Luboeinski, T.; Korfei, M.; Schmidt, R.; Wygrecka, M.; Mahavadi, P.; Mayer, K.; Wilhelm, J.; Seeger, W.; Guenther, A.; et al. Alveolar Oxidative Stress Is Associated with Elevated Levels of Nonenzymatic Low-Molecular-Weight Antioxidants in Patients with Different Forms of Chronic Fibrosing Interstitial Lung Diseases. *Antioxid. Redox Signal.* **2009**, *11*, 227–240. [CrossRef] [PubMed]
137. Walters, D.M.; Cho, H.Y.; Kleeberger, S.R. Oxidative Stress and Antioxidants in the Pathogenesis of Pulmonary Fibrosis: A Potential Role for Nrf2. *Antioxid. Redox Signal.* **2008**, *10*, 321–332. [CrossRef] [PubMed]
138. Fois, A.G.; Paliogiannis, P.; Sotgia, S.; Mangoni, A.A.; Zinellu, E.; Pirina, P.; Carru, C.; Zinellu, A. Evaluation of Oxidative Stress Biomarkers in Idiopathic Pulmonary Fibrosis and Therapeutic Applications: A Systematic Review. *Respir. Res.* **2018**, *19*, 51. [CrossRef] [PubMed]
139. Scotet, V.; Gutierrez, H.; Farrell, P.M. Newborn Screening for CF across the Globe-Where Is Itworthwhile? *Int. J. Neonatal Screen.* **2020**, *6*, 18. [CrossRef] [PubMed]
140. Galli, F.; Battistoni, A.; Gambari, R.; Pompella, A.; Bragonzi, A.; Pilolli, F.; Iuliano, L.; Piroddi, M.; Dechecchi, M.C.; Cabrini, G. Oxidative Stress and Antioxidant Therapy in Cystic Fibrosis. *Biochim. Biophys. Acta* **2012**, *1822*, 690–713. [CrossRef] [PubMed]
141. Fanen, P.; Wohlhuter-Haddad, A.; Hinzpeter, A. Genetics of Cystic Fibrosis: CFTR Mutation Classifications toward Genotype-Based CF Therapies. *Int. J. Biochem. Cell Biol.* **2014**, *52*, 94–102. [CrossRef]
142. Bareil, C.; Bergougnoux, A. CFTR Gene Variants, Epidemiology and Molecular Pathology. *Arch. Pediatr.* **2020**, *27*, eS8–eS12. [CrossRef]
143. Farrell, P.M.; White, T.B.; Ren, C.L.; Hempstead, S.E.; Accurso, F.; Derichs, N.; Howenstine, M.; McColley, S.A.; Rock, M.; Rosenfeld, M.; et al. Diagnosis of Cystic Fibrosis: Consensus Guidelines from the Cystic Fibrosis Foundation. *J. Pediatr.* **2017**, *181*, S4–S15.e1. [CrossRef] [PubMed]
144. Cheng, S.H.; Gregory, R.J.; Marshall, J.; Paul, S.; Souza, D.W.; White, G.A.; O'Riordan, C.R.; Smith, A.E. Defective Intracellular Transport and Processing of CFTR Is the Molecular Basis of Most Cystic Fibrosis. *Cell* **1990**, *63*, 827–834. [CrossRef]

145. Younger, J.M.; Ren, H.Y.; Chen, L.; Fan, C.Y.; Fields, A.; Patterson, C.; Cyr, D.M. A Foldable CFTRΔF508 Biogenic Intermediate Accumulates upon Inhibition of the Hsc70-CHIP E3 Ubiquitin Ligase. *J. Cell Biol.* **2004**, *167*, 1075–1085. [CrossRef]
146. Gilbert, A.; Jadot, M.; Leontieva, E.; Wattiaux-De Coninck, S.; Wattiaux, R. ΔF508 CFTR Localizes in the Endoplasmic Reticulum—Golgi Intermediate Compartment in Cystic Fibrosis Cells. *Exp. Cell Res.* **1998**, *242*, 144–152. [CrossRef]
147. Kerbiriou, M.; Le Drévo, M.A.; Férec, C.; Trouvé, P. Coupling Cystic Fibrosis to Endoplasmic Reticulum Stress: Differential Role of Grp78 and ATF6. *Biochim. Biophys. Acta Mol. Basis Dis.* **2007**, *1772*, 1236–1249. [CrossRef]
148. Wang, Y.; Shen, J.; Arenzana, N.; Tirasophon, W.; Kaufman, R.J.; Prywes, R. Activation of ATF6 and an ATF6 DNA Binding Site by the Endoplasmic Reticulum Stress Response. *J. Biol. Chem.* **2000**, *275*, 27013–27020. [CrossRef]
149. Haze, K.; Yoshida, H.; Yanagi, H.; Yura, T.; Mori, K. Mammalian Transcription Factor ATF6 Is Synthesized as a Transmembrane Protein and Activated by Proteolysis in Response to Endoplasmic Reticulum Stress. *Mol. Biol. Cell* **1999**, *10*, 3787–3799. [CrossRef]
150. Tang, A.C.; Saferali, A.; He, G.; Sandford, A.J.; Strug, L.; Turvey, S.E. Endoplasmic Reticulum Stress and Chemokine Production in Cystic Fibrosis Airway Cells: Regulation by STAT3 Modulation. *J. Infect. Dis.* **2017**, *215*, 293–302. [CrossRef]
151. Stutts, M.J.; Knowles, M.R.; Gatzy, J.T.; Boucher, R.C. Oxygen Consumption and Ouabain Binding Sites in Cystic Fibrosis Nasal Epithelium. *Pediatr. Res.* **1986**, *20*, 1316–1320. [CrossRef] [PubMed]
152. Worlitzsch, D.; Tarran, R.; Ulrich, M.; Schwab, U.; Cekici, A.; Meyer, K.C.; Birrer, P.; Bellon, G.; Berger, J.; Weiss, T.; et al. Effects of Reduced Mucus Oxygen Concentration in Airway Pseudomonas Infections of Cystic Fibrosis Patients. *J. Clin. Investig.* **2002**, *109*, 317–325. [CrossRef]
153. Colarusso, C.; Terlizzi, M.; Molino, A.; Pinto, A.; Sorrentino, R. Role of the Inflammasome in Chronic Obstructive Pulmonary Disease (COPD). *Oncotarget* **2017**, *8*, 81813–81824. [CrossRef]
154. Kelly-Aubert, M.; Trudel, S.; Fritsch, J.; Nguyen-Khoa, T.; Baudouin-Legros, M.; Moriceau, S.; Jeanson, L.; Djouadi, F.; Matar, C.; Conti, M.; et al. GSH Monoethyl Ester Rescues Mitochondrial Defects in Cystic Fibrosis Models. *Hum. Mol. Genet.* **2011**, *20*, 2745–2759. [CrossRef] [PubMed]
155. Laval, J.; Ralhan, A.; Hartl, D. Neutrophils in Cystic Fibrosis. *Biol. Chem.* **2016**, *397*, 485–496. [CrossRef] [PubMed]
156. Thomson, E.; Brennan, S.; Senthilmohan, R.; Gangell, C.L.; Chapman, A.L.; Sly, P.D.; Kettle, A.J. Identifying Peroxidases and Their Oxidants in the Early Pathology of Cystic Fibrosis. *Free Radic. Biol. Med.* **2010**, *49*, 1354–1360. [CrossRef] [PubMed]
157. Kettle, A.J.; Chan, T.; Osberg, I.; Senthilmohan, R.; Chapman, A.L.P.; Mocatta, T.J.; Wagener, J.S. Myeloperoxidase and Protein Oxidation in the Airways of Young Children with Cystic Fibrosis. *Am. J. Respir. Crit. Care Med.* **2004**, *170*, 1317–1323. [CrossRef] [PubMed]
158. Fischer, H. Mechanisms and Function of DUOX in Epithelia of the Lung. *Antioxid. Redox Signal.* **2009**, *11*, 2453–2465. [CrossRef] [PubMed]
159. Roum, J.H.; Buhl, R.; McElvaney, N.G.; Borok, Z.; Crystal, R.G. Systemic Deficiency of Glutathione in Cystic Fibrosis. *J. Appl. Physiol.* **1993**, *75*, 2419–2424. [CrossRef]
160. Linsdell, P.; Hanrahan, J.W. Glutathione Permeability of CFTR. *Am. J. Physiol. Cell Physiol.* **1998**, *275*, C323–C326. [CrossRef]
161. Grasemann, H.; Michler, E.; Wallot, M.; Ratjen, F. Decreased Concentration of Exhaled Nitric Oxide (NO) in Patients with Cystic Fibrosis. *Pediatr. Pulmonol.* **1997**, *24*, 173–177. [CrossRef]
162. Grasemann, H.; Al-Saleh, S.; Scott, J.A.; Shehnaz, D.; Mehl, A.; Amin, R.; Rafii, M.; Pencharz, P.; Belik, J.; Ratjen, F. Asymmetric Dimethylarginine Contributes to Airway Nitric Oxide Deficiency in Patients with Cystic Fibrosis. *Am. J. Respir. Crit. Care Med.* **2011**, *183*, 1363–1368. [CrossRef]
163. Chen, J.; Kinter, M.; Shank, S.; Cotton, C.; Kelley, T.J.; Ziady, A.G. Dysfunction of Nrf-2 in CF Epithelia Leads to Excess Intracellular H_2O_2 and Inflammatory Cytokine Production. *PLoS ONE* **2008**, *3*, e3367. [CrossRef]
164. Causer, A.J.; Shute, J.K.; Cummings, M.H.; Shepherd, A.I.; Gruet, M.; Costello, J.T.; Bailey, S.; Lindley, M.; Pearson, C.; Connett, G.; et al. Circulating Biomarkers of Antioxidant Status and Oxidative Stress in People with Cystic Fibrosis: A Systematic Review and Meta-Analysis. *Redox Biol.* **2020**, *32*, 101436. [CrossRef]
165. Collins, C.E.; Quaggiotto, P.; Wood, L.; O'Loughlin, E.V.; Henry, R.L.; Garg, M.L. Elevated Plasma Levels of F2(α) Isoprostane in Cystic Fibrosis. *Lipids* **1999**, *34*, 551–556. [CrossRef] [PubMed]
166. Back, E.I.; Frindt, C.; Nohr, D.; Frank, J.; Ziebach, R.; Stern, M.; Ranke, M.; Biesalski, H.K. Antioxidant Deficiency in Cystic Fibrosis: When Is the Right Time to Take Action? *Am. J. Clin. Nutr.* **2004**, *80*, 374–384. [CrossRef] [PubMed]
167. Kharitonov, S.A.; Corradi, M.; van Rensen, L.; Geddes, D.M.; Hodson, M.E.; Barnes, P.J.; Montuschi, P.; Ciabattoni, G. Exhaled 8-Isoprostane as a New Non-Invasive Biomarker of Oxidative Stress in Cystic Fibrosis. *Thorax* **2000**, *55*, 205–209. [CrossRef]
168. Iuliano, L.; Monticolo, R.; Straface, G.; Zullo, S.; Galli, F.; Boaz, M.; Quattrucci, S. Association of Cholesterol Oxidation and Abnormalities in Fatty Acid Metabolism in Cystic Fibrosis. *Am. J. Clin. Nutr.* **2009**, *90*, 477–484. [CrossRef] [PubMed]
169. Lucas, J.S.; Davis, S.D.; Omran, H.; Shoemark, A. Primary Ciliary Dyskinesia in the Genomics Age. *Lancet Respir. Med.* **2020**, *8*, 202–216. [CrossRef]
170. Baz-Redón, N.; Rovira-Amigo, S.; Paramonov, I.; Castillo-Corullón, S.; Cols Roig, M.; Antolín, M.; García Arumí, E.; Torrent-Vernetta, A.; de Mir Messa, I.; Gartner, S.; et al. Implementation of a Gene Panel for Genetic Diagnosis of Primary Ciliary Dyskinesia. *Arch. Bronconeumol.* **2020**. [CrossRef]
171. Cockx, M.; Gouwy, M.; Van Damme, J.; Struyf, S. Chemoattractants and Cytokines in Primary Ciliary Dyskinesia and Cystic Fibrosis: Key Players in Chronic Respiratory Diseases. *Cell. Mol. Immunol.* **2018**, *15*, 312–323. [CrossRef]

172. Güney, E.; Emiralioğlu, N.; Cinel, G.; Yalçın, E.; Doğru, D.; Kiper, N.; Uğur Özçelik, H. Nasal Nitric Oxide Levels in Primary Ciliary Dyskinesia, Cystic Fibrosis and Healthy Children. *Turk. J. Pediatr.* **2019**, *61*, 20–25. [CrossRef]
173. Lucas, J.S.; Barbato, A.; Collins, S.A.; Goutaki, M.; Behan, L.; Caudri, D.; Dell, S.; Eber, E.; Escudier, E.; Hirst, R.A.; et al. European Respiratory Society Guidelines for the Diagnosis of Primary Ciliary Dyskinesia. *Eur. Respir. J.* **2017**, *49*, 1601090. [CrossRef]
174. Collins, S.A.; Gove, K.; Walker, W.; Lucas, J.S.A. Nasal Nitric Oxide Screening for Primary Ciliary Dyskinesia: Systematic Review and Meta-Analysis. *Eur. Respir. J.* **2014**, *44*, 1589–1599. [CrossRef]
175. Zihlif, N.; Paraskakis, E.; Tripoli, C.; Lex, C.; Bush, A. Makers of Airway Inflammation in Primary Ciliary Dyskinesia Studied Using Exhaled Breath Condensate. *Pediatr. Pulmonol.* **2006**, *41*, 509–514. [CrossRef]
176. Reula, A.; Pellicer, D.; Castillo, S.; Banyuls, L.; Magallón, M.; Navarro, M.M.; Escribano, A.; Armengot, M.; Dasí, F. Caracterización del perfil oxidativo en células epiteliales nasales de pacientes con discinesia ciliar primaria desarrollo de un nuevo algoritmo diagnóstico. In Proceedings of the 52° Congreso SEPAR, Santiago de Compostela, Spain, 13–16 June 2019; p. 476.
177. Janciauskiene, S. The Beneficial Effects of Antioxidants in Health and Diseases. *Chronic Obstr. Pulm. Dis. J. COPD Found.* **2020**, *7*, 182–202. [CrossRef] [PubMed]
178. Otoupalova, E.; Smith, S.; Cheng, G.; Thannickal, V.J. Oxidative Stress in Pulmonary Fibrosis. *Compr. Physiol.* **2020**, *10*, 509–547. [CrossRef] [PubMed]
179. Ciofu, O.; Smith, S.; Lykkesfeldt, J. Antioxidant Supplementation for Lung Disease in Cystic Fibrosis. *Cochrane Database Syst. Rev.* **2019**, *2019*, CD007020. [CrossRef]
180. Tonelli, A.R.; Brantly, M.L. Augmentation Therapy in Alpha-1 Antitrypsin Deficiency: Advances and Controversies. *Ther. Adv. Respir. Dis.* **2010**, *4*, 289–312. [CrossRef]
181. Chapman, K.R.; Burdon, J.G.W.; Piitulainen, E.; Sandhaus, R.A.; Seersholm, N.; Stocks, J.M.; Stoel, B.C.; Huang, L.; Yao, Z.; Edelman, J.M.; et al. Intravenous Augmentation Treatment and Lung Density in Severe A1 Antitrypsin Deficiency (RAPID): A Randomised, Double-Blind, Placebo-Controlled Trial. *Lancet* **2015**, *386*, 360–368. [CrossRef]
182. Barnes, P.J. Oxidative Stress-Based Therapeutics in COPD. *Redox Biol.* **2020**, *33*, 101544. [CrossRef] [PubMed]
183. Bals, R. Alpha-1-Antitrypsin Deficiency. *Best Pract. Res. Clin. Gastroenterol.* **2010**, *24*, 629–633. [CrossRef]
184. Ronzoni, R.; Berardelli, R.; Medicina, D.; Sitia, R.; Gooptu, B.; Fra, A.M. Aberrant Disulphide Bonding Contributes to the ER Retention of Alpha1-Antitrypsin Deficiency Variants. *Hum. Mol. Genet.* **2016**, *25*, 642–650. [CrossRef]
185. Alam, S.; Li, Z.; Janciauskiene, S.; Mahadeva, R. Oxidation of Z α 1 -Antitrypsin by Cigarette Smoke Induces Polymerization. *Am. J. Respir. Cell Mol. Biol.* **2011**, *45*, 261–269. [CrossRef] [PubMed]
186. Shahzeidi, S.; Sarnstrand, B.; Jeffery, P.K.; McAnulty, R.J.; Laurent, G.J. Oral N-Acetylcysteine Reduces Bleomycin-Induced Collagen Deposition in the Lungs of Mice. *Eur. Respir. J.* **1991**, *4*, 845–852. [PubMed]
187. Hagiwara, S.I.; Ishii, Y.; Kitamura, S. Aerosolized Administration of N-Acetylcysteine Attenuates Lung Fibrosis Induced by Bleomycin in Mice. *Am. J. Respir. Crit. Care Med.* **2000**, *162*, 225–231. [CrossRef]
188. Berend, N. Inhibition of Bleomycin Lung Toxicityby N-Acetyl Cysteine in the Rat. *Pathology* **1985**, *17*, 108–110. [CrossRef]
189. Sun, T.; Liu, J.; Zhao, D.W. Efficacy of N-Acetylcysteine in Idiopathic Pulmonary Fibrosis: A Systematic Review and Meta-Analysis. *Medicine* **2016**, *95*, e3629. [CrossRef]
190. Oldham, J.M.; Ma, S.F.; Martinez, F.J.; Anstrom, K.J.; Raghu, G.; Schwartz, D.A.; Valenzi, E.; Witt, L.; Lee, C.; Vij, R.; et al. TOLLIP, MUC5B, and the Response to N-Acetylcysteine among Individuals with Idiopathic Pulmonary Fibrosis. *Am. J. Respir. Crit. Care Med.* **2015**, *192*, 1475–1482. [CrossRef]
191. Tanaka, K.I.; Ishihara, T.; Azuma, A.; Kudoh, S.; Ebina, M.; Nukiwa, T.; Sugiyama, Y.; Tasaka, Y.; Namba, T.; Ishihara, T.; et al. Therapeutic Effect of Lecithinized Superoxide Dismutase on Bleomycin-Induced Pulmonary Fibrosis. *Am. J. Physiol.-Lung Cell. Mol. Physiol.* **2010**, *298*, 348–360. [CrossRef]
192. Kamio, K.; Azuma, A.; Ohta, K.; Sugiyama, Y.; Nukiwa, T.; Kudoh, S.; Mizushima, T. Double-Blind Controlled Trial of Lecithinized Superoxide Dismutase in Patients with Idiopathic Interstitial Pneumonia—Short Term Evaluation of Safety and Tolerability. *BMC Pulm. Med.* **2014**, *14*, 86. [CrossRef]
193. Hecker, L.; Logsdon, N.J.; Kurundkar, D.; Kurundkar, A.; Bernard, K.; Hock, T.; Meldrum, E.; Sanders, Y.Y.; Thannickal, V.J. Reversal of Persistent Fibrosis in Aging by Targeting Nox4-Nrf2 Redox Imbalance. *Sci. Transl. Med.* **2014**, *6*, 231ra47. [CrossRef]
194. Sato, N.; Takasaka, N.; Yoshida, M.; Tsubouchi, K.; Minagawa, S.; Araya, J.; Saito, N.; Fujita, Y.; Kurita, Y.; Kobayashi, K.; et al. Metformin Attenuates Lung Fibrosis Development via NOX4 Suppression. *Respir. Res.* **2016**, *17*, 1–12. [CrossRef]
195. Tsubouchi, K.; Araya, J.; Minagawa, S.; Hara, H.; Ichikawa, A.; Saito, N.; Kadota, T.; Sato, N.; Yoshida, M.; Kurita, Y.; et al. Azithromycin Attenuates Myofibroblast Differentiation and Lung Fibrosis Development through Proteasomal Degradation of NOX4. *Autophagy* **2017**, *13*, 1420–1434. [CrossRef] [PubMed]
196. Wuyts, W.A.; Willems, S.; Vos, R.; Vanaudenaerde, B.M.; De Vleeschauwer, S.I.; Rinaldi, M.; Vanhooren, H.M.; Geudens, N.; Verleden, S.E.; Demedts, M.G.; et al. Azithromycin Reduces Pulmonary Fibrosis in a Bleomycin Mouse Model. *Exp. Lung Res.* **2010**, *36*, 602–614. [CrossRef] [PubMed]
197. Kawamura, K.; Ichikado, K.; Yasuda, Y.; Anan, K.; Suga, M. Azithromycin for Idiopathic Acute Exacerbation of Idiopathic Pulmonary Fibrosis: A Retrospective Single-Center Study. *BMC Pulm. Med.* **2017**, *17*, 94. [CrossRef]
198. Xu, Y.; Tai, W.; Qu, X.; Wu, W.; Li, Z.K.; Deng, S.; Vongphouttha, C.; Dong, Z. Rapamycin Protects against Paraquat-Induced Pulmonary Fibrosis: Activation of Nrf2 Signaling Pathway. *Biochem. Biophys. Res. Commun.* **2017**, *490*, 535–540. [CrossRef] [PubMed]

199. Yan, B.; Ma, Z.; Shi, S.; Hu, Y.; Ma, T.; Rong, G.; Yang, J. Sulforaphane Prevents Bleomycin-Induced Pulmonary Fibrosis in Mice by Inhibiting Oxidative Stress via Nuclear Factor Erythroid 2-Related Factor-2 Activation. *Mol. Med. Rep.* **2017**, *15*, 4005–4014. [CrossRef]
200. Liu, Y.; Lu, F.; Kang, L.; Wang, Z.; Wang, Y. Pirfenidone Attenuates Bleomycin-Induced Pulmonary Fibrosis in Mice by Regulating Nrf2/Bach1 Equilibrium. *BMC Pulm. Med.* **2017**, *17*, 63. [CrossRef]
201. Tang, H.; Gao, L.; Mao, J.; He, H.; Liu, J.; Cai, X.; Lin, H.; Wu, T. Salidroside Protects against Bleomycin-Induced Pulmonary Fibrosis: Activation of Nrf2-Antioxidant Signaling, and Inhibition of NF-KB and TGF-B1/Smad-2/-3 Pathways. *Cell Stress Chaperones* **2016**, *21*, 239–249. [CrossRef]
202. Liu, M.; Xu, H.; Zhang, L.; Zhang, C.; Yang, L.; Ma, E.; Liu, L.; Li, Y. Salvianolic Acid B Inhibits Myofibroblast Transdifferentiation in Experimental Pulmonary Fibrosis via the Up-Regulation of Nrf2. *Biochem. Biophys. Res. Commun.* **2018**, *495*, 325–331. [CrossRef] [PubMed]
203. Zhao, H.; Qin, H.Y.; Cao, L.F.; Chen, Y.H.; Tan, Z.X.; Zhang, C.; Xu, D.X. Phenylbutyric Acid Inhibits Epithelial-Mesenchymal Transition during Bleomycin-Induced Lung Fibrosis. *Toxicol. Lett.* **2015**, *232*, 213–220. [CrossRef]
204. Griese, M.; Kappler, M.; Eismann, C.; Ballmann, M.; Junge, S.; Rietschel, E.; Van Koningsbruggen-Rietschel, S.; Staab, D.; Rolinck-Werninghaus, C.; Mellies, U.; et al. Inhalation Treatment with Glutathione in Patients with Cystic Fibrosis: A Randomized Clinical Trial. *Am. J. Respir. Crit. Care Med.* **2013**, *188*, 83–89. [CrossRef]
205. Kariya, C.; Leitner, H.; Min, E.; Van Heeckeren, C.; Van Heeckeren, A.; Day, B.J. A Role for CFTR in the Elevation of Glutathione Levels in the Lung by Oral Glutathione Administration. *Am. J. Physiol.-Lung Cell. Mol. Physiol.* **2007**, *292*, 1590–1597. [CrossRef]
206. Conrad, C.; Lymp, J.; Thompson, V.; Dunn, C.; Davies, Z.; Chatfield, B.; Nichols, D.; Clancy, J.; Vender, R.; Egan, M.E.; et al. Long-Term Treatment with Oral N-Acetylcysteine: Affects Lung Function but Not Sputum Inflammation in Cystic Fibrosis Subjects. A Phase II Randomized Placebo-Controlled Trial. *J. Cyst. Fibros.* **2015**, *14*, 219–227. [CrossRef]
207. Niki, E. Evidence for Beneficial Effects of Vitamin E. *Korean J. Intern. Med.* **2015**, *30*, 571–579. [CrossRef] [PubMed]
208. Sagel, S.D.; Khan, U.; Jain, R.; Graff, G.; Daines, C.L.; Dunitz, J.M.; Borowitz, D.; Orenstein, D.M.; Abdulhamid, I.; Noe, J.; et al. Effects of an Antioxidant-Enriched Multivitamin in Cystic Fibrosis. *Am. J. Respir. Crit. Care Med.* **2018**, *198*, 639–647. [CrossRef]
209. Harding, H.P.; Zeng, H.; Zhang, Y.; Jungries, R.; Chung, P.; Plesken, H.; Sabatini, D.D.; Ron, D. Diabetes Mellitus and Exocrine Pancreatic Dysfunction in Perk-/- Mice Reveals a Role for Translational Control in Secretory Cell Survival. *Mol. Cell* **2001**, *7*, 1153–1163. [CrossRef]
210. Zhang, K.; Wong, H.N.; Song, B.; Miller, C.N.; Scheuner, D.; Kaufman, R.J. The Unfolded Protein Response Sensor IRE1α Is Required at 2 Distinct Steps in B Cell Lymphopoiesis. *J. Clin. Investig.* **2005**, *115*, 268–281. [CrossRef]
211. Lee, A.H.; Chu, G.C.; Iwakoshi, N.N.; Glimcher, L.H. XBP-1 Is Required for Biogenesis of Cellular Secretory Machinery of Exocrine Glands. *EMBO J.* **2005**, *24*, 4368–4380. [CrossRef]
212. Reimold, A.M.; Etkin, A.; Clauss, I.; Perkins, A.; Friend, D.S.; Zhang, J.; Horton, H.F.; Scott, A.; Orkin, S.H.; Byrne, M.C.; et al. An Essential Role in Liver Development for Transcription Factor XBP-1. *Genes Dev.* **2000**, *14*, 152–157. [CrossRef] [PubMed]
213. Liu, S.H.; Yang, C.C.; Chan, D.C.; Wu, C.T.; Chen, L.P.; Huang, J.W.; Hung, K.Y.; Chiang, C.K. Chemical Chaperon 4-Phenylbutyrate Protects against the Endoplasmic Reticulum Stress-Mediated Renal Fibrosis in Vivo and in Vitro. *Oncotarget* **2016**, *7*, 22116–22127. [CrossRef] [PubMed]
214. Tanaka, Y.; Ishitsuka, Y.; Hayasaka, M.; Yamada, Y.; Miyata, K.; Endo, M.; Kondo, Y.; Moriuchi, H.; Irikura, M.; Tanaka, K.I.; et al. The Exacerbating Roles of CCAAT/Enhancer-Binding Protein Homologous Protein (CHOP) in the Development of Bleomycin-Induced Pulmonary Fibrosis and the Preventive Effects of Tauroursodeoxycholic Acid (TUDCA) against Pulmonary Fibrosis in Mice. *Pharmacol. Res.* **2015**, *99*, 52–62. [CrossRef] [PubMed]
215. Rani, S.; Sreenivasaiah, P.K.; Kim, J.O.; Lee, M.Y.; Kang, W.S.; Kim, Y.S.; Ahn, Y.; Park, W.J.; Cho, C.; Kim, D.H. Tauroursodeoxycholic Acid (TUDCA) Attenuates Pressure Overload-Induced Cardiac Remodeling by Reducing Endoplasmic Reticulum Stress. *PLoS ONE* **2017**, *12*, e0176071. [CrossRef] [PubMed]

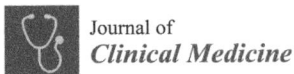

Article

Alpha-1 Antitrypsin Screening in a Selected Cohort of Patients Affected by Chronic Pulmonary Diseases in Naples, Italy

Anna Annunziata [1,*], Ilaria Ferrarotti [2], Antonietta Coppola [1], Maurizia Lanza [1], Pasquale Imitazione [1], Sara Spinelli [1], Pierpaolo Di Micco [3] and Giuseppe Fiorentino [1]

1. Unit of Respiratory Physiopathology, Department of Critic Area, Monaldi Hospital, 80131 Naples, Italy; antonietta.coppola84@gmail.com (A.C.); maurizia.lanza85@gmail.com (M.L.); pasqualeimitazione@gmail.com (P.I.); spinelli.sara@outlook.it (S.S.); giuseppefiorentino1@gmail.com (G.F.)
2. Center for Diagnosis of Inherited Alpha1-Antitrypsin Deficiency, Pneumology Unit, Department of Internal Medicine and Therapeutics, IRCCS San Matteo Hospital Foundation, University of Pavia, 27100 Pavia, Italy; i.ferrarotti@smatteo.pv.it
3. Department of Medicine, Buon Consiglio Fatebenefratelli Hospital of Naples, 80128 Naples, Italy; pdimicco@libero.it
* Correspondence: anna.annunziata@gmail.com

Abstract: Introduction. Alpha-1 antitrypsin deficiency (AATD) is a genetic condition associated with several respiratory diseases in patients with severe protein deficiency. AATD is often late diagnosed or underdiagnosed. Diagnosis frequently occurs in patients with chronic obstructive pulmonary disease and emphysema characterized by frequent exacerbations and over ten years' duration. The purpose of this study was to evaluate the incidence of alpha-1 antitrypsin deficiency in patients with the chronic pulmonary disease after a thorough screening in the city of Naples in southern Italy. Materials and methods. Two hundred patients suffering from respiratory pathology (chronic obstructive pulmonary disease (COPD), emphysema, asthma, or bronchiectasis) were examined and evaluated in our outpatients' clinic and tested for serum levels of AAT. Patients who had a respiratory disease suspected of AATD and/or serum AAT < 120 mg/dL underwent genetic testing. Genetic screening was performed on samples from 141 patients. Results. A total of 36 patients had an intermediate deficiency of AAT levels. Among them, 8 were PI*MZ, 6 were PI*MS and 22 had rare pathological mutations. Five patients had a severe AATD, all were composite heterozygous with S or Z allele, while the other allele had a rare pathological mutation. Conclusions. The incidence of genetic defects as AATD in the population of patients affected by chronic respiratory disorders is always a matter of discussion because of the frequent interaction between genes and environmental causes. In our series, numerous rare variants and compound heterozygosity have been described. No homozygous patients have been described. The present is one of few studies available on the incidence of rare variants in the geographic area of the city of Naples. So, our results could be considered interesting not only to know the incidence of AATD and its related rare mutations but also to support early diagnosis and treatments for patients with chronic pulmonary disease and frequent exacerbation and to fight the association with environmental causes of pulmonary damages as smoking.

Keywords: alpha1 antitrypsin deficiency; chronic obstructive pulmonary disease; bronchiectasis; asthma; emphysema

Citation: Annunziata, A.; Ferrarotti, I.; Coppola, A.; Lanza, M.; Imitazione, P.; Spinelli, S.; Micco, P.D.; Fiorentino, G. Alpha-1 Antitrypsin Screening in a Selected Cohort of Patients Affected by Chronic Pulmonary Diseases in Naples, Italy. *J. Clin. Med.* **2021**, *10*, 1546. https://doi.org/10.3390/jcm10081546

Academic Editor: Francisco Dasí

Received: 14 February 2021
Accepted: 31 March 2021
Published: 7 April 2021

Publisher's Note: MDPI stays neutral with regard to jurisdictional claims in published maps and institutional affiliations.

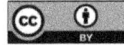

Copyright: © 2021 by the authors. Licensee MDPI, Basel, Switzerland. This article is an open access article distributed under the terms and conditions of the Creative Commons Attribution (CC BY) license (https://creativecommons.org/licenses/by/4.0/).

1. Introduction

Alpha-1 antitrypsin (AAT) is a circulating glycoprotein, and its main function is to inhibit neutrophil elastase and other serine proteases in blood and tissues [1–3].

AAT is the most prevalent protease inhibitor in human serum (90–200 mg/dL), and it is also coded as SERPINA1 (serine protease inhibitor, group A, member 1) gene. AAT deficiency (AATD) was first identified in 1963 by Laurell and Eriksson. From a clinical point of view, the absence of the AAT in the alpha-1 electrophoresis band was observed in patients who had developed emphysema at a young age [4].

Epidemiologically, AATD deficiency is a relatively common genetic disorder [5,6]. In a study compiling data from 97 countries, approximately 190 million cases of AATD were estimated out of a total population of 5.2 billion or a prevalence of about 3.6% [7]. Of these 190 million estimated cases of AATD, approximately 75% will have a mild deficiency that does not increase their risk of the onset of the clinical disease. Serum protein deficiency can be severe when both alleles are pathological, or intermediate when one of the two alleles is pathological. The serological decrease may be due to genetic alteration. AATD is an autosomal codominant genetic condition that mainly affects Caucasians of European heritage due to the presence of a deficient allele that could be identified as S allele or Z allele according to the type of genetic mutation. Of the remaining 25%, almost all (24%) are heterozygous with one normal allele (M) and one deficient allele (S or Z). There are data of increased disease risk in the presence of these mutations. The SZ (0.7%) phenotype and the ZZ (0.1%) genotypes have a well-documented increase in their risk of AATD-associated diseases [7]. Furthermore, although S and Z are the most common mutations, 150 different mutations of SERPINA1 have been reported [8,9].

Currently, the World Health Organization, the American Thoracic Society, and the European Respiratory Society recommend screening for AATD in patients suffering from the chronic obstructive pulmonary disease (COPD), emphysema, bronchiectasis and asthma. The clinical course of the following respiratory diseases in homozygous patients with AATD is severe [10]. Typically, patients show an early onset of COPD and emphysema in adults and liver disease. Less frequently, AAT deficiency is associated with asthma, systemic vasculitis, neutrophilic panniculitis, and other inflammatory, autoimmune and neoplastic diseases.

Some individuals with genetic variants manifest overt clinical diseases, while others have only minor symptoms [11,12]. Often the diagnosis is made in patients with COPD and emphysema with frequent exacerbations of over 10 years duration. Of course, early diagnosis of these patients could be beneficial to improve the outcome and also to provide additional motivation for smoking cessation and avoidance of second-hand smoke, which could reduce the risk of lung damage. Diagnosis of AATD could also provide an additional avenue for treatment of lung dysfunction with AAT replacement therapy. The first step in diagnosing AATD is the measurement of AAT level in plasma or serum. This is a simple, inexpensive, and widely available test. AAT level can be determined by radial immunodiffusion, nephelometry, or turbidimetry. Currently, the preferred method is nephelometry, because radial immunodiffusion tends to overestimate the AAT concentration [13]. The reference range for serum AAT concentrations in adults is usually 90–200 mg/dL, corresponding to 20–60 μmol/dL. Sensitive, specific quantification of plasma AAT by immunoturbidimetry or nephelometry is followed by isoelectric focusing to determine the phenotypic variants and/or by genotyping. Phenotyping and genotyping are carried out by only a few specialized laboratories. Homozygous or compound heterozygous patients generally have a severely deficient serum level, <50 mg/dL; heterozygotes, depending on the different mutations, may have a serum level of alpha 1 antitrypsin, sometimes even higher than 90 mg/dL. The clinical significance of these intermediate levels of AAT has always been debated.

Yet, AATD remains underdiagnosed, despite the recommendations of international health organizations for broader screening. So, the purpose of this study is to evaluate the incidence of AATD in a cohort of 200 patients in our specialist outpatients' clinic for pulmonary diseases in the geographic area of the city of Naples in Southern Italy.

2. Materials and Methods

From October 2018 to May 2019, 200 patients who were examined in our clinic (Division of Respiratory Physiopathology, Monaldi Hospital, Naples, Italy) for various respiratory diseases were also screened for serum AAT and the C-reactive protein.

The patients suffered from one of the following conditions for at least five years: COPD, emphysema, asthma, bronchiectasis of unknown etiology, or obstructive sleep apnea syndrome with persistent diurnal dyspnea.

Familial anamnesis was negative for AATD in first degree relatives, and all patients never measured their serum AAT levels before this study.

All patients quantified plasma AAT by nephelometry. Patients who had a suspected clinical picture associated with serum AAT levels <120 mg/dL with normal C-reactive protein (normal value < 1) underwent further testing. These patients performed high-resolution CT lung scan.

Furthermore, samples underwent subjected qualitative analysis of the SERPINA1 gene and AAT protein by the specialized Center in Pavia [14].

3. Results

Out of 200 pulmonary patients screened, 141 were found to have alpha1-antitrypsin (AAT) levels less than 120 mg/dL and were subjected to isoelectric focusing for phenotyping of the most common variants and genotyping, while 41 patients presented mutations of the SERPINA1 gene. The mean age of the 41 patients was 56.6 ± 15.7 years old. The majority of these patients were non-smokers (51.0%) and former smokers (46%). Only one patient was an active smoker.

After the clinical evaluation, the high-resolution CT lung scan showed no findings in 12 patients (29%). Most of the patients with CT abnormalities showed evidence of emphysema (46% panlobular and 17% centrilobular) or other pathological findings. The most common clinical pictures were emphysema (44%) and COPD (39%); bronchiectasis was also found in six patients (14.6%), while pulmonary fibrosis in two patients (2.8%). Some patients had multiple pathological findings together (Table 1).

Table 1. Patients' characteristics. Out of 200 pulmonary patients screened, 141 were found to have alpha1-antitrypsin (AAT) levels less than 120 mg/dL and were subjected to isoelectric focusing for phenotyping of the most common variants and genotyping, while 41 patients presented mutations of the SERPINA1 gene. The demographics and patient characteristics of these 41 patients are listed in this table. COPD = chronic obstructive pulmonary disease; CT = computed tomography.

Female/Male, n (%)	15/26 (36.5%/63.5%)
Age (years, mean ± SD)	56.6 ± 15.7
Smoking History	
Active Smokers, n (%)	1 (2.4%)
Former Smokers, n (%)	19 (46.3%)
Never Smokers, n (%)	21 (51.0%)
Clinical pattern	
Dyspnea, n (%)	4 (9.7%)
COPD, n (%)	16 (39.0%)
Bronchiectasis, n (%)	1 (2.4%)
Asthma, n (%)	3 (7.0%)
Emphysema, n (%)	18 (44%)
CT Features	
No findings, n (%)	12 (29.0%)
Panlobular Emphysema, n (%)	19 (46.0%)
Centrilobular Emphysema, n (%)	7 (17.0%)
Bronchiectasis, n (%)	6 (14.6%)
Fibrosis, n (%)	2 (2.8%)

A total of 141 patients had serum levels of AAT < 120 mg/dL and were subjected to qualitative analysis. Among them, 36 showed an intermediate deficiency of AAT and five showed a severe deficiency of AAT. Subgroup analysis was performed for these 41 patients. Most of them showed an intermediate deficit of AAT with a mean value of 86.37

+/− 16.46 mg/dL, while the average serum AAT level in patients with the severe deficit was 49.50 +/− 31.02 mg/dL. Twelve patients had a serum alpha 1 antitrypsin value greater than 90 mg/dL, the maximum value was 119 mg/dL in two patients. No differences were found in other laboratory values as C reactive protein.

Molecular analysis was conducted on 141 patients with AAT < 120 mg/dL. Of them, 41 were heterozygous or compound heterozygous for pathological mutations of the SERPINA1 gene, as reported in Figure 1. Commonly, the M allele is the most common allele and is associated with normal serum levels of AAT. The S allele produces moderate levels of AAT, and the Z allele produces very little AAT. The genotype PI*MS is associated with AAT levels about 80% of normal, while PI*MZ is associated with levels ≈50–70% of normal. The rare alleles determine a variable serum level depending on the variant of AAT.

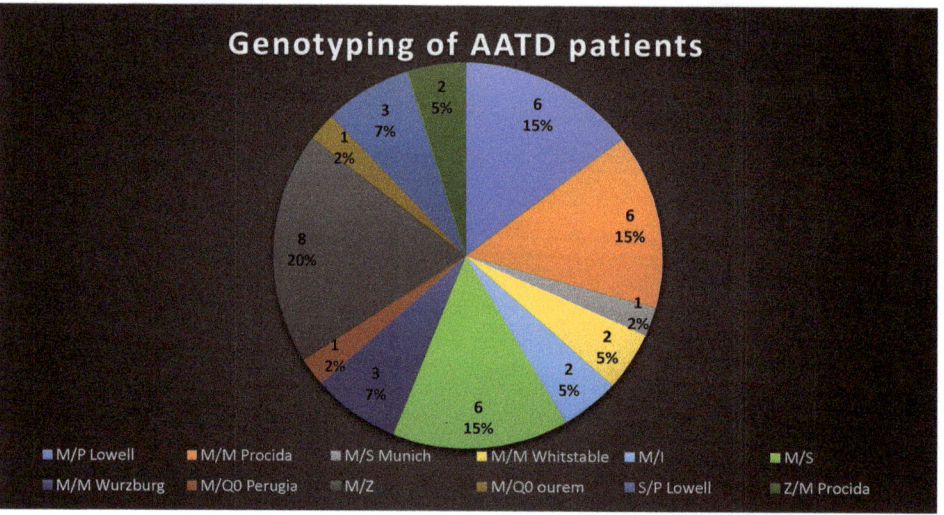

Figure 1. Genotyping of alpha-1 antitrypsin deficiency (AATD) patients. Samples from 41 patients with intermediate or low levels of AAT were subjected to genotyping, and the mutations identified are shown in this table.

Among 36 patients that showed an intermediate deficiency of AAT, 8 showed genotype PI*MZ and 6 showed PI*MS, while 22 showed other genotypes.

Six patients carried the mutation P_{lowell} [15]. These patients had emphysema and COPD. Six patients were identified with the mutation $M_{procida}$ [16]; these patients were affected by COPD, obstructive sleep apnea syndrome, and fibromyalgia. One COPD patients had the mutation S_{munich} [17]. Three patients with emphysema had $M_{Wurzburg}$ mutation [18]. Two patients had the mutation $M_{Whitestable}$ [19]: one with pulmonary emphysema and the other with combined emphysema and pulmonary fibrosis pattern. Two patients were heterozygous for mutation I [20], and they had emphysema and bronchiectasis. One patient with COPD and lung cancer had the mutation $Q0_{ourem}$ [21] and one with respiratory failure and emphysema had the mutation $Q0_{perugia}$ [22] (Table 2).

Five patients had a severe AATD in serum (i.e., AAT levels <50 mg/dL).

4. Discussion

Alpha/1 antitrypsin deficiency is an autosomal codominant genetic condition that predisposes to the early onset of chronic pulmonary disease and liver disease. Even if AATD is one of the most widespread inherited diseases in Caucasian populations, identifying and diagnosing affected patients is still unsatisfactory, with only a minority of affected individuals being detected. Although WHO recommends that all patients with a diagnosis of COPD or adult-onset asthma should be tested [23], these recommendations are often disregarded [24]. Accurate and complete identification of the AATD geno/phenotype is clinically fundamental when deciding on potential treatment options for individual patients [25]. Methodological advances have facilitated the more widespread application of rapid, convenient, and cost-effective AATD tests, leading to an increase in the number of individual diagnosed with the disorder [26]. Laboratory diagnosis of AATD currently consists of serum biochemical analysis to evaluate protein deficiency and electrophoretic abnormalities, as well as genetic analysis to identify gene variants responsible for the protein deficiency [14].

Table 2. The M allele is the most common, and homozygosity (MM) is associated with normal alpha1-antitrypsin levels. The S, Z, and rare alleles are associated with varying degrees of AAT deficiency. The AAT variants are indicated with the corresponding mutation, the consequent anomaly, and the clinical data detected in our population.

Variant Name	Mutation	Consequences	Clinical Manifestation
Z	Glu 342 > Lys c. 1096G > A	Polymerization, decreased inhibitory activity; protein deficiency	Emphysema, COPD
S	Glu 264 > Val c. 863A > T	increased turnover; decreased inhibitory activity; mild protein deficiency	Emphysema, Asthma
P$_{Lowell}$	Asp 256 > Val c. 839A > T	Polymerization, degraded in liver cells; protein deficiency	Emphysema, COPD
M$_{Procida}$	Leu 41 > Pro c.194T > C	Intracellular proteolysis, decreased inhibitory activity; protein deficiency	COPD, Asthma
S$_{Munich}$	Ser330Phe c. 1061C > T	Mild protein deficiency	COPD
M$_{Whitstable}$	Intron mutation, 26 bp detection and 2 bp insertion in intron IV	Truncated protein, protein deficiency	Emphysema and fibrosis
I	Arg 39 > Cys c. 187C > T	Polymerization, slightly decreased inhibitory activity; mild protein deficiency	Emphysema, bronchiectasis
M$_{Wurzburg}$	Pro369Ser c. 1177C > T	Degradation, protein deficiency	Emphysema
Q0$_{Perugia}$	Val239→ DelG→STOP CODON241 V239GTG−delG > T ter241TGA	No detectable protein	Emphysema
Q0$_{ourem}$	IVS1C + 1G→A exon5L352TTA, insT > Ter376TGA	No detectable protein	COPD, Lung cancer

The first step in diagnosing AATD is the quantitative test to determine the AAT concentration in plasma. It is a simple, inexpensive, and widely available test in most biochemical laboratories [27]. To interpret the result of an isolated quantitative determination, it must be considered that AAT is also an acute phase reactant. Therefore, infectious or inflammatory processes increase levels of AAT and give false normal or high values in patients with moderate deficiency. High levels of serum AAT during pregnancy and after the consumption of oral contraceptives have also been reported [28].

Indeed, the World Health Organization, the American Thoracic Society, and the European Respiratory Society recommend screening for AATD in patients with recurrent re-exacerbation pulmonary diseases and to test AAT level in a different moment from acute infection/inflammation. For the current study, 120 mg/dL accompanied by clinical evidence of lung disease was used as the decisional value to suspect AATD to address patients for further testing.

According to this selection, several SERPINA1 genotypes with different clinical features have been described. Nevertheless, the measurement of protein levels can identify patients with protein deficiency, but it cannot differentiate between the various AATD genetic subtypes. Therefore, molecular analysis of the AAT gene is the reference method to identify allelic variants.

Among 200 patients screened, 141 had AAT levels <120 mg/dL and underwent genetic testing. Of these, 36 (25.5%) were found to have an intermediate deficiency, and five (3.5%) were found to have severe AATD. This incidence is slightly higher than recent data based on the case-finding program in COPD in Spain, Ireland, and Argentina [29–31], but it is lower than those reported in the German population [32]. Therefore, since South Italy is a low AATD prevalence area, the frequencies of intermediate and severe AATD reported in the present study is higher than expected, thus supporting the correct approach in selecting patients for AATD testing.

The most prevalent SERPINA1 genotypes in the general Italian population were MS and MZ (5.8% and 1.5%, respectively) [16]. Accordingly, in the current study on patients with chronic pulmonary disease, MS and MZ mutations were the most common genotypes at 3.0% and 4.0% of the screened population and 14.6% and 19.0% of the population with reduced AAT, respectively [33].

PI*SS and PI*ZZ genotypes together are further rare pathological mutations that have a prevalence of 0.1% in the general population. Moreover, a study on the Italian population showed that the rare AATD variants displayed a different geographic distribution, peaking in some regions, for example in Sardinia. The authors also considered that the nomenclature of many rare AATD variants reflects their probable southern Italian origin (e.g., MProcida, MPalermo, Q0isola di Procida, Q0trastevere) [34]. Furthermore, concerning the distribution of rare mutations, another study focused on a North Italian area known to have a high incidence of AATD, showed that the prevalence of combined rare mutations was 0.5% [35].

As expected, we found a relative main difference in the distribution of AATD in the general population with a high incidence of AATD. In fact, in this study, in our cohort of 200 pulmonary patients, the prevalence in the overall patient population was 9.0%. Of course, the patients who were screened were selected patients with chronic pulmonary disease, and so this would explain the difference with the general population. A further selection analyzing patients with AAT levels <120 mg/dL found a combined global incidence of 20% (i.e., including MS, MZ and other rare alleles).

The main findings of our study are the high incidence of AATD in a selected cohort of patients tested in a specialist division of pulmonary disease as far as the identification of a considerable number of rare mutations causing AATD. Actually, there are only a few case reports on Italian cohorts [36,37], and this is the first report that looked for the prevalence of AATD in the geographic area of the city of Naples in Southern Italy.

From a clinical point of view, although the clinical condition most frequently associated with AATD is pulmonary emphysema [25], there are little data on the clinical presentation of rare mutations. In our study, patients with rare mutations showed frequently asthma and bronchiectasis as a main clinical feature.

Finally, our screening program enables us to diagnose a great number of rare mutations among patients with AATD, 27 rare alleles out of a total of 40 AAT alleles (67.5%), thus supporting the importance of an accurate molecular diagnosis that does not limit the testing to the S and Z variant. A recent paper showed a high prevalence of M_{malton} mutation in a small Italian cohort of patients admitted to the outpatient lung clinic in Parma [38]. In the present paper, we detected even eight different variants ($M_{procida}$, P_{lowell}, I, $M_{whitstable}$, Q0$_{ourèm}$, S_{munich}, $M_{wurzburg}$, Q0$_{peerugia}$). This finding enables us to speculate about the genetic inhomogeneity of the Neapolitan population, which was historically submitted to migratory and conquest movements.

Further larger studies are needed to give improved information not only from an epidemiological point of view but also regarding the outcome of this clinical setting, in particular on our geographic area. For this objective, it should be fundamental to approach, as in our study, clinical data together with radiological findings and genetic screening to better understand the gene–environmental interactions and their influence on the clinical outcome.

Author Contributions: Conceptualization, A.A., I.F., A.C., P.I., S.S. and G.F.; methodology, A.A., I.F., A.C., M.L., G.F.; validation A.A., I.F., A.C. and P.D.M.; formal analysis, A.A., A.C. and M.L.; investigation, A.A., I.F., A.C., P.I., S.S. and G.F.; data curation, A.A., I.F., A.C., P.I., S.S., G.F. and P.D.M.; writing—original draft preparation, A.A., I.F., A.C., P.I., S.S. and G.F.; writing—review and editing, A.A., I.F., A.C., M.L., P.I., P.D.M. and G.F.; visualization, A.A., I.F., A.C., M.L., P.I. and S.S.; supervision, M.L., P.D.M. and G.F.; project administration, A.A., I.F., A.C., M.L., P.I., S.S., P.D.M. and G.F.; All authors have read and agree to the published version of the manuscript.

Funding: This research received no external funding.

Institutional Review Board Statement: The study was conducted according to the guidelines of the Declaration of Helsinki, and approved by the Institutional Review Board Università degli Studi della Campania "Luigi Vanvitelli" e Azienda Ospedaliera dei Colli, approval number 0016428/2019, 27 July 2019.

Informed Consent Statement: Informed consent was obtained from all subjects involved in the study.

Data Availability Statement: Data is contained within the article.

Acknowledgments: We thank Luisa, Anita, Silvana and Teresa for their support.

Conflicts of Interest: Authors declare no conflict of interest.

References

1. Ohlsson, K. Neutral Leucocyte Proteases and Elastase Inhibited by Plasma Alpha 1-Antitrypsin. *Scand. J. Clin. Lab. Investig.* **1971**, *28*, 251–253. [CrossRef]
2. Beatty, K.; Bieth, J.; Travis, J. Kinetics of Association of Serine Proteinases with Native and Oxidized Alpha-1-Proteinase Inhibitor and Alpha-1-Antichymotrypsin. *J. Biol. Chem.* **1980**, *255*, 3931–3934. [CrossRef]
3. Rao, N.V.; Wehner, N.G.; Marshall, B.C.; Gray, W.R.; Gray, B.H.; Hoidal, J.R. Characterization of Proteinase-3 (PR-3), a Neutrophil Serine Proteinase. Structural and Functional Properties. *J. Biol. Chem.* **1991**, *266*, 9540–9548. [CrossRef]
4. Laurell, C.-B.; Eriksson, S. The Electrophoretic A1-Globulin Pattern of Serum in A1-Antitrypsin Deficiency. 1963. *COPD* **2013**, *10* (Suppl. 1), 3–8. [CrossRef] [PubMed]
5. Bornhorst, J.A.; Calderon, F.R.O.; Procter, M.; Tang, W.; Ashwood, E.R.; Mao, R. Genotypes and Serum Concentrations of Human Alpha-1-Antitrypsin "P" Protein Variants in a Clinical Population. *J. Clin. Pathol.* **2007**, *60*, 1124–1128. [CrossRef]
6. Abboud, R.T.; Nelson, T.N.; Jung, B.; Mattman, A. Alpha1-Antitrypsin Deficiency: A Clinical-Genetic Overview. *Appl. Clin. Genet.* **2011**, *4*, 55–65. [CrossRef]
7. de Serres, F.J.; Blanco, I. Prevalence of A1-Antitrypsin Deficiency Alleles PI*S and PI*Z Worldwide and Effective Screening for Each of the Five Phenotypic Classes PI*MS, PI*MZ, PI*SS, PI*SZ, and PI*ZZ: A Comprehensive Review. *Ther. Adv. Respir. Dis.* **2012**, *6*, 277–295. [CrossRef]
8. Ottaviani, S.; Barzon, V.; Buxens, A.; Gorrini, M.; Larruskain, A.; El Hamss, R.; Balderacchi, A.M.; Corsico, A.G.; Ferrarotti, I. Molecular Diagnosis of Alpha1-Antitrypsin Deficiency: A New Method Based on Luminex Technology. *J. Clin. Lab. Anal.* **2020**, *34*, e23279. [CrossRef]
9. Giacopuzzi, E.; Laffranchi, M.; Berardelli, R.; Ravasio, V.; Ferrarotti, I.; Gooptu, B.; Borsani, G.; Fra, A. Real-World Clinical Applicability of Pathogenicity Predictors Assessed on SERPINA1 Mutations in Alpha-1-Antitrypsin Deficiency. *Hum. Mutat.* **2018**, *39*, 1203–1213. [CrossRef]
10. American Thoracic Society; European Respiratory Society. American Thoracic Society/European Respiratory Society Statement: Standards for the Diagnosis and Management of Individuals with Alpha-1 Antitrypsin Deficiency. *Am. J. Respir. Crit. Care Med.* **2003**, *168*, 818–900. [CrossRef]
11. Stoller, J.K.; Aboussouan, L.S. A Review of A1-Antitrypsin Deficiency. *Am. J. Respir. Crit. Care Med.* **2012**, *185*, 246–259. [CrossRef]
12. de Serres, F.; Blanco, I. Role of Alpha-1 Antitrypsin in Human Health and Disease. *J. Intern. Med.* **2014**, *276*, 311–335. [CrossRef]
13. Brantly, M.L.; Wittes, J.T.; Vogelmeier, C.F.; Hubbard, R.C.; Fells, G.A.; Crystal, R.G. Use of a Highly Purified Alpha 1-Antitrypsin Standard to Establish Ranges for the Common Normal and Deficient Alpha 1-Antitrypsin Phenotypes. *Chest* **1991**, *100*, 703–708. [CrossRef] [PubMed]
14. Ferrarotti, I.; Ottaviani, S. Laboratory diagnosis. In α_1-*Antitrypsin Deficiency (ERS Monograph)*; Strnad, P., Brantly, M.L., Bals, R., Eds.; European Respiratory Society: Sheffield, UK, 2019; pp. 39–51. [CrossRef]
15. Faber, J.P.; Weidinger, S.; Olek, K. Sequence Data of the Rare Deficient Alpha 1-Antitrypsin Variant PI Zaugsburg. *Am. J. Hum. Genet.* **1990**, *46*, 1158–1162.
16. Takahashi, H.; Nukiwa, T.; Satoh, K.; Ogushi, F.; Brantly, M.; Fells, G.; Stier, L.; Courtney, M.; Crystal, R.G. Characterization of the Gene and Protein of the Alpha 1-Antitrypsin "Deficiency" Allele Mprocida. *J. Biol. Chem.* **1988**, *263*, 15528–15534. [CrossRef]
17. Faber, J.P.; Poller, W.; Weidinger, S.; Kirchgesser, M.; Schwaab, R.; Bidlingmaier, F.; Olek, K. Identification and DNA Sequence Analysis of 15 New Alpha 1-Antitrypsin Variants, Including Two PI*Q0 Alleles and One Deficient PI*M Allele. *Am. J. Hum. Genet.* **1994**, *55*, 1113–1121.

18. Poller, W.; Merklein, F.; Schneider-Rasp, S.; Haack, A.; Fechner, H.; Wang, H.; Anagnostopoulos, I.; Weidinger, S. Molecular Characterisation of the Defective Alpha 1-Antitrypsin Alleles PI Mwurzburg (Pro369Ser), Mheerlen (Pro369Leu), and Q0lisbon (Thr68Ile). *Eur. J. Hum. Genet. EJHG* **1999**, *7*, 321–331. [CrossRef]
19. Ambrose, H.J.; Chambers, S.M.; Mieli-Vergani, G.; Ferrie, R.; Newton, C.R.; Robertson, N.H. Molecular Characterization of a New Alpha-1-Antitrypsin M Variant Allele, Mwhitstable: Implications for DNA-Based Diagnosis. *Diagn. Mol. Pathol. Am. J. Surg. Pathol. Part B* **1999**, *8*, 205–210. [CrossRef]
20. Graham, A.; Kalsheker, N.A.; Newton, C.R.; Bamforth, F.J.; Powell, S.J.; Markham, A.F. Molecular Characterisation of Three Alpha-1-Antitrypsin Deficiency Variants: Proteinase Inhibitor (Pi) Nullcardiff (Asp256—Val); PiMmalton (Phe51—Deletion) and PiI (Arg39-Cys). *Hum. Genet.* **1989**, *84*, 55–58. [CrossRef] [PubMed]
21. Vaz Rodrigues, L.; Costa, F.; Marques, P.; Mendonça, C.; Rocha, J.; Seixas, S. Severe α-1 Antitrypsin Deficiency Caused by Q0(Ourém) Allele: Clinical Features, Haplotype Characterization and History. *Clin. Genet.* **2012**, *81*, 462–469. [CrossRef]
22. Ferrarotti, I.; Carroll, T.P.; Ottaviani, S.; Fra, A.M.; O'Brien, G.; Molloy, K.; Corda, L.; Medicina, D.; Curran, D.R.; McElvaney, N.G.; et al. Identification and Characterisation of Eight Novel SERPINA1 Null Mutations. *Orphanet J. Rare Dis.* **2014**, *9*, 172. [CrossRef]
23. Tsechkovski, M.; Boulyjenkov, V.; Heuck, C. Alpha 1-Antitrypsin Deficiency: Memorandum from a WHO Meeting. *Bull. World Health Organ.* **1997**, *75*, 397–415.
24. Greulich, T.; Weist, B.J.D.; Koczulla, A.R.; Janciauskiene, S.; Klemmer, A.; Lux, W.; Alter, P.; Vogelmeier, C.F. Prevalence of Comorbidities in COPD Patients by Disease Severity in a German Population. *Respir. Med.* **2017**, *132*, 132–138. [CrossRef]
25. Miravitlles, M.; Dirksen, A.; Ferrarotti, I.; Koblizek, V.; Lange, P.; Mahadeva, R.; McElvaney, N.G.; Parr, D.; Piitulainen, E.; Roche, N.; et al. European Respiratory Society Statement: Diagnosis and Treatment of Pulmonary Disease in A1-Antitrypsin Deficiency. *Eur. Respir. J.* **2017**, *50*. [CrossRef] [PubMed]
26. Balderacchi, A.M.; Barzon, V.; Ottaviani, S.; Corino, A.; Zorzetto, M.; Wencker, M.; Corsico, A.G.; Ferrarotti, I. Comparison of Different Algorithms in Laboratory Diagnosis of Alpha1-Antitrypsin Deficiency. *Clin. Chem. Lab. Med.* **2021**. [CrossRef]
27. Prinsen, J.H.; Schweisfurth, H.; Rasche, B.; Breuer, J. Comparison of Three Methods for the Determination of Serum Alpha-1-Antitrypsin in Patients with Pulmonary Diseases. *Clin. Physiol. Biochem.* **1989**, *7*, 198–202.
28. Lopes, A.P.; Mineiro, M.A.; Costa, F.; Gomes, J.; Santos, C.; Antunes, C.; Maia, D.; Melo, R.; Canotilho, M.; Magalhães, E.; et al. Portuguese Consensus Document for the Management of Alpha-1-Antitrypsin Deficiency. *Pulmonology* **2018**, *24* (Suppl. 1), 1–21. [CrossRef]
29. da Costa, C.H.; Noronha Filho, A.J.; Marques, E.; Silva, R.M.F.; da Cruz, T.F.; de Oliveira Monteiro, V.; Pio, M.; Rufino, R.L. Alpha 1-Antitrypsin Deficiency in Patients with Chronic Obstructive Pulmonary Disease Patients: Is Systematic Screening Necessary? *BMC Res. Notes* **2019**, *12*, 10. [CrossRef] [PubMed]
30. Menga, G.; Fernandez Acquier, M.; Echazarreta, A.L.; Sorroche, P.B.; Lorenzon, M.V.; Fernández, M.E.; Saez, M.S.; grupo de estudio DAAT.AR. Prevalence of Alpha-1 Antitrypsin Deficiency in COPD Patients in Argentina. The DAAT.AR Study. *Arch. Bronconeumol.* **2020**, *56*, 571–577. [CrossRef]
31. Carroll, T.P.; O'Connor, C.A.; Floyd, O.; McPartlin, J.; Kelleher, D.P.; O'Brien, G.; Dimitrov, B.D.; Morris, V.B.; Taggart, C.C.; McElvaney, N.G. The Prevalence of Alpha-1 Antitrypsin Deficiency in Ireland. *Respir. Res.* **2011**, *12*, 91. [CrossRef]
32. Veith, M.; Tüffers, J.; Peychev, E.; Klemmer, A.; Kotke, V.; Janciauskiene, S.; Wilhelm, S.; Bals, R.; Koczulla, A.R.; Vogelmeier, C.F.; et al. The Distribution of Alpha-1 Antitrypsin Genotypes Between Patients with COPD/Emphysema, Asthma and Bronchiectasis. *Int. J. Chron. Obstruct. Pulmon. Dis.* **2020**, *15*, 2827–2836. [CrossRef]
33. de Serres, F.J.; Blanco, I.; Fernández-Bustillo, E. Genetic Epidemiology of Alpha-1 Antitrypsin Deficiency in Southern Europe: France, Italy, Portugal and Spain. *Clin. Genet.* **2003**, *63*, 490–509. [CrossRef]
34. Ferrarotti, I.; Baccheschi, J.; Zorzetto, M.; Tinelli, C.; Corda, L.; Balbi, B.; Campo, I.; Pozzi, E.; Faa, G.; Coni, P.; et al. Prevalence and Phenotype of Subjects Carrying Rare Variants in the Italian Registry for Alpha1-Antitrypsin Deficiency. *J. Med. Genet.* **2005**, *42*, 282–287. [CrossRef]
35. Corda, L.; Medicina, D.; La Piana, G.E.; Bertella, E.; Moretti, G.; Bianchi, L.; Pinelli, V.; Savoldi, G.; Baiardi, P.; Facchetti, F.; et al. Population Genetic Screening for Alpha1-Antitrypsin Deficiency in a High-Prevalence Area. *Respir. Int. Rev. Thorac. Dis.* **2011**, *82*, 418–425. [CrossRef]
36. Mosella, M.; Accardo, M.; Molino, A.; Maniscalco, M.; Zamparelli, A.S. Description of a New Rare Alpha-1 Antitrypsin Mutation in Naples (Italy): PI*M S-Napoli. *Ann. Thorac. Med.* **2018**, *13*, 59–61. [CrossRef] [PubMed]
37. Annunziata, A.; Ferrarotti, I.; Lanza, M.; Cauteruccio, R.; Spirito, V.D.; Fiorentino, G. Alpha 1 antitrypsin deficiency and intermediate risk: The case of a heterozygote for the MWurzburg allele. *Ital. Rev. Respir. Dis.* **2020**, *35*, 115–117. [CrossRef]
38. Aiello, M.; Fantin, A.; Longo, C.; Ferrarotti, I.; Bertorelli, G.; Chetta, A. Clinical Manifestations in Patients with PI*MMMalton Genotypes. A Matter Still Unsolved in Alpha-1 Antitrypsin Deficiency. *Respirol. Case Rep.* **2020**, *8*, e00528. [CrossRef] [PubMed]

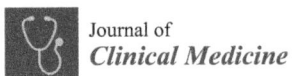

Article

Utility of Transient Elastography for the Screening of Liver Disease in Patients with Alpha1-Antitrypsin Deficiency

Mònica Pons [1,†], Alexa Núñez [2,3,†], Cristina Esquinas [2,3], María Torres-Durán [4], Juan Luis Rodríguez-Hermosa [5], Myriam Calle [5], Ramón Tubio-Pérez [4], Irene Belmonte [2], Francisco Rodríguez-Frías [6,7], Esther Rodríguez [2], Joan Genescà [1,7], Marc Miravitlles [2,3,8,*] and Miriam Barrecheguren [2]

1. Liver Unit, Department of Internal Medicine, Hospital Universitari Vall d'Hebron, Vall d'Hebron Institut de Recerca (VHIR), Vall d'Hebron Barcelona Hospital Campus, 08035 Barcelona, Spain; monica_xina@hotmail.com (M.P.); jgenesca@vhebron.net (J.G.)
2. Pneumology Department, Hospital Universitari Vall d'Hebron/Vall d'Hebron Institut de Recerca (VHIR), Vall d'Hebron Barcelona Hospital Campus, 08035 Barcelona, Spain; alexagnd01@hotmail.com (A.N.); crise4@hotmail.com (C.E.); irbelmu@gmail.com (I.B.); estherod@vhebron.net (E.R.); mbarrech@vhebron.net (M.B.)
3. Department of Medicine, Universitat Autònoma de Barcelona, 08193 Barcelona, Spain
4. Pneumology Department, University Hospital Complex of Vigo, Instituto de Investigación Biomédica Galicia Sur, 36213 Vigo, Spain; mtordur@yahoo.es (M.T.-D.); ramon.antonio.tubio.perez@sergas.es (R.T.-P.)
5. Pneumology Department, Instituto de Investigación Sanitaria del Hospital Clínico San Carlos (IdISSC), Hospital Clínico de San Carlos, Departamento de Medicina, Facultad de Medicina, Universidad Complutense de Madrid, 28040 Madrid, Spain; jlrhermosa@yahoo.es (J.L.R.-H.); mcallerubio@gmail.com (M.C.)
6. Department of Clinical Biochemistry, Hospital Universitari Vall d'Hebron, Vall d'Hebron Barcelona Hospital Campus, 08035 Barcelona, Spain; frarodri@gmail.com
7. Centro de Investigación Biomédica en Red de Enfermedades Hepáticas y Digestivas (CIBEREHD), 28029 Madrid, Spain
8. Centro de Investigación Biomédica en Red de Enfermedades Respiratorias (CIBERES), 28029 Madrid, Spain
* Correspondence: marcm@separ.es
† Both authors have contributed equally and should be considered first authors.

Abstract: Screening of liver disease in alpha-1 antitrypsin deficiency (AATD) is usually carried out with liver enzymes, with low sensitivity. We conducted a multicenter cross-sectional study aiming to describe the utility of transient elastography for the identification of liver disease in patients with AATD. A total of 148 AATD patients were included. Among these, 54.7% were Pi*ZZ and 45.3% were heterozygous for the Z allele. Between 4.9% and 16.5% of patients had abnormal liver enzymes, without differences among genotypes. Liver stiffness measurement (LSM) was significantly higher in Pi*ZZ individuals than in heterozygous Z (5.6 vs. 4.6 kPa; $p = 0.001$). In total, in 8 (5%) individuals LSM was >7.5 kPa, considered significant liver fibrosis, and $\geq$10 kPa in 3 (1.9%) all being Pi*ZZ. Elevated liver enzymes were more frequently observed in patients with LSM > 7.5 kPa, but in 5 out of 8 of these patients all liver enzymes were within normal range. In patients with AATD, the presence of abnormal liver enzymes is frequent; however, most of these patients do not present significant liver fibrosis. Transient elastography can help to identify patients with liver fibrosis even with normal liver enzymes and should be performed in all Z-allele carriers to screen for liver disease.

Keywords: alpha1-antitrypsin deficiency; liver disease; transient elastography

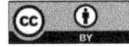

1. Introduction

Alpha1-antitrypsin deficiency (AATD) is caused by a specific mutation of the SER-PINA 1 gene which results in abnormal production and low circulating levels of alpha1-antitrypsin (AAT). It is one of the most common genetic diseases in adulthood and is associated with an increased risk of developing pulmonary emphysema and liver disease [1,2].

AAT is a protein synthesized and secreted mainly by hepatocytes, the main function of which is to protect lung tissue from damage caused by proteolytic enzymes such as neutrophil elastase [2]. AAT is a highly polymorphic protein with more than 120 variants, including about 60 deficient alleles. The normal allele, present in more than 95% of normal subjects, is called M [1,2]. The most frequent deficient alleles are S and Z, and they are found in 10% and 2% of the Spanish population, respectively [3–6].

The Z variant presents an alteration in its tertiary structure that facilitates misfolding of the protein and gives rise to the spontaneous formation of polymers, leading to the accumulation of the protein in the endoplasmic reticulum of the hepatocytes [7,8]. Liver damage is then caused by this protein accumulation, inducing apoptosis of the hepatocytes and a compensatory hepatocyte proliferation that eventually produces liver fibrosis that can evolve to cirrhosis or hepatocellular carcinoma [8,9]. Most patients with liver disease are homozygous for the deficient Z allele (Pi*ZZ), although different degrees of liver involvement have been described in heterozygotes (Pi*SZ and Pi*MZ), especially if associated with other co-factors such as alcohol consumption or metabolic syndrome [10,11].

Currently there is no non-invasive gold standard technique for the screening and early diagnosis of liver disease in patients with AATD [12]. In clinical practice, liver enzymes are routinely checked, while liver ultrasound is performed if necessary. However, it has been observed that transaminase levels have a low sensitivity to identify liver disease, and they correlate little with the degree of liver disease, especially in adulthood [13]. Serum biomarkers and image devices based on elastography technique have been developed to overcome this problem and to assess the presence of fibrosis in liver diseases of different etiologies [14,15].

Recently, there has been increasing interest in the use of elastographic methods, such as transient elastography, for screening liver disease in AATD patients [16–18]. However, the screening and management of asymptomatic liver disease in AATD can differ among centers due to a lack of consensus or guidelines. Therefore, the aim of our study was to describe the utility of transient elastography for the identification of liver disease in patients with AATD.

2. Materials and Methods

This was a multicenter cross-sectional study including patients older than 18 years with mild, moderate, and severe AATD (Pi*MS, SS, MZ, SZ, ZZ, and rare variants) consecutively recruited from the outpatient Pneumology Clinics of three AATD reference centers in Spain (Vall d'Hebron University Hospital, Barcelona, University Hospital Complex of Vigo, and Hospital Clínico San Carlos, Madrid) from 1 April 2017 to 1 January 2020. As part of the assessment of patients with AATD, all of them were offered blood analysis, full lung function tests, and transient elastography, and the only exclusion criterion was to refuse to sign informed consent. The study was approved by the Vall d'He- bron Hospital Ethics Committee (Barcelona, Spain), number PR(AG)335/2016, and all patients provided written informed consent.

2.1. Variables

During the first visit, a complete physical examination was performed in all patients with special interest in signs of chronic liver disease such as splenomegaly, jaundice, or palmar erythema. Sociodemographic and clinical characteristics were collected and other parameters such as body mass index (BMI), lung function tests (forced expiratory volume in the first second (FEV1), FEV1/forced ventilatory capacity (FVC), and carbon monoxide transfer coefficient (KCO)), comorbidities, treatments, and AAT augmentation therapy were reported. Diagnosis of chronic obstructive pulmonary disease (COPD) was established when the post-bronchodilator FEV1/FVC ratio was below 0.7.

Blood samples were obtained for determination of liver function tests: Aspartate aminotransferase (AST), alanine aminotransferase (ALT), gamma-glutamyl transferase (GGT), alkaline phosphatase (ALP), international normalized ratio (INR), platelet count, and albumin. In addition, the Fibrosis-4 (FIB-4) score was calculated as age (years) × AST [IU/L]/(platelet count [10⁹/L] × √ALT [IU/L]) and AST-to-platelet ratio index (APRI) as (AST [IU/L]/40 IU/L)/platelet count [10⁹/L] × 100. Patients were classified according to the previously established FIB-4 cut-offs of <1.45 with a high negative predictive value for ruling out advanced fibrosis and >3.25 with a high specificity and a 65% positive predictive value for ruling in advanced fibrosis [19]. For APRI, we used the cut-off <0.5 for excluding cirrhosis (high negative predictive value) and >1.0 as a high specific cut-off for predicting cirrhosis [20].

The Enhanced Liver Fibrosis (ELF) test (Siemens Healthcare Diagnostics, Vienna, Austria) was available as a biomarker of liver fibrosis in one of the centers. The ELF test is a panel of markers that consists of 3 components: Type III procollagen peptide, hyaluronic acid, and tissue inhibitor of metalloproteinase-1. We explored the manufacturer-recommended 9.8 cut-off to rule in advanced fibrosis [21].

2.2. Liver Stiffness Measurement by Transient Elastography

Liver stiffness measurements (LSM) were performed in a fasting state using a Fibroscan 502 Touch (Echosens, Paris, France) using the M or XL probe as per device indication. Quality criteria used in all centers were at least 10 valid measurements and an interquartile-to-median ratio ≤ 30%. The LSM technique was carried out in accordance with the European Association for Study of the Liver (EASL) clinical guidelines [22].

Results were expressed in kilopascals (kPa). Normal liver stiffness values are around 5 kPa. Transient elastography has good re-producibility and has good diagnostic performance for estimating liver fibrosis. However, the accuracy is not as good for detecting significant fibrosis compared to advanced fibrosis or cirrhosis [22,23]. Since there are no specific LSM cut-offs for AATD liver disease, a LSM > 7.5 kPa was used as suggestive of significant fibrosis and ≥10 kPa was suggestive of advanced fibrosis according to previously established cut-offs in other liver diseases (mainly viral etiologies and alcoholic liver disease) [22,24].

The presence of steatosis was assessed by the controlled attenuation parameter (CAP) and results were expressed in decibel per meter (dB/m). The cut-off >268 dB/m was used as an indicator of moderate steatosis, and for severe steatosis the cut-off was >280 dB/m [25].

2.3. Statistical Analysis

Qualitative variables were described with absolute frequencies and percentages. The description of quantitative variables was performed using the mean, standard deviation (SD) or median, and interquartile range (IQR). The Kolmogorov–Smirnov test was used to assess the normality of distributions.

Patient characteristics were compared according to genotypes and other clinical conditions. In the case of quantitative variables, the Student's *t*-test for normally distributed variables or the Mann–Whitney U-test if normality was not assumed was used, while ANOVA tests were performed in the case of variables with more than 2 categories. The Chi-squared test (Fisher test for frequencies < 5) was used for the comparison of categorical variables. A linear relationship between quantitative variables, in particular between surrogates of liver disease (LSM, CAP and FIB-4) and spirometric markers of airflow obstruction (FEV1(%) and FEV1/FVC), were analyzed using Spearman tests. For all the tests, *p*-values < 0.05 were considered statistically significant. The statistical package R Studio (V2.5.1) was used for the analyses.

3. Results

3.1. Demographic and Clinical Findings

A total of 148 AATD patients were included from January 2017 to December 2019. Among these, 81 (54.7%) were homozygous Pi*ZZ and 67 (45.3%) were heterozygous for the Z allele (29 Pi*SZ, 35 Pi*MZ, 1 Pi*FZ, 1 Pi*PlowellZ, 1 Pi*MmaltonZ).

The mean age was 52.5 and 57 years for heterozygous and Pi*ZZ, respectively, and 50% of the patients were male. Liver disease in infancy was reported as the cause of the diagnosis of AATD in 19.4% and 11.1% of heterozygous and homozygous patients, although there were no patients with an active diagnosis of liver disease at the time of the study. COPD was diagnosed in 22.7% of heterozygous subjects and up to 70% for Pi*ZZ patients. Consequently, the mean FEV1 (%) was significantly lower in Pi*ZZ compared with heterozygous (69% (SD: 30.5%) versus 92.9% (SD: 27.6%); $p < 0.001$). The baseline characteristics of the global population and the two genotype groups are shown in Table 1.

Table 1. Baseline characteristics of the patients included by AAT genotype.

	ZZ (n = 81)	Heterozygous Z (n = 67)	p-Value
Age	57.0 (14.4)	52.5 (14.5)	0.051 [1]
Sex, men	41 (50.6%)	34 (50.7%)	0.985 [2]
BMI	25.1 (3.9)	24.0 (7.0)	0.398 [1]
Smoking exposure:			0.010 [2]
Active	43 (53.1%)	22 (32.8%)	
Former smoker	7 (8.6%)	16 (23.9%)	
Never smoker	31 (38.3%)	29 (43.3%)	
Alcohol consumption	19 (23.5%)	19 (28.4%)	0.991 [2]
Diabetes mellitus	0 (0%)	2 (3.0%)	0.203 [2]
Hypertension	14 (17.5%)	16 (23.9%)	0.453 [2]
AAT levels, mg/dL	33.3 (61.9)	71.9 (20.8)	<0.001 [1]
Reason for diagnosis:			0.002 [2]
Liver disease	9 (11.1%)	13 (19.4%)	
Lung disease	52 (64.2%)	23 (34.3%)	
Family study	17 (21.0%)	28 (41.8%)	
Other	3 (3.7%)	3 (4.5%)	
COPD	57 (70.4%)	15 (22.7%)	<0.001 [2]
Asthma	5 (7.8%)	14 (21.2%)	0.056 [2]
Neonatal jaundice	6 (7.4%)	3 (4.5%)	0.513 [2]
FVC, L	3.6 (1.5)	3.9 (1.1)	0.197 [1]
FVC, %	90.0 (28.5)	99.8 (19.8)	0.033 [1]
FEV1, L	2.1 (1.2)	3.0 (1.2)	<0.001 [1]
FEV1, %	69.0 (30.5)	92.9 (27.6)	<0.001 [1]
FEV1/FVC	0.6 (0.2)	0.7 (0.2)	0.001 [1]
KCO, %	51.0 (32.5)	58.9 (36.7)	0.231 [1]

Footnote: BMI: Body mass index; COPD: Chronic obstructive pulmonary disease; FVC: Forced ventilatory capacity; FEV1: Forced expiratory volume in 1 s; KCO: Transfer coefficient of the lung for carbon monoxide; AAT: Alpha-1 antitrypsin. [1] Mann–Whitney U-test p-value, [2] Chi-squared p-value.

3.2. Clinical and Laboratory Signs of Liver Disease

Thirty-two patients (21.6%) had abnormal liver enzymes. The distribution of values showed significant differences only in AST values, which were significantly higher in Pi*ZZ patients (29.2 UI/L (SD: 15.4) vs. 25.0 UI/L (SD: 8.0); $p = 0.029$). The most frequent pattern was an elevation in GGT (14.9% of patients). Pi*ZZ patients had a higher FIB-4 score compared to heterozygous Z (1.6 (SD: 0.8) vs. 1.2 (SD:0.5); $p < 0.001$). Only 5 patients had FIB-4 > 3.25 and all were Pi*ZZ. The APRI score was higher in Pi*ZZ patients than in heterozygous Z (0.35 (SD: 0.18) vs. 0.27 (SD: 0.09); p = 0.007), but most of the patients had APRI values < 0.5, excluding advanced fibrosis or cirrhosis, and only one Pi*ZZ patient had an APRI score > 1.0. The ELF score was obtained in 52 patients (27 Pi*ZZ and 25 Pi*Z patients). Pi*ZZ had significantly higher values compared to Pi*Z phenotypes (8.6 (SD: 0.8) vs. 8 (SD: 0.6); p = 0.007). Only 1 Pi*ZZ patient showed values above the cut-off of 9.8 (Table 2).

Table 2. Results of blood analysis and transient elastography in patients with different AAT genotypes.

	ZZ (n = 81)	Heterozygous Z (n = 67)	p-Value
Laboratory findings			
Platelet count, $\times 10^9$/L	222 (59)	239 (61)	0.074 [1]
INR	1.0 (0.2)	1.0 (0.1)	0.067 [1]
Bilirubin, mg/dL	0.8 (0.5)	0.7 (0.3)	0.158
AST, IU/L	29.2 (15.4)	25.0 (8.0)	0.029 [1]
AST > ULN	4 (4.9%)	4 (6%)	0.869 [2]
ALT, IU/L	26.6 (22.6)	26.1 (13.4)	0.967 [1]
ALT > ULN	6 (7.4%)	5 (7.5%)	0.952 [2]
ALP, IU/L	78.2 (29.6)	81.8 (21)	0.412 [1]
ALP > ULN	6 (7.4%)	2 (3%)	0.294 [2]
GGT, IU/L	36.2 (33.9)	31.1 (29.4)	0.336 [1]
GGT > ULN	13 (16.5%)	9 (13.6%)	0.637 [2]
Albumin, g/dL	4.3 (0.6)	4.4 (0.3)	0.044 [1]
Cholesterol, mg/dL	207 (35)	198 (36)	0.161
FIB-4	1.6 (0.8)	1.2 (0.5)	<0.001
FIB-4 < 1.45	38 (47.5%)	51 (78.5%)	<0.001 [2]
FIB-4 > 3.25	5 (6.2%)	0	0.065 [2]
APRI	0.35 (0.18)	0.27 (0.09)	<0.001 [1]
APRI < 0.5	67 (83)	64 (91)	0.023 [2]
APRI > 1.0	1 (1.2)	0	0.956
ELF, n = 60	8.6 (0.8)	8 (0.6)	0.007 [1]
Transient elastography			
LSM	5.6 (2.4)	4.6 (1.2)	0.001 [1]
LSM > 7.5 kPa	8 (9.9%)	0	0.040 [2]
LSM $\geq$ 10 kPa	3 (3.7%)	0	
CAP	256 (59)	253 (50)	0.252 [1]
CAP 268–280 dB/m	7 (8.6%)	4 (6%)	0.807 [2]
CAP > 280 dB/m	26 (32.1%)	21 (31.3%)	

Footnote: INR: International normalized ratio; ULN: Upper limit of normal; AST: Aspartate aminotransferase; ALT: Alanine aminotransferase; ALP: Alkaline phosphatase; GGT: Gamma-glutamyl transferase; FIB-4: Fibrosis 4; APRI: AST to platelet ratio index; ELF: Enhanced liver fibrosis; LSM: Liver stiffness measurement; CAP: Controlled attenuation parameter. [1] Mann–Whitney U-test p-value, [2] Chi-squared p-value.

3.3. Transient Elastography

The mean LSM was significantly higher in Pi*ZZ individuals than in heterozygous Z (5.6 (SD: 2.5) kPa vs. 4.6 (SD:1.2) kPa, respectively; $p = 0.007$). In total, LSM was >7.5 kPa in 8 (5%) individuals and $\geq$10 kPa in 3 (1.9%), all being Pi*ZZ (Figure 1). By lowering the cut-off of LSM to >7.1 kPa as suggested in other studies [11], we found 10 Pi*ZZ patients (12.3%) and 3 heterozygous patients (4.5%), two of whom were Pi*SZ patients with LSM 7.3 kPa, and one was a Pi*MZ patient with LSM 7.5 kPa.

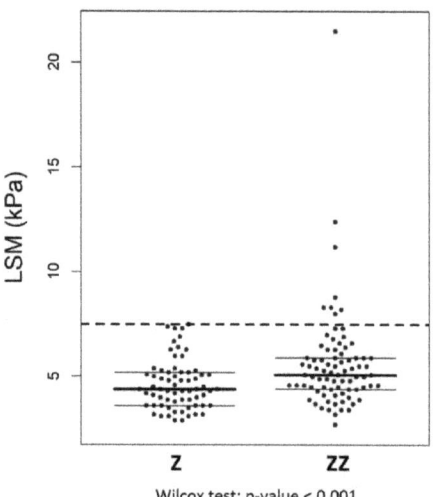

Figure 1. Comparison of mean LSM values by phenotype.

Using the LSM > 8.45 kPa cut-off of the study by Clark et al. [13], we would have identified 4 Pi*ZZ patients (4.9%) suggestive of having F $\geq$ 3.

Almost one-third of the patients had severe steatosis according to CAP values > 280 dB/m, with no significant differences between homozygous and heterozygous patients. (Table 2).

3.4. Characteristics of Pi*ZZ Patients According to LSM Values

Pi*ZZ individuals with LSM > 7.5 kPa were older and had a higher BMI. Two-thirds consumed alcohol, and all had COPD (versus 67% in patients with LSM $\leq$ 7.5 kPa; $p = 0.097$).

Elevated liver enzymes were more frequently observed in patients with LSM > 7.5 kPa. Twenty-five percent of patients with LSM > 7.5 kPa had elevated AST values compared to 2.7% in patients with LSM $\leq$ 7.5 kPa ($p = 0.048$), and 37.5% of patients with LSM > 7.5 kPa had elevated GGT compared to 14.1% of patients with LSM $\leq$ 7.5 kPa ($p = 0.120$) (Table 3, Figure 2). Conversely, 11/61 patients (18%) had at least one elevated liver enzyme but with normal LSM values (LSM < 6 kPa). Correlations between LSM and liver enzymes were only significant, albeit weakly, between LSM and AST (0.311 ($p < 0.001$)), and LSM and GGT (0.389 ($p < 0.001$)).

Table 3. Comparison between Pi*ZZ individuals based on liver stiffness (LSM) and diagnosis of chronic obstructive pulmonary disease (COPD).

	LSM ≤ 7.5 (n = 73)	LSM > 7.5 (n = 8)	p-Value	No COPD (n = 24)	COPD (n = 57)	p-Value
Age	56.2 (14.5)	64.9 (11.4)	0.076	46.2 (14.5)	61.6 (11.7)	<0.001 [1]
Sex, men	37 (50.7%)	4 (50%)	1.00	11 (45.8%)	30 (52.6%)	0.752 [2]
BMI	24.6 (3.4)	29.0 (5.3)	0.056	24.2 (3.7)	25.4 (3.9)	0.186 [1]
Smoking exposure:			0.527			<0.001 [2]
Active	37 (50.7%)	6 (75%)		7 (29.2%)	36 (63.2%)	
Former smoker	7 (9.6%)	0 (0%)		0 (0%)	7 (12.3%)	
Never smoker	29 (39.7%)	2 (25%)		17 (70.8%)	14 (24.6%)	
Alcohol consumption	16 (24.2%)	3 (60%)	0.115	5 (25%)	14 (27.2)	1.000 [2]
Hypertension	10 (13.9%)	4 (50%)	0.028	1 (4.2%)	13 (23.2%)	0.054 [2]
COPD	49 (67.1%)	8 (100%)	0.097	0	57 (100%)	0.001 [2]
Neonatal jaundice	6 (8.2%)	0 (0%)	1.000	4 (16.7%)	2 (3.5%)	0.060 [2]
FEV1, %	70.4 (30.7)	56.4 (27.3)	0.205	99.6 (13.1)	56.2 (26.3)	<0.001 [1]
Laboratory findings:						
Platelet count, $\times 10^9$/L	224 (60)	202 (49)	0.267	210 (48)	226 (62)	0.214 [1]
INR	1.0 (0.2)	1.1 (0.1)	0.378	1.0 (0.1)	1.1 (0.2)	0.040 [1]
Bilirubin, mg/dL	0.8 (0.5)	0.6 (0.2)	0.262	1.0 (0.9)	0.7 (0.2)	0.143 [1]
AST, UI/L	27.2 (10.1)	47.6 (34.7)	0.141	27.2 (10.6)	30.0 (16.9)	0.375 [1]
AST > ULN *	2 (2.7%)	2 (25%)	0.048	1 (4.2%)	3 (5.3%)	0.675 [2]
ALT, UI/L	24.2 (14.2)	48.8 (55.8)	0.254	25.5 (14.4)	27.1 (25.3)	0.719 [1]
ALT > ULN *	4 (5.5%)	2 (25.0%)	0.108	3 (12.5%)	3 (5.3%)	0.226 [2]
ALP, UI/L	78.5 (30.9)	75.9 (14.8)	0.816	70.3 (31)	81.4 (28.7)	0.130 [1]
ALP > ULN *	6 (8.5%)	0 (0%)	1.000	2 (8.3%)	4 (7.0%)	1.000 [2]
GGT, UI/L	31.8 (19.3)	75.6 (84.1)	<0.001	33.2 (22.2)	37.2 (37.7)	0.685 [1]
GGT > ULN *	10 (14.1%)	3 (37.5%)	0.120	5 (20.8%)	8 (14%)	0.589 [2]
Albumin, g/dL	4.3 (0.6)	4.4 (0.3)	0.615	4.5 (0.3)	4.2 (0.6)	0.004 [1]
Cholesterol, mg/dL	206 (35)	208 (39)	0.901	205 (39)	207 (34)	0.824 [1]
FIB-4	1.5 (0.8)	2.2 (0.7)	0.032	1.3 (0.8)	1.7 (0.8)	0.046 [1]
FIB-4 < 1.45:	37 (50.7%)	1 (12.5%)	0.059	15 (62.5%)	23 (40.4%)	0.077 [2]
FIB-4 > 3.25:	4 (5.5%)	1 (12.5%)	0.418	1 (4.2%)	4 (7%)	1.000 [2]
APRI	0.33 (0.1)	0.56 (0.3)	<0.001	0.35 (0.17)	0.35 (0.19)	0.992 [1]
Transient elastography						
LSM	5.0 (1.1)	10.8 (4.6)	0.009	5.3 (1.1)	5.7 (2.8)	0.361 [1]
CAP	249 (56)	318 (48)	0.004	233 (56)	266 (58)	0.023 [1]
LSM > 7.5 kPa:	0	8 (100%)	NA	0	8 (14.0%)	0.097 [2]

Footnote: BMI: Body mass index; COPD: Chronic obstructive pulmonary disease; FEV1: Forced expiratory volume in 1 s; AAT: Alpha-1 antitrypsin; INR: International normalized ratio; AST: Aspartate aminotransferase; ALT: Alanine aminotransferase; ALP: Alkaline phosphatase; GGT: Gamma-glutamyl transferase; ULN: Upper limit of normal; FIB-4: Fibrosis 4; APRI: AST to platelet ratio index; ELF: Enhanced liver fibrosis; LSM: Liver stiffness measurement; CAP: Controlled attenuation parameter. *: Upper limit of normal according to sex-specific cut-offs: For AST and ALT: >35 IU/L in female, >50 IU/L in male; for ALP: >120 IU/L for both genders; for GGT: >38 IU/L in females and >55 IU/L in males. [1] Mann–Whitney U-test p-value, [2] Chi-squared p-value.

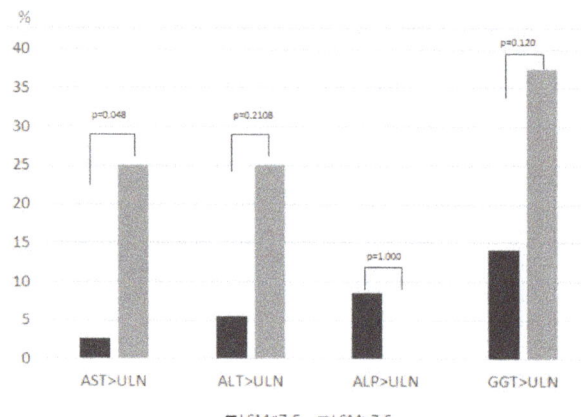

Figure 2. All individuals from the cohort with liver enzymes above the highest level of normal based on LSM values. UPN: Upper limit of normal for GGT: >38 IU/L in females and >55 IU/L in males.

Among the 8 patients with LSM > 7.5, 3 had GGT above the normal limit and 1 also had a FIB-4 score > 3.25 (Figure 3). The FIB-4 score (2.2 (SD: 0.7) versus 1.5 (SD: 0.8); $p = 0.032$), as well as CAP measurement (317.9 (SD: 48) dB/m vs. 249.6 (SD: 56.5) dB/m; $p = 0.004$), were also higher in Pi*ZZ patients with LSM > 7.5 kPa (Table 3). Severe steatosis, with CAP > 280 dB/m, was present in 6 patients (75%) with LSM > 7.5 kPa compared to 20 patients (27.4%) with LSM < 7.5 kPa ($p = 0.041$).

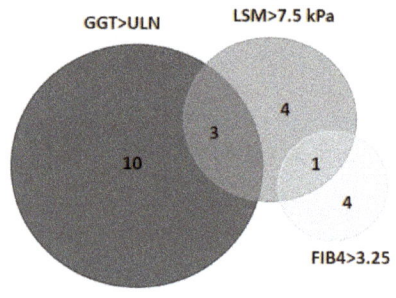

Figure 3. Relation between elevated GGT, FIB4, and LSM in Pi*ZZ patients. GGT: Gamma-glutamyl transferase; FIB-4: Fibrosis 4; LSM: Liver stiffness measurement; UPL: Upper limit of normal (according to sex-specific cut-offs: for GGT: >38 IU/L in females and >55 IU/L in males).

The APRI was higher in Pi*ZZ patients with LSM > 7.5 kPa than in those with LSM ≤ 7.5 kPa (0.56 vs. 0.33, $p < 0.001$). The APRI had a significant correlation with LSM ($r = 0.353$, $p = 0.030$).

3.5. Comparison between Pi*ZZ Patients with or without COPD

Fifty-seven Pi*ZZ patients (70.4%) had COPD. Pi*ZZ patients with COPD were older and more frequently had a history of smoking compared with non-COPD individuals. As expected, they had worse lung function with a lower FEV1 (1.6 (SD: 0.8) L vs. 3.5 (SD: 1) L; $p < 0.001$) and KCO (%) (43.7% (SD: 30.8%) vs. 68% (SD: 30.4%); $p = 0.003$).

Regarding the liver study, no differences were observed in transaminase levels, but the FIB-4 score was higher in COPD patients (1.7 (SD: 0.8) vs. 1.2 (SD: 0.8); $p = 0.046$). More individuals in the COPD group had a LSM > 7.5 kPa (14% vs. 0%; p = 0.097) and they also had higher CAP values (265.9 (SD: 58.3) dB/m vs. 233.5 (SD: 55.8) dB/m; p = 0.023) (Table 3). Significant, albeit weak, correlations were found between FIB-4 and FEV1 (mL) (r = −0.350, p = 0.002), and CAP and FEV1 (mL) and FEV1(%) (r = −0.391, p < 0.001 and r = −0.306, p = 0.006, respectively). No significant correlations were found between LSM or ELF and measures of airflow obstruction.

4. Discussion

In our study population, we found that 10% of Pi*ZZ individuals had transient elastography results suggestive of liver fibrosis, but none of the heterozygous individuals reached the suggested threshold. Although individuals with higher LSM had higher transaminase levels and FIB-4 scores, normal levels of these biomarkers did not reliably rule out liver disease, since some of the patients with normal values had high LSM values. All patients with high LSM also had COPD.

Transient elastography is a non-invasive tool that has proven to be useful in the diagnosis of liver fibrosis of different etiologies. More recently, its utility has also been explored in AATD-related liver disease with promising results [16–18,26]. Although different cut-offs have been proposed, there is no validated cut-off of LSM for AATD liver disease. In a study including 94 Pi*ZZ patients with paired LSM and liver biopsies, Clark et al. [26] observed that cut-offs of 5.54 and 8.45 kPa had the highest accuracy for detecting significant fibrosis (≥F2) and advanced fibrosis (≥F3), respectively. However, these cut-offs had a low specificity and a low positive predictive value. Hamesch et al. [17] increased the cut-off for significant fibrosis to >7.1 kPa in order to increase the positive predictive value, confirming the presence of ≥F2 in 22 out of 23 patients with liver biopsies [27], while Guillaud et al. [16] suggested an LSM > 7.2 kPa for significant fibrosis and LSM > 14 kPa for cirrhosis. In another study in 75 patients with AATD, the investigators offered a liver biopsy to all individuals with a LSM > 6 or altered liver enzymes in combination with an abnormal ultrasound. Among the 11 biopsies analyzed, they found that the LSM scores in patients with moderate or severe fibrosis were >8 kPa [18]. According to these results and the cut-offs previously established in other etiologies, we chose an arbitrary cut-off of LSM > 7.5 kPa as suggestive of significant fibrosis, and LSM ≥ 10 kPa as advanced fibrosis/cirrhosis. In our sample, there were two Pi*SZ patients with LSM = 7.3 kPa, one of whom was overweight and had diabetes mellitus and increased GGT values, and the other was a Pi*MZ patient with LSM = 7.5 kPa without other identified risk factors of liver disease. Since the etiology of liver disease has an impact on LSM and the data on AATD induced liver disease are limited [28], further studies are needed to validate the best LSM cut-off for screening of liver disease in AATD.

Ten percent of Pi*ZZ patients in our cohort had LSM > 7.5 kPa, similar to the prevalence of liver fibrosis reported in initial studies in AATD patients, which varied from 10–15% in clinical studies [29,30] to 37% in autopsy studies [31]. More recently, with the development of transient elastography, there has been growing interest in the early detection of liver disease in AATD. The study by Guillaud et al. [16] described 5 patients (18%) with LSM suggestive of significant fibrosis and 2 patients (7%) with LSM suggestive of advanced liver fibrosis/cirrhosis. Other studies have reported a higher prevalence; Hamesch et al. [17] described a prevalence of liver fibrosis of 23.6% among 403 Pi*ZZ individuals and observed that liver disease was 9 to 20 times more frequent in this population compared to non-AAT-deficient individuals. In a cohort of COPD Pi*ZZ patients referred for lung transplantation, Morer et al. [32] found that 13% of patients had significant fibrosis (F2) and 8% advanced fibrosis (≥F3). Similar to these numbers, 8 (14%) of our COPD Pi*ZZ patients had LSM > 7.5 kPa, while in 3 (5.7%) LSM was higher than 10 kPa, suggesting the presence of advanced fibrosis.

In our cohort, Pi*MZ individuals had lower values of LSM compared to Pi*ZZ individuals. The mean LSM was 4.7 kPa for the 34 Pi*MZ patients included. None of these patients had values above 7.5, and only one had LSM = 7.5 kPa. In this patient, other co-factors for liver disease such as obesity, alcohol consumption, or metabolic syndrome were not found. The incidence of liver disease could be higher in heterozygous Z than in the general population, although some authors have hypothesized that while the Pi*MZ genotype acts as a disease modifier, it is not sufficient per se to trigger clinically relevant liver impairment [33]. In a study that analyzed 1184 individuals with non-alcoholic fatty liver disease (NAFLD) and 2462 with chronic alcohol misuse, the Z variant increased the risk of patients with NAFLD to develop cirrhosis and was more frequently present in alcohol misusers with cirrhosis compared to those without significant liver injury [34]. In contrast, a recent analysis of data from the European alpha-1 liver cohort showed that 10% out 419 Pi*MZ had LSM values $\geq$ 7.1 kPa compared with 4% of non-Z carriers. After adjusting for potential confounders, Pi*MZ individuals still had significantly higher odds for LSM $\geq$ 7.1 kPa [12]. There is agreement that, in coexistence with other risk factors, and especially in the context of alcohol misuse or NAFLD, Z carriage is a strong risk factor for the development of cirrhosis [17,18] and may also lead to faster hepatic decompensations [35]. In our cohort, 60% of Pi*ZZ patients with LSM > 7.5 kPa had some alcohol consumption and had a higher BMI than those with LSM $\leq$ 7.5 kPa, and, therefore, these factors could have contributed to the progression of liver disease.

Liver enzymes have often been used to screen liver disease in AATD in clinical practice [36]. In our cohort, elevated liver enzymes and FIB-4 were more frequently observed in patients with LSM > 7.5 kPa, but normal levels were also frequently present in patients with high LSM. In fact, liver enzyme alterations ranged from only 25% of cases for AST and ALT to 37.5% for GGT in Pi*ZZ patients with LSM > 7.5 kPa. Patients with fibrosis or even cirrhosis may present normal serum liver enzymes [11], and this has also been observed in Pi*ZZ individuals [13,17]. On the other hand, up to 10% of AATD patients with normal liver function tests and ultrasound may have increased LSM values [16]. Furthermore, an increase in ALT has a low sensitivity for identifying liver disease in AATD individuals [13,15]. In the European alpha-1 liver cohort, heterozygous Pi*MZ carriers also had higher serum transaminases compared to non-carriers, although this percentage varied from 5.4% to 28.6% and was higher in individuals older than 50 years [12].

The relationship between lung and liver disease in individuals with AATD is controversial. The first series of patients with the deficiency suggested that lung and liver disease rarely coexisted in AATD, and liver disease was more frequently reported in AATD never smokers compared to smokers [37,38]. However, more recent studies using new diagnostic techniques have reported more frequent coexistence of the alterations in both organs [39]. In this line, all of our patients with elevated LSM also had COPD, although the correlation between lung function and LSM was not significant. Moreover, recruiting patients from respiratory departments may have influenced the high prevalence of COPD among patients with elevated LSM; although they were also older, with higher BMI and with a higher frequency of alcohol misuse compared with patients with normal LSM. Therefore, a clear relationship between elevated LSM and lung disease cannot be established from our results.

Our study had some limitations. First, the identification of liver fibrosis was only made by transient elastography as we did not perform liver biopsies. However, as there are no specific treatments for AATD liver disease to date, the performance of an invasive diagnostic technique in otherwise asymptomatic patients may not be justified. Second, this was a cross-sectional study, and data on the evolution of LSM over time were not available. Third, the design of our study did not allow us to investigate a causal relationship between AATD and liver alterations. Our sample size was not big enough for a multivariate analysis adjusted for known confounders of increased liver fibrosis. However, the study had some strengths: We recruited individuals from three reference centers, and, considering that AATD is a rare disease, we reported information from a large series of patients with homozygous and heterozygous AATD.

In conclusion, the results of this study support the assessment of liver disease in all AATD Pi*ZZ individuals and heterozygous Pi*Z individuals with additional liver risk factors. Transient elastography has been shown to be a valuable tool to screen for AATD liver disease, and collaboration between hepatologists and pneumologists is crucial for providing the best care to AATD patients. Due to the poor correlation between liver enzymes and other serum biomarkers and the underlying liver disease, all Z-allele carriers, even those with normal serum biomarker values, should be screened with transient elastography. Since AATD is a rare disease, international collaboration in large registries is needed to investigate the best screening strategy for lung and liver disease [12,17,40].

Author Contributions: Conceptualization, M.P., A.N., C.E., M.M., and M.B.; methodology, M.P., A.N., and C.E.; formal analysis, C.E.; investigation, M.P., A.N., C.E., M.T.-D., J.L.R.-H., M.C., R.T.-P., I.B., F.R.-F., J.G., M.M., and M.B.; resources, M.T.-D., J.L.R.-H., M.C., R.T.-P., J.G., and M.M.; data curation, M.P., A.N., C.E., M.T.-D., J.L.R.-H. and E.R.; writing—original draft preparation, M.P., A.N., M.M., and M.B.; writing—review and editing, C.E., M.T.-D., J.L.R.-H., M.C., R.T.-P., I.B., F.R.-F., and J.G.; supervision, J.G., M.M., and M.B.; project administration, M.M.; funding acquisition, M.T.-D., J.L.R.-H., M.C., and M.M. All authors have read and agreed to the published version of the manuscript.

Funding: This research was funded by Grifols through an unrestricted grant from the Catalan Center for Research in Alpha-1 antitrypsin deficiency of the Vall d'Hebron Research Institute (VHIR) in the Vall d'Hebron Barcelona Hospital Campus, Barcelona, Spain; from the Madrid Center for Research in Alpha-1 antitrypsin deficiency of the Hospital Clínico San Carlos, Madrid, Spain; from the Galicia Center for Research in Alpha-1 antitrypsin deficiency of the University Hospital Complex of Vigo, Spain; as well as a research grant from Fundació Catalana de Pneumologia (FUCAP).

Institutional Review Board Statement: The study was approved by the Vall d'Hebron Hospital Ethics Committee (Barcelona, Spain), number PR(AG)335/2016 (28 October 2016).

Informed Consent Statement: Informed consent was obtained from all subjects involved in the study.

Data Availability Statement: Data are available from the authors upon request.

Acknowledgments: Mònica Pons was the recipient of a Rio Hortega contract in the 2018 Strategic Action Health Call from the Instituto de Salud Carlos III for the years 2019–2020. Alexa Núñez was the recipient of a Rio Hortega contract in the 2019 Strategic Action Health Call from the Instituto de Salud Carlos III for the years 2020–2022. We thank Ignacio Martín Granizo and Montserrat Figueira Alvarez for their collaboration in the elastography in the University Hospital Complex of Vigo.

Conflicts of Interest: Myriam Calle received speaking or consulting fees from Boehringer Ingelheim, Grifols, Chiesi, CSL Behring, AstraZeneca, GlaxoSmithKline, Menarini, Gebro Pharma, Zambon, and Novartis. There is no real or perceived conflict of interest between these sources and the present paper. Juan Luis Rodríguez-Hermosa received speaking fees from Boehringer Ingelheim, GlaxoSmithKline, Grifols, CSL Behring, Zambon, and Gebro Pharma. There is no real or perceived conflict of interest between these sources and the present paper. Cristina Esquinas received speaker fees from CSL Behring. Marc Miravitlles received speaker or consulting fees from AstraZeneca, Bial, Boehringer Ingelheim, Chiesi, Cipla, CSL Behring, Laboratorios Esteve, Gebro Pharma, Kamada, GlaxoSmithKline, Grifols, Menarini, Mereo Biopharma, Novartis, pH Pharma, Rovi, TEVA, Spin Therapeutics, Verona Pharma, and Zambon, and research grants from Grifols. Miriam Barrecheguren received speaker fees from Grifols, Menarini, CSL Behring, and GSK, and consulting fees from GSK, Novartis, Boehringer Ingelheim, and Gebro Pharma. The remaining authors report no conflict of interest.

References

1. Miravitlles, M.; Dirksen, A.; Ferrarotti, I.; Koblizek, V.; Lange, P.; Mahadeva, R.; MacElvaney, N.G.; Parr, D.; Piitulainen, E.; Roche, N.; et al. European Respiratory Society Statement: Diagnosis and treatment of pulmonary disease in alpha-1 antitrypsin deficiency. *Eur. Respir. J.* **2017**, *50*, 1700610. [CrossRef]
2. Strnad, P.; McElvaney, N.G.; Lomas, D.A. Alpha1-Antitrypsin Deficiency. *N. Engl. J. Med.* **2020**, *382*, 1443–1455. [CrossRef]
3. Blanco, I.; Bueno, P.; Diego, I.; Pérez-Holanda, S.; Casas-Maldonado, F.; Esquinas, C.; Miravitlles, M. Alpha-1 antitrypsin Pi*Z gene frequency and Pi*ZZ genotype numbers worldwide: An update. *Int. J. Chron. Obstruct. Pulmon. Dis.* **2017**, *12*, 561–569. [CrossRef]

4. Blanco, I.; Bueno, P.; Diego, I.; Pérez-Holanda, S.; Lara, B.; Casas-Maldonado, F.; Esquinas, C.; Miravitlles, M. Alpha-1 antitrypsin Pi*SZ genotype: Estimated prevalence and number of SZ subjects worldwide. *Int. J. Chron. Obstruct. Pulmon. Dis.* **2017**, *12*, 1683–1694. [CrossRef]
5. Janciauskiene, S.; DeLuca, D.S.; Barrecheguren, M.; Welte, T.; Miravitlles, M. Serum Levels of Alpha1-antitrypsin and Their Relationship with COPD in the General Spanish Population. *Arch. Bronconeumol.* **2020**, *56*, 76–83. [CrossRef]
6. Ellis, P.; Turner, A. What Do Alpha-1 Antitrypsin Levels Tell Us About Chronic Inflammation in COPD? *Arch. Bronconeumol.* **2020**, *56*, 72–73. [CrossRef] [PubMed]
7. Lomas, D.A. Twenty years of polymers: A personal perspective on alpha-1 antitrypsin deficiency. *COPD* **2013**, *10*, 17–25. [CrossRef] [PubMed]
8. Mela, M.; Smeeton, W.; Davies, S.E.; Miranda, E.; Scarpini, C.; Coleman, N.; Alexander, G.J.M. The Alpha-1 Antitrypsin Polymer Load Correlates with Hepatocyte Senescence, Fibrosis Stage and Liver-Related Mortality. *Chronic. Obstr. Pulm. Dis.* **2020**, *7*, 151–162. [CrossRef] [PubMed]
9. Bouchecareilh, M. Alpha-1 Antitrypsin Deficiency-Mediated Liver Toxicity: Why Do Some Patients Do Poorly? What Do We Know So Far? *Chronic. Obstr. Pulm. Dis.* **2020**, *7*, 172–181. [CrossRef]
10. Teckman, J.H.; Jain, A. Advances in alpha-1-antitrypsin deficiency liver disease. *Curr. Gastroenterol. Rep.* **2014**, *16*, 367. [CrossRef]
11. Hamesch, K.; Strnad, P. Non-Invasive Assessment and Management of Liver Involvement in Adults with Alpha-1 Antitrypsin Deficiency. *Chronic. Obstr. Pulm. Dis.* **2020**, *7*, 260–271.
12. Schneider, C.V.; Hamesch, K.; Gross, A.; Mandorfer, M.; Moeller, L.S.; Pereira, V.; Pons, M.; Kuca, P.; Reichert, M.C.; Benini, F.; et al. European Alpha-1 Liver Study Group. Liver Phenotypes of European Adults Heterozygous or Homozygous for Pi*Z Variant of AAT (Pi*MZ vs Pi*ZZ genotype) and Noncarriers. *Gastroenterology* **2020**, *159*, 534–548. [CrossRef]
13. Clark, V.C.; Dhanasekaran, R.; Brantly, M.; Rouhani, F.; Schreck, P.; Nelson, D.R. Liver test results do not identify liver disease in adults with α(1)-antitrypsin deficiency. *Clin. Gastroenterol. Hepatol.* **2012**, *10*, 1278–1283. [CrossRef] [PubMed]
14. Del Poggio, P.; Colombo, S. Is transient elastography a useful tool for screening liver disease? *World J. Gastroenterol.* **2009**, *15*, 1409–1414. [CrossRef] [PubMed]
15. Kim, R.G.; Nguyen, P.; Bettencourt, R.; Dulai, P.S.; Haufe, W.; Hooker, J.; Minocha, J.; Valasek, M.A.; Aryafar, H.; Brenner, D.A.; et al. Magnetic resonance elastography identifies fibrosis in adults with alpha-1 antitrypsin deficiency liver disease: A prospective study. *Aliment. Pharmacol. Ther.* **2016**, *44*, 287–299. [CrossRef]
16. Guillaud, O.; Dumortier, J.; Traclet, J.; Restier, L.; Joly, P.; Chapuis-Cellier, C.; Lachaux, A.; Mornex, J.F. Assessment of Liver Fibrosis by Transient Elastography (Fibroscan®) in Patients with A1AT Deficiency. *Clin. Res. Hepatol. Gastroenterol.* **2019**, *43*, 77–81. [CrossRef] [PubMed]
17. Hamesch, K.; Mandorfer, M.; Pereira, V.M.; Moeller, L.S.; Pons, M.; Dolman, G.E.; Reichert, M.C.; Heimes, C.V.; Woditsch, V.; Voss, J.; et al. European Alpha1-Liver Study Group. Liver Fibrosis and Metabolic Alterations in Adults with Alpha1 Antitrypsin Deficiency Caused by the Pi*ZZ Mutation. *Gastroenterology* **2019**, *157*, 705–719. [CrossRef]
18. Abbas, S.H.; Pickett, E.; Lomas, D.A.; Thorburn, D.; Gooptu, B.; Hurst, J.R.; Marshall, A. Non-invasive testing for liver pathology in alpha-1 antitrypsin deficiency. *BMJ Open. Respir. Res.* **2020**, *7*, e000820. [CrossRef] [PubMed]
19. Sterling, R.K.; Lissen, E.; Clumeck, N.; Sola, R.; Correa, M.C.; Montaner, J.; Sulkowski, M.S.; Torriani, F.J.; Dieterich, D.T.; Thomas, D.L.; et al. Development of a simple noninvasive index to predict significant fibrosis patients with HIV/HCV co-infection. *Hepatology* **2006**, *43*, 1317–1325. [CrossRef]
20. Lin, Z.H.; Xin, Y.N.; Dong, Q.J.; Wang, Q.; Jiang, X.J.; Zhan, S.H.; Sun, Y.; Xuan, S.Y. Performance of the aspartate aminotransferase-to-platelet ratio index for the staging of hepatitis C-related fibrosis: An updated meta-analysis. *Hepatology* **2011**, *53*, 726–736. [CrossRef] [PubMed]
21. Lichtinghagen, R.; Pietsch, D.; Bantel, H.; Manns, M.P.; Brand, K.; Bahr, M.J. The Enhanced Liver Fibrosis (ELF) score: Normal values, influence factors and proposed cut-off values. *J. Hepatol.* **2013**, *59*, 236–242. [CrossRef] [PubMed]
22. European Association for Study of Liver. EASL-ALEH Clinical Practice Guidelines: Non-invasive Tests for Evaluation of Liver Disease Severity and Prognosis. *J. Hepatol.* **2015**, *63*, 237–264. [CrossRef] [PubMed]
23. Mulabecirovic, A.; Mjelle, A.B.; Gilja, O.H.; Vesterhus, M.; Havre, R.F. Liver elasticity in healthy individuals by two novel shear-wave elastography systems—Comparison by age, gender, BMI and number of measurements. *PLoS ONE* **2018**, *13*, e0203486. [CrossRef] [PubMed]
24. Castera, L. Non-invasive tests for liver fibrosis in NAFLD: Creating pathways between primary healthcare and liver clinics. *Liver Int.* **2020**, *40* (Suppl. 1), 77–81. [CrossRef] [PubMed]
25. Karlas, T.; Petroff, D.; Sasso, M.; Fan, J.G.; Mi, Y.Q.; de Lédinghen, V.; Kumar, M.; Lupsor-Platon, M.; Han, K.H.; Cardoso, A.C.; et al. Individual patient data meta-analysis of controlled attenuation parameter (CAP) technology for assessing steatosis. *J. Hepatol.* **2017**, *66*, 1022–1030. [CrossRef] [PubMed]
26. Clark, V.C.; Marek, G.; Liu, C.; Collinsworth, A.; Shuster, J.; Kurtz, T.; Nolte, J.; Brantly, M. Clinical and histologic features of adults with alpha-1 antitrypsin deficiency in a non-cirrhotic cohort. *J. Hepatol.* **2018**, *69*, 1357–1364. [CrossRef] [PubMed]
27. Kümpers, J.; Fromme, M.; Schneider, C.V.; Trautwein, C.; Denk, H.; Hamesch, K.; Strnad, P. Assessment of liver phenotype in adults with severe alpha-1 antitrypsin deficiency (Pi*ZZ genotype). *J. Hepatol.* **2019**, *71*, 1272–1274. [CrossRef]

28. Behairy, B.-S.; Sira, M.M.; Zalata, K.R.; Salama, E.-S.E.; Abd-Allah, M.A. Transient elastography compared to liver biopsy and morphometry for predicting fibrosis in pediatric chronic liver disease: Does etiology matter? *World J. Gastroenterol.* **2016**, *22*, 4238–4249. [CrossRef] [PubMed]
29. Cox, D.W.; Smyth, S. Risk for liver disease in adults with alpha 1-antitrypsin deficiency. *Am. J. Med.* **1983**, *74*, 221–227. [CrossRef]
30. Tanash, H.A.; Piitulainen, E. Liver disease in adults with severe alpha-1-antitrypsin deficiency. *J. Gastroenterol.* **2019**, *54*, 541–548. [CrossRef] [PubMed]
31. Fairbanks, K.D.; Tavill, A.S. Liver disease in alpha 1-antitrypsin deficiency: A review. *Am. J. Gastroenterol.* **2008**, *103*, 2136–2141. [CrossRef] [PubMed]
32. Morer, L.; Choudat, L.; Dauriat, G.; Durand, F.; Cazals-Hatem, D.; Thabut, G.; Brugière, O.; Castier, Y.; Mal, H. Liver involvement in patients with PiZZ-emphysema, candidates for lung transplantation. *Am. J. Transplant.* **2017**, *17*, 1389–1395. [CrossRef]
33. Fromme, M.; Oliverius, M.; Strnad, P. DEFI-ALFA: The French key to the alpha1 mystery? *Liver Int.* **2019**, *39*, 1019–1021. [CrossRef] [PubMed]
34. Strnad, P.; Buch, S.; Hamesch, K.; Fischer, J.; Rosendahl, J.; Schmelz, R.; Brueckner, S.; Brosch, M.; Heimes, C.V.; Woditsch, V. Heterozygous carriage of the alpha1-antitrypsin Pi*Z variant increases the risk to develop liver cirrhosis. *Gut* **2019**, *68*, 1099–1107. [CrossRef] [PubMed]
35. Schaefer, B.; Mandorfer, M.; Viveiros, A.; Finkenstedt, A.; Ferenci, P.; Schneeberger, S.; Tilg, H.; Zoller, H. Heterozygosity for the alpha-1-antitrypsin Z allele in cirrhosis is associated with more advanced disease. *Liver Transpl.* **2018**, *24*, 744–751. [CrossRef]
36. Hernández Pérez, J.M.; Blanco, I.; Sánchez Medina, J.A.; Díaz Hernández, L.; Pérez Pérez, J.A. Serum Levels of Glutamate-Pyruvate Transaminase, Glutamate-Oxaloacetate Transaminase and Gamma-Glutamyl Transferase in 1494 Patients with Various Genotypes for the Alpha-1 Antitrypsin Gene. *J. Clin. Med.* **2020**, *9*, 3923. [CrossRef] [PubMed]
37. Stoller, J.K.; Tomashefski, J., Jr.; Crystal, R.G.; Arroliga, A.; Strange, C.; Killian, D.N.; Schluchter, M.D.; Wiedemann, H.P. Mortality in individuals with severe deficiency of alpha1-antitrypsin: Findings from the National Heart, Lung, and Blood Institute Registry. *Chest* **2005**, *127*, 1196–1204. [PubMed]
38. Tanash, H.A.; Nilsson, P.M.; Nilsson, J.A.; Piitulainen, E. Clinical course and prognosis of never-smokers with severe alpha-1-antitrypsin deficiency (PiZZ). *Thorax* **2008**, *63*, 1091–1095. [CrossRef] [PubMed]
39. Dawwas, M.F.; Davies, S.E.; Griffiths, W.J.H.; Lomas, D.A.; Alexander, G.J. Prevalence and risk factors for liver involvement in individuals with PiZZ-related lung disease. *Am. J. Respir. Crit. Care Med.* **2013**, *187*, 502–508. [CrossRef] [PubMed]
40. Barrecheguren, M.; Torres-Duran, M.; Casas-Maldonado, F.; Miravitlles, M. Spanish implementation of the new international alpha-1 anitrypsin deficiency international registry: The European Alpha-1 Research Collaboration (EARCO). *Arch. Bronconeumol.* **2021**, *57*, 81–82. [CrossRef] [PubMed]

MDPI
St. Alban-Anlage 66
4052 Basel
Switzerland
Tel. +41 61 683 77 34
Fax +41 61 302 89 18
www.mdpi.com

Journal of Clinical Medicine Editorial Office
E-mail: jcm@mdpi.com
www.mdpi.com/journal/jcm

www.ingramcontent.com/pod-product-compliance
Lightning Source LLC
LaVergne TN
LVHW070432100526
838202LV00014B/1580